FOODSERVICE MANAGEMENT— BY DESIGN

FOODSERVICE MANAGEMENT—
BY DESIGN

Dee Legvold, MPH, RD
Co-Owner, *dk Foodservice* Solutions, LLC
Apple Valley, MN

Kristi Salisbury, CDM, CFPP, RD
Co-Owner, *dk Foodservice* Solutions, LLC
Mendota Heights, MN

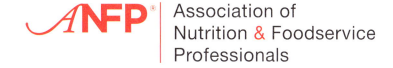

ANFP® | Association of
Nutrition & Foodservice
Professionals

Association of Nutrition & Foodservice Professionals
406 Surrey Woods Dr.
St. Charles, IL 60174
800.323.1908
www.ANFPonline.org

ISBN 0-9825884-3-7

Printed in the United States of America.

Dedication

We dedicate this book to all those dietary managers who strive to better themselves through increased education. We have met many Certified Dietary Managers throughout our careers who have inspired us to learn and improve our own skills.

This book is written as a textbook for students and as a future reference for working managers. We are proud of how it turned out and look forward to seeing more Certified Dietary Managers meet the evolving needs of our senior living, hospitals, schools and other creative foodservice careers.

We thank the authors of the past editions who laid the groundwork for us. It was our goal to build upon the foundation they established and to provide operators with a hands-on working resource.

Finally, we thank our families who have supported our time over the last year of writing, discussing the best options, talking about the book and finally completing the book. We appreciate the opportunity provided by the Association of Nutrition & Foodservice Professionals to share our experiences as operators and management consultants with you.

Table of Contents

Preface

Non-commercial food service is changing rapidly. The lines between commercial and non-commercial food service are blurring as hospitals, schools, and long-term care facilities provide more choice for their clientele. In hospitals, retail sales are becoming an increasingly important part of the overall foodservice budget. In schools, more options are available to students. Long-term care facilities are preparing for the next generation resident that is demanding more choices than ever before.

Today, Certified Dietary Managers, Certified Food Protection Professionals (CDM, CFPP)—noted throughout the text as Certified Dietary Managers or CDMs—are responsible for the daily operations of their department while helping the facility fulfill its mission and goals. They coordinate the service of food and nourishments among various departments, such as dining services and nursing. Certified Dietary Managers ensure that clients are satisfied with their dining experience and that the meals meet their nutritional and emotional needs. In addition, they oversee food safety, the inventory and ordering of food, equipment, and supplies, and arrange for the routine maintenance and upkeep of the foodservice equipment and facilities. Certified Dietary Managers are generally responsible for all administrative and human resource functions of the foodservice department, including recruiting new employees and monitoring employee performance and training.

The authors' design in writing this textbook is based on tasks that a team of Certified Dietary Managers has identified as common to most foodservice operations. These tasks represent current practice in the United States. As the driving force of any foodservice department, "The Menu" is the starting point of the *Foodservice Management—By Design* textbook. The authors have structured the content and flow of material to build from that central concept. This book is intended to be both a student's textbook and a reference for working managers in operating a foodservice department. The textbook is based upon and integrates the 2016 Blueprint Content Outline.

In addition, *Supplemental Materials—Foodservice* is included as an online resource for the student. The supplement offers supporting documents, articles, and forms to assist in learning to become a Certified Dietary Manager.

Foodservice is referenced in the Preface, however within the body of the book, foodservice may be interchanged with Dining Services. Foodservice is used primarily as a generic term including all types of meal and food preparation, from fast food and food trucks to white linen fine dining and room service. The term Dining Services generally refers more to quantity food production and meal service in care centers, schools, correctional facilities, hospitals and employee feeding venues. All terms are correct. Dining Services, however, is more specific to the segments of the foodservice departments that many Certified Dietary Managers are employed.

Acknowledgements

We would like to express our appreciation to many individuals who have contributed to the development of this textbook throughout the years and set the standard that we strive to follow, including Susan Davis Allen, Sue Grossbauer, James Kinneer, John Knight, Jack Ninemeier and Ruby Puckett. Some original work has been retained in this edition.

In addition, we would like to recognize the contribution of the review team who generously invested their professional expertise and valuable time:

Betty Barton, MS, RD, LD

Linda Boire, MS, RDN, CDN

Michael Braun, MS, RD

Pam Brummit, MA, RD/LD

Linda Hittleman, MS, RD, CDN, CDE

Judith Kaplan, MS, RDN,LD

Debbie Kern, MEd, RDN, LDN

Tama Krause, MS, RDN, LMNT

Linda S. Eck Mills, MBA, RDN, LDN, FADA

Ruby Puckett, MA, FCSI

Monica Pyzia, MS, RDN, LDN, CDE

Tim Roberts, PhD, RD, LD

Brenda Rubash, RD, LD

Becky Rude, MS, RD, CDM, CFPP

Jillian Schafer, RD

Sarah Terrio, BS, DTR, CDM, CFPP

Mary Ann Turlington, RD, LDN

Collen Zenk, MS, CDM, CFPP

Furthermore, we wish to recognize the ongoing efforts of the developers of the Nutrition and Foodservice Professional Training Curriculum; Susan Davis Allen, MS, RD and Sue Moen; the Certifying Board for Dietary Managers®; and the ANFP staff for their commitment to the profession and members.

Technical Content Reviewer: Renee Zonka, CEC, MBA, RD, CHE

Graphic Designer: Mercy Ehrler

Editing Team: The Shamrock Companies

ANFP Staff: Anna Shlachter, MS, RDN, LDN and Pam Himrod, MS, RD, CDM, CFPP

A Personal Invitation

As a student enrolled in the Nutrition & Foodservice Professional Training Program, we invite you to join the Association of Nutrition & Foodservice Professionals (ANFP) as a Pre-Professional member.

ANFP is the premier resource for foodservice managers, directors and those aspiring towards careers in foodservice management, with more than 14,000 professionals dedicated to the mission of providing optimum nutritional care through foodservice management and food safety.

Pre-Professional membership is a stepping stone for professional growth. Network and connect with members in all practice areas, understand the profession, and gain valuable tools and resources at your fingertips.

Enjoy benefits such as:

- 24/7 Members-only access to website, online community and social media and receive an electronic version of *Nutrition & Foodservice Edge* magazine
- Scholarship opportunities
- eNews monthly online newsletter
- Special discounted member pricing for ANFP products and services
- Network nationally, locally, and even globally with peers

You are the future of our profession. Take the first step in nourishing your career. Join ANFP today! For more information, visit www.ANFPonline.org or call 800-323-1908.

Meal Service and Menu Style

Overview and Objectives

How do you provide meals to your clients? The decision depends upon the dining venues, equipment available and needs of the clientele. This chapter will take you through the steps of accessing your options and recognizing that no one style is always best for the clientele. After completing this chapter, you should be able to:

✓ Describe different Styles of Service commonly used in the industry

✓ Discuss the changing culture of meal delivery services

✓ Relate how the Style of Service impacts the Style of Menu

Certified Dietary Managers (CDM) are working in an increasing number of service venues. The days of the traditional "nursing home" manager have been replaced with opportunities in School Foodservice, Corrections Food Managers, and Business Restaurant Manager. Healthcare now includes the **Continuous Care Retirement Communities (CCRC)** with country club style dining rooms and steakhouse concepts. The population or audience served by a CDM may include patients, students, toddlers, prisoners, seniors, tenants, restaurant patrons and catering attendees. Given the broad spectrum of the term, clients will be used for the purposes of this textbook.

Dining services in the senior living communities range from the traditional large dining room to the smaller neighborhood concept with room-service meals offered to the Transitional Care Unit "patients." Hospitals are recognizing the value of trained CDMs as part of their supervisory and management team. Meal services can span from the typical trayline and cart delivery to high-end room service and specialty dining options.

Today's food technology and equipment development have allowed for centralized production centers such as cook-chill and satelliting of meals in bulk or as pre-plated trays. Meals services are planned and managed for congregate dining, home delivered meals and remote meal service where there are limited food production facilities.

There is no one definition for today's dining services.

Glossary

CCRC
Continuous Care Retirement Communities

Style of Service

How you provide food in your facility is considered your Style of Service. There are many different methods for delivering meals to your clientele. A Certified Dietary Manager needs to use judgment to design and/or revise systems. In addition to the needs of clients, the manager must consider:

- The physical design of the kitchen
- Locations of dining rooms or service areas
- Requirements for off-site service (if any)
- Mission and goals of the organization
- Staffing resources
- Budget and operating costs
- Timing requirements for service

Centralized Versus Decentralized Meal Service

Prior to considering the point of service or Style of Service, it is important to consider the preparation of the meal to be served. In a **Centralized Production Center,** food is prepared in large quantities for service either satellited to multiple locations or time delayed through a cook-chill process. More commonly seen is one kitchen for the building that produces the meals to be served on-site; a **Main or Centralized Kitchen**. The **Decentralized Kitchen** receives much of its food from a Production Center or Main Kitchen and provides finishing or reheating (**rethermalizing**) prior to service, often supplementing food items from a pantry or short order grill. (Production systems are further explored in Chapter 5.)

Similarly, **Centralized Meal Service** means that food is portioned onto trays in a central location, such as the dining services department. An alternative is **Decentralized Meal Service**, in which food is distributed to other locations for plating at the point of service, such as Table-Side service in senior living.

Cook-Chill is a production system that has been available for over 20 years. The food is prepared in advance, often in a Production Center, and either "blast chilled" or frozen and held for service at a later time. Food items may be distributed for reheating in bulk and served in a satellite dining room such as congregate meals or a remote facility. Individual meals may be pre-plated COLD on a trayline system and reheated in specialty equipment prior to service. Meals are shipped to other buildings, or transported by carts to nursing units for rethermalizing "on the unit floor". Often, cook-chill is a model used by school systems, where food production is centralized and food is transported to individual school cafeterias for plating at the time of service.

In both centralized and decentralized systems, the equipment used must support the service and delivery model. Temperature control from the time of assembly to actual delivery is of paramount concern. To help ensure food safety, as well as quality, food must be kept out of the danger zone (41° - 135°F).

For a **Cook-Serve** tray service, when meals will be produced and served immediately, some of the most basic temperature control systems are:

- Insulated trays
  - > Each compartment is separated and insulated.
  - > Keeps hot food hot and cold food cold.
  - > Tray lid may cover all or part of the tray.

> The tray on the left in Figure 1.1 illustrates a typical insulated tray.
- Heated base systems
  > Wax filled bases are pre-heated prior to meal plating
  > The tray on the right in Figure 1.1 illustrates a heated base tray
- An instant heating system is also available from a number of manufacturers
  > Transfer heat into a base plate while keeping the edges cool
  > Figure 1.2 illustrates a Heat-On-Demand base heater
- Insulated transportation carts
  > The cart is insulated and may even be heated to help maintain hot food temperatures
  > Figure 1.3 illustrates an insulated cart for transportation of completed trays

Figure 1.1 Insulated Tray and Dinnerware

Insulated Tray	Insulated Dinnerware

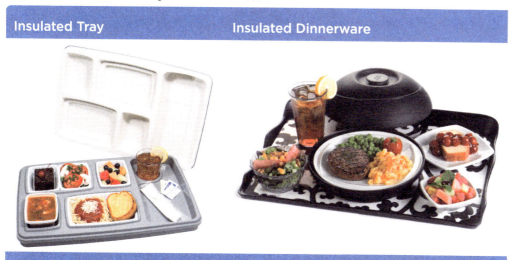

Figure 1.2 Heat-On-Demand

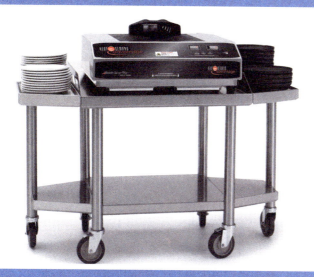

Aladdin-Temprite® Reprinted with permission.

Putting It Into Practice

1. When working in a large hospital, you decide that food will be prepared in a central kitchen and then shipped in bulk to the other wings/floors to reheat and serve. What type of meal delivery system is this?

Figure 1.3 Insulated Carts for Transporting Completed Trays

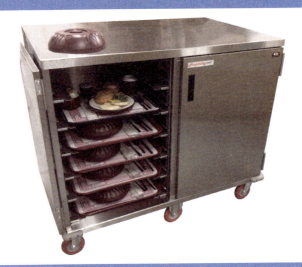

Carter-Hoffmann Reprinted with permission.

Not all meals are served from pre-plated meal trays. In today's marketplace, "Table-Side" meal selection is fairly common in senior dining where the client is served a meal from a hot-cart located within the dining room. Typically heated bases, transport carts and insulated trays are not viewed by CMS (Centers for Medicare & Medicaid Services) as part of the home-like dining experience.

Service Options—The Traditional Trayline and Beyond

Trayline Service

A **Trayline**, or the modified version **POD system**, is still the most common meal assembly process in acute care and many senior living communities. Trayline systems are also common in correctional facilities.

A trayline system moves trays through an assembly line where employees place items on trays. During this process, trays may move along a straight line or a circular platform, often with the help of a conveyor belt. Some conveyor belt systems are powered by electric motors with speeds that can be regulated. Other facilities operate skate wheel systems where trays are manually slid along the wheels. In a POD system, all of the serving stations are compressed into a small wrap-around space so everything is within easy reach of the server.

The individual trays are typically transported by carts and delivered to clients. Serving meals through a trayline system involves a number of steps that are tightly integrated with the diet order system and a menu management process. How these steps are implemented varies from one operation to another. Figure 1.4 provides a sample flow for a traditional trayline service.

Glossary

POD System
A small serving station with all items within reach of the server

Figure 1.4 Trayline Service—The Steps

1 Prior to the meal service time, either an individual Meal Ticket or Tray Identification Card is prepared for each client.

2 The Meal Tickets are grouped by unit or dining room location.

3 Staff send the Meal Tickets or Tray Identification Cards down the trayline for assembly.

4 Food items and supplies are organized by stations on the trayline.

5 Items seleted or appropriate for the diet are added to the tray.

6 Staff place the tray on a cart or traveyor (an elevator belt with platforms for transporting trays to higher floors).

7 Nursing or Dining Services staff deliver trays to the client.

Tray Delivery Options

Typically meal trays are transported throughout the facility in enclosed "food only" carts. Tray transport carts are designed to securely hold the trays while going up ramps, over bumps in the flooring, etc. Some carts are designed to provide thermostatically maintained heat, while others include a refrigeration section.

For temperature controlled cart systems, Figure 1.5, during assembly, employees place hot foods on the "hot" side of the tray and cold foods on the "cold" side. A dividing seal helps maintain temperature control. Some units can plug into a controller unit to rethermalize hot foods on trays immediately prior to service. Although this system can be very successful in maintaining temperatures, the "high tech" appearance of the tray becomes visually institutional looking.

Figure 1.5 Temperature Controlled Cart System

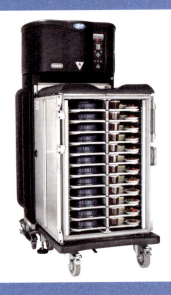

Aladdin-Temprite® Reprinted with permission.

Figure 1.6 Rethermalization Systems

Bulk Rethermalization System

Tray Rethermalization System

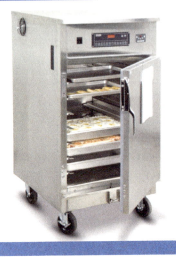
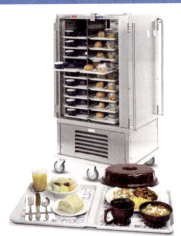

Dinex. Reprinted with permission.

If an operation is using a cook-chill pre-plated tray system, in which foods are delivered cold and rethermalized just before service, trays are pre-assembled and delivered in carts. The carts and related technologies are designed to heat the food quickly using induction or convection heat. Figure 1.6 illustrates some rethermalization systems. Note that tray rethermalization can occur in a centralized location (in the dining services department just before tray distribution), or in a decentralized location (on the nursing units). Also, specialized rethermalization systems generally require specialized dinnerware to integrate with the systems. In selecting equipment, it is important to review related needs and costs for dinnerware. Many are available in a range of colors and designs.

With today's service equipment, a manager can use software support for meal delivery systems to track temperature data, program rethermalization features, control and monitor remote delivery systems and generate reports through a desktop computer. Each style of service has its benefits and its compromises.

Pantry Service—Made to Order

In an effort to better meet client expectations, some facilities have implemented a **Pantry** mini service on the unit. Typically food is prepared in a central kitchen and supplied to kitchenettes or pantries on the unit for plating and service to the clients. The pantry servery can support any menu format, from non-select to room service meal on demand, with what is expected to be hotter and fresher meal service.

Room Service

Many definitions of **Room Service** have been brought forward over the past 10-15 years. Originally conceived as a hotel style of room service, the process has evolved to reflect the needs of the healthcare setting and delivery of meals in a business account. Menus are often altered to provide options that are known to function better on a room service format.

In hotels and commercial dining locations, a service or delivery charge is typically added to the bill to cover the cost of labor related to special delivery of the meal. In healthcare, although the added cost of labor is a factor, implementing a service charge is not an option.

Room Service, or some variation of the concept, is now a common element in healthcare from the large metropolitan acute care hospital to the Transitional Care Unit services in a community health center. Typically the room service concept is one of several styles of service within a given facility from:

- a non-select meal served at a defined time for clients unable or unwilling to select their meal; to
- menus selected by the client served from a traditional trayline at defined meal times in some units; to
- a meals on demand room service concept.

Table-Side In-Dining Room Service

In an effort to provide a more "homelike" atmosphere in the senior living and congregate dining setting, many communities have turned to a **Table-Side** service using a hot well service station in the dining room. Plating and delivery of the meal to the client is completed in front of the clients. The meal served is often a select menu with two or more choices for the entrées and side-dishes.

A number of communities have established the "neighborhood" concept for the senior living environment. Typically, in this setting, the clients live within a small group and share their meals around a family style dining table. Meals supplied from dining services are plated and served to the clients from a home or residential looking kitchen. Often special services, such as eggs made to order or sandwiches prepared upon request, are offered in the neighborhood dining room.

Glossary

Pantry
A small serving station or kitchenette

Room Service
Meals selected and served upon request

Table-Side Service
Serving clients from a hot well cart present in the dining venue

Buffet Style
Meals selected to the client from buffet style serving line

Buffet Style Service

Buffet Style service is offered in some long-term care facilities as a way to create an atmosphere of choice. Facilities offer the same number of choices as with restaurant style service (further discussed below), only clients can serve themselves. Be prepared to offer extra help for those clients who may not be able to manage walking a buffet line, handle their tray/plate, serve themselves and carry the meal to the table.

The buffet style of service is commonly used in a catered function whether in healthcare or the business setting. Catered events can be anything from coffee and donuts for a staff meeting of six to a full holiday meal for the board of directors.

Restaurant Style Service

Restaurant Style is another way of implementing a new culture in residential dining. Your regular menu cycle entrée can be the daily special with an option of sandwiches, grilled items, vegetables and salads. Restaurant style dining might include the following:

- Dining Service staff waiting on tables
- Food ordered and delivered in courses
- Food plated in the dining room
- Specials such as sandwiches, salads or desserts offered tableside from a cart

In many CCRC and corporate dining rooms, a high-end or white linen dining service is the norm. Meal options are more extensive and also upscaled with an emphasis on presentation. Training of staff on the correct service techniques in formal dining is essential to completing the fine dining experience.

Cafeteria Service

School or dormitory foodservice, employee dining rooms, commercial feeding, and correctional facilities all use a variation of the **Cafeteria** model. Whether the straight-line tray slides or the more popular scramble concept, the cafeteria is designed to move a large number of customers through the meal selection process quickly.

Typically the actual plating of the food is provided by a cafeteria server with some self-serve or "grab-n-go" items available. Often the cafeteria includes a grill and some made-to-order items like sandwiches and specialty salads. Other than the correctional or dormitory setting, cafeterias are a cash based operation.

C-Store—Sandwich Counters and Kiosks

Many of the CCRC and independent senior living communities offer a C-Store (Convenience Store) with frequently needed staples and supplies. Often a sandwich counter is an added service for a simple lunch meal when the main dining room is not available. A coffee kiosk or sandwich counter may be available in the lobby of an office complex, hospital out-patient surgery unit or campus walk-way.

Multiple Venues

Dining services are being offered in more locations and with different "personalities" all within a single facility. Senior living communities may have a traditional dining room seating 50-100 residents, plus a wellness smoothie bar, a coffee kiosk with fresh bakery items and sandwiches, a white linen steakhouse, and a lounge with a full-service bar and appetizers—all on the same campus.

Glossary

Restaurant Style
A set menu of multiple options that does not change from day to day

Cafeteria Model
Straight-line or scramble system offers cafeteria style options

Satelliting Foodservice

Equipping and staffing a food production kitchen is expensive and requires a lot of space and utilities support. Sometimes organizations decide to obtain their food items from a production center. Whether the food is delivered in bulk for reheating and serviced in a dining room, such as congregate dining, or pre-plated meals for individual clients in a school or care center, satelliting of meals is becoming more common.

One type of satellited meal that has been employed across the country is Home Delivered Meals for the homebound and the elderly.

Beyond equipment, there are additional service considerations related to the trayline system, particularly in healthcare. We will examine delivery to clients in a trayline system.

Service Concerns and Issues

Even with well-designed equipment and well-planned systems, foodservice departments sometimes face delivery challenges with trayline systems. For example, in a healthcare facility, if trays reach their destinations through a cart service, staff then need to distribute trays to clients. This task may be the responsibility of either nursing or dining services staff.

Staff who deliver trays need to accomplish several things:

- Be available as trays arrive and distribute trays promptly
- Verify that each tray is reaching the right client
  - > Two "patient identifiers" is a guideline by The Joint Commission (TJC) and recommended by World Health Organization (WHO) and Centers for Medicare & Medicaid Services (CMS)
  - > Verify a Client Name and Medical Record Number, or Date of Birth against the name on the menu or ticket on the tray. Some tray tickets include client photos for easier verification
- Be alert to any diet changes that have just occurred
- Help the client set up the tray and open any packaging
- Help the client with feeding, as needed and approved by nursing
- Obtain substitutes or make adjustments if a client has any difficulties with the meal
- Make sure food is arriving to the client at the appropriate temperature and accurate to the menu ticket

These tasks require training. In addition, they can take a lot of time. When nursing staff are required to assist, there can be time conflicts. A nurse may be involved in another clinical task at the time that trays arrive and this can cause delays. Furthermore, the Certified Dietary Manager needs to review schedules carefully to assure that they are reasonable and feasible with respect to client schedules. An effective staffing plan takes into account the skills and timing requirements of the job. In addition, it involves coordination between nursing, rehab and dining services departments.

Delays in the distribution process are a common reason for complaints about food temperature and/or quality. In addition, there is a food safety concern with trays that sit at room temperature too long. How can a Certified Dietary Manager tackle this challenge?

There is no single best answer. Some healthcare organizations have begun using additional auxiliary staff to assist with tray distribution and client feeding. Some have begun switching tray distribution from nursing to dining services staff to avoid timing conflicts. In addition, some of the rethermalization systems described allow staff to control temperature much closer to the time of service. A temperature control cart that holds food temps may help provide a longer window of time in which to accomplish the job without sacrificing safety and quality. Also, to facilitate delivery, sequence the menus or tray tickets to ensure that trays are assembled and grouped in a meaningful order.

Meal delivery schedules must also comply with additional regulations to assure that frequency and timing fit prescribed needs. For example, in healthcare, the time frame between supper and breakfast cannot be more than 14 hours (i.e., 5:30 supper and 7:30 breakfast).

If delivery problems arise, it is up to the Certified Dietary Manager to review them with a nursing supervisor or administrator to help ensure that the entire meal delivery system functions effectively.

Culture Change in Healthcare Dining Services

IThe choices for healthcare communities for older Americans are expanding and the type of food and nutrition care will need to expand as well. With 2010 CMS regulations, F242, "your facility has to demonstrate that it's allowing residents' choice and self-determination in dining." At the same time, it is important to tailor a menu to the dietary requirements of the client. How do we accomplish this? This section will describe the culture change movement around the dining experience and the menu options to support the change.

Culture Change in Language

Culture change begins with the language we use. Karen Schoeneman wrote about this in an editorial for the Pioneer Network Culture Change project. She asked people to come up with alternative words for bibs, feeder, elderly, etc. Figure 1.8 lists samples of dining terms that were suggested to help older adults maintain their dignity and healthcare facilities to become more person-centered.

Figure 1.8 Terminology of Culture Change

OLD TERMINOLOGY	SUGGESTED TERMINOLOGY
Elderly	Elder, older adult, individual
Wing, unit	Household, neighborhood, street
Institutional care	Individual care
Feeder table	Dining table
Feeder	Person who needs help eating
Facility, institution, nursing home	Home life center, living center
Foodservice worker, Hey You	The person's name
Dietary service, food service	Dining services
Tray line	Fine dining
Nourishment	Snack
Bib	Napkin, clothing protector
Diabetic	Person who has diabetes
Mechanical soft food	Chopped food
Trays are here	It's dinner time; dinner is served

Source: http://www.pioneernetwork.net Used with permission.

Culture Change in Dining

The culture change movement in dining is driven, in part, by the large numbers of Americans who are aging and who will be entering the various healthcare communities as they age. It is also being driven by the change in regulations to implement more person-centered, resident-driven dining programs. This is indeed an opportune time to showcase dining services and your ability to enhance the quality of life through food and dining choices. One service option change is to offer restaurant or in-dining room table-side service instead of the traditional trayline.

As with any change, there is resistance based on concerns about cost, staffing, and coordinating the changes with regulations.

As you begin to adopt a new culture, there are many questions that need to be answered. Start with questioning clients to help decide what they want for dining services. You might ask questions such as:

- What time of day do you like to eat your meals?
- Do you snack regularly?
- How frequently during the day do you want coffee, tea, or water?
- Where do you prefer to eat your meals?
- What foods do you usually eat at breakfast, lunch, and dinner?
- Where should you begin with the culture change? (expanded snack program, restaurant services, selective menu)

Next, you will want to choose appropriate resources for changing your dining and/or menu options. You could survey other facilities in your area to determine how/if they have begun to implement a culture change in their dining services. The Association of Nutrition & Foodservice Professionals (ANFP) published a position paper in 2011: *The Role of Certified Dietary Manager in Person-Directed Dining.* This position paper is available in the online *Supplemental Textbook Material—Foodservice.* Remember, the changes you make need to reflect your clients' food and dining preferences.

Once you have data for what you want to do and why, the next step is to work with all departments in your facility. This will be a change for them as well, and you want them to support your efforts. Other departments that are likely to be affected are maintenance and nursing. You will want to develop a policy and procedure that outlines every department's responsibility for each type of change you initiate. Communication and training will be key steps. It is important to note that a culture change is a process that takes some time to implement.

While the changes outlined in *Person-Directed Dining* are directed at the healthcare field, they apply to any dining service. Dignity in dining is a concern in all marketplaces. Providing customer choice, quality products and trained staff are hallmarks of good management.

Your menu and the style of the menu are major components in developing a new dining culture. The equipment available defines many of the meal delivery options available to you. Decisions to transition away from a set trayline/ no choice meal system to a more accommodating meal service and options take planning and forethought.

Putting It Into Practice

2. List at least three steps you would take to implement a culture change in your facility.

Menu Options

Two of the most common options are selective and nonselective. Whether you have a select or non-select format, you need to have a defined number of days over which the menu is used. This is referred to as the **menu cycle**—how fast you return to day 1 of the cycle. You do not want to write a new menu every week and end up with a cycle 365 days long.

In the acute care setting, the average length of stay is now around 4 days. Many hospitals have gone to a cycle of 5-8 days so that the same items do not always fall on a Tuesday.

In the residential segment of business (senior living, rehab and group homes) the cycle is more likely going to be 3–6 weeks. Often using an odd number of weeks works better for these communities and employee cafeterias. Typically staff work every other weekend and when the menu is set to a 2 or 4 week cycle the staff see the same thing every weekend. By using a 5 week cycle a nurse will work 10 weeks before they see the Oven Roasted Turkey and Dressing on Sunday again.

Business and Industry dining rooms and school foodservice also benefit from a longer menu cycle of 3-5 weeks just to avoid the repetition of items on the serving line. The presence of the daily standard items in the grill, sandwich service and salad bars allows for an ever present and popular set of alternatives.

Selective Menus

A **selective menu** is the way to implement current federal regulations, and more importantly, enhance the quality of life and quality of care for your clients. A selective menu is one in which clients have the opportunity to make choices or selections in advance of meal service. For example, it usually offers at least two choices for an entrée and multiple choices for most items.

Computer-based selective menu systems may use handheld computers and/or telephone systems for entry of choices into an automated system. Typically, a selective menu is distributed to clients in advance of the meal.

Select menus generally fit one of the following types:

Pre-Select

- Typically a printed menu with choices for Breakfast, Lunch and Dinner.
- Often distributed to the client the morning of or the day before service for selection and return to the meal preparation area.
- The selection maybe limited to two entrées with the same side dishes or, more commonly, offers two to three entrées, two to three starches and vegetables .
- Family members may pre-select the meals for a week in advance knowing the client's preferences.
- No matter how many options are offered, a defined menu is set for each day as the non-select meal for those who choose not to make their selections.
  - > The defined menu ensures nutritional adequacy of the default meal being provided.

Glossary

Menu Cycle
The number of days over which a menu is used

Selective Menu
A menu designed with multiple choices

Putting It Into Practice

3. You have a long-term patient (16 days) complaining about their meals. You have a non-select seven day menu cycle. What can you offer the patient?

Table-Side Select

- This may be the same base menu designed for the Pre-Select with a selection made in the dining room at the time of service.
- The menu is typically posted in and around the dining room so clients can see in advance what the choices will be for the meal.
- There is also a non-select menu for those who choose not to make their selections.

Spoken

- This may be the same base menu designed for the Pre-Select.
- The menu is presented to the client by a Dining Services staff member by speaking. For example: "Good morning Mrs. Jones, today for lunch we have a garden salad, spaghetti with meat sauce, green beans and lemon sorbet for dessert. How does that sound to you?"… "I did not realize that you don't like green beans, would you prefer broccoli or chopped spinach?"
- By placing the first or non-select default item as "today for lunch we have…" leads the client to the preferred choice but leaves them with the option to request an alternative.
- The printed version of the menu may be available to clients to see in advance what the choices will be for the meal.
- There is also a non-select option for those who choose not to select their menu.

Restaurant Variation

- Typically this menu format is set up with a list of items that are always available as standard choices.
- Additionally a daily feature or chef's choice is presented as the preferred or default option for the meal.
- Standard items tend to be a short order type that can be finished quickly, such as baked fish or chicken stir-fry.
- The featured selection is often one that takes more time to prepare and would not be available every day, such as pot roast or pork chops.
- The printed version of the restaurant menu is available to clients to see in advance what the choices will be for the meal and the daily features may be printed for the day or the week for client review.
- There is also a non-select meal (typically the daily feature item) for those who choose not to make their selection.

Cafeteria

- Typically this menu format is set up with a list of items that are always available as a set or standard choices.
- Additionally a daily feature or chef's choice is also presented.
- Standard items tend to be a short order type that can be finished quickly, such as baked fish or chicken stir-fry.
- Featured menu selections are often ones that take more time to prepare and would not be available every day, such as pot roast or pork chops.

Buffet

- Generally a buffet menu is planned for a self-serve line.
- This style is often centered around single-serve or portion-controlled items like baked chicken breast or lower-cost products where over portioning does not negatively impact financial performance.

Menus can be printed in a number of formats but typically start out as a Week-At-A-Glance (WAG) layout with Breakfast, Lunch and Dinner (or Supper) planned for the week. This allows the manager and coordinator of the meal services to see in one place all of the meals planned for several days. Problems with repeating food items are easier to spot when looking at the WAG version. The WAG meets the needs of the "back of the house" production team but does not market well to your customers. For the "front of the house" or customer facing menu, most organizations prefer to jazz up the appearance and highlight the specials. The following 2 examples demonstrate the typical WAG for a healthcare facility, Figure 1.9, and a sample select menu for the day, Figure 1.10.

Figure 1.9 Sample Week-At-A-Glance Menu Layout

	SUN	MON	TUES	WED	THUR	FRI	SAT
BREAKFAST	Choice of Juice	Choice of Juice	Choice of Juice	Choice of Juice	Choice of Juice	Choice of Juice	Choice of Juice
	Choice of Cold Cereal	Choice of Cold Cereal	Choice of Cold Cereal	Choice of Cold Cereal	Choice of Cold Cereal	Choice of Cold Cereal	Choice of Cold Cereal
	Scrambled Eggs						
	Oatmeal	Malt-O-Meal	Cream of Wheat	Oatmeal	Malt-O-Meal	Cream of Wheat	Malt-O-Meal
	Ham Patty	Poached Egg	Fried Egg	Hard Cooked Egg	Scrambled Egg	Omelet	Scrambled Egg
	Caramel Roll	Wheat Toast	Wheat Toast	Pancake & Syrup	Muffin	Wheat Toast	Waffle
	Milk	Milk	Milk	Milk	Milk	Milk	Milk
	Coffee	Coffee	Coffee	Coffee	Coffee	Coffee	Coffee
LUNCH			Tomato Soup	Wild Rice Soup			
	Pork Roast	Shepherd's Pie	Grilled Cheese	Bratwurst	Beef Lasagna	Chicken Tacos	Baked Pork Chop
	Mashed Potatoes with Gravy			Potato Salad		Spanish Rice	Oven Brown Potatoes
	Nantucket Vegetables	Vegetable Medley	Mixed Vegetable Salad	Baked Beans	French Style Green Beans	Shredded Lettuce Diced Tomatoes	Winter Blend
	Bread/Dinner Roll	Bread/Dinner Roll	Crackers	Bread/Bun	Garlic Bread		Bread/Dinner Roll
	Fruit Pie	Fresh Fruit	Bananas or Fruit Cocktail Topped with Pudding	Mandarin Oranges	Diced Peaches and Pears	Homemade Bars	Pumpkin Crunch
	Baked Fish with Rice Pilaf	Chicken (Strip or Salad) Wrap	Turkey Burger on a Bun	Roast Beef Sandwich	Chef Salad	Egg Salad Sandwich	Tuna Salad Wrap
	Iced Tea/Coffee	Iced Tea/Coffee	Iced Tea/Coffee	Iced Tea/Coffee	Iced Tea/Coffee	Iced Tea/Coffee	Iced Tea/Coffee
SUPPER	Hearty Vegetable Soup				V8		
	Turkey Sandwich	Tuna Rice Bake with Peas	Beef Stroganoff	Grilled Chicken Breast	Breakfast Ham	Breaded Fish Fillet	Goulash
			Noodles	Scalloped Potatoes	French Toast	Potato Wedges	
	Three Bean Salad	Garden Salad	Dilled Carrots	Asparagus	Fresh Fruit	Cheesy Broccoli	Cut Corn
	Crackers	Bread/Dinner Roll	Bread/Dinner Roll	Bread/Dinner Roll		Dinner Roll/Muffin	Bread/Dinner Roll
	Diced Pears	Brownie	Cobbler	Better Than Anything Cake	Sherbet	Fruited Red Gelatin	Custard
	Pizza	Scrambled Eggs and English Muffin	Chicken Salad Stuffed Tomato	Cube Steak and Gravy	Grilled Cheese Sandwich	Hot Dog on Bun	Soup and Deli Sandwich
	Milk	Milk	Milk	Milk	Milk	Milk	Milk
	Coffee	Coffee	Coffee	Coffee	Coffee	Coffee	Coffee

Figure 1.10 Sample Select Menu for a Day

BREAKFAST	LUNCH	SUPPER
Assorted Juice Hot or Cold Cereal Egg of Choice Breakfast Ham Slice	Fried Chicken Mashed Potatoes Chicken Gravy Green Beans	BBQ Riblette Mixed Vegetables Pasta Salad
English Muffin Jelly or Honey Margarine, Salt & Pepper Milk Coffee or Hot Tea	Fruit Cobbler Dinner Roll Margarine, Salt & Pepper Milk Coffee or Iced Tea	Brownie Cornbread Muffin Margarine, Salt & Pepper Milk Coffee or Iced Tea
Other Menu Selections Breakfast Fruit of the Day Toast Mini Danish	**Other Menu Selections** Cheeseburger on Bun Chef's Salad Loaded Baked Potato	**Other Menu Selections** Grilled Chicken Breast Tuna Salad Stuffed Tomato Lemon Baked Fish
Room: _____ Diet Order: _____ Name: _____	Room: _____ Diet Order: _____ Name: _____	Room: _____ Diet Order: _____ Name: _____

In healthcare facilities, or in any environment where the dining services department is responsible for honoring therapeutic diets, it is standard practice to review meal choices before they are served. If clients make choices on a selective menu, a member of the dining services team then reviews these choices against the medical diet of record and the nutrition guidelines for the diet. Common adjustments that may need to be made are:

- Portion sizes of products that count as fluid, for a fluid-restricted diet.
- Portion sizes of high-carbohydrate foods, for a carbohydrate counting diet.
- Consistency of foods and liquids for specific dysphagia diets.
- Special adjustments for diets with multiple restrictions.
- Adjustments to incorporate a standing order, such as the addition of a liquid nutritional supplement to meals.

What happens if the client does not request enough food on a selective menu? What if the client selects food that is not on his/her diet? Dining Services staff should be trained to address a client's diet when they drop off the menu, for example:

- "Good morning Mrs. Smith. I know that you are on a sodium restricted diet and here are your menu selections for today." This helps remind the client of their diet and sets the stage for their choices.
- If they see that the client has not selected very much food, the Dining Services staff might say, "Oh, Mrs. Smith, our roast chicken is very tender and moist today. May I add that to your selection?"
- If the client insists on selecting something that is not on their menu, such as bacon on a salt restricted diet, gently remind the client that their diet does not allow them to have bacon.

Always treat clients with respect and respond in such a way that they don't become defensive. Keep in mind that you need to educate clients on the limits of their medically ordered diet, however, their resident/patient rights may overrule the dietary restrictions. Refer diet conflicts like these to the clinical nutrition staff for intervention and documentation in the medical record.

Figure 1.11 Examples of Food Substitutions*

FOOD ITEM	FOOD CHOICES	VITAMIN A CONTENT (per 1/2 cup serving)	VITAMIN C CONTENT (per 1/2 cup serving)
Dark Green Vegetables	Asparagus, boiled	905 IU	7 mg
	Broccoli, frozen, boiled	1,208 IU	50 mg
	Brussels sprouts, frozen, boiled	1435 IU	70 mg
	Green beans, canned	54 IU	8 mg
	Green peppers, boiled	194 IU	28 mg
	Kale (use in soups)	8853 IU	265 mg
	Mixed vegetables, frozen	1944 IU	1.5 mg
	Pea pods, boiled	532 IU	17 mg
	Peas, frozen and boiled	824 IU	38 mg
	Romaine lettuce, 1 cup	2098 IU	1 mg
Bright Orange Vegetables	Carrots, frozen	9094 IU	1.6 mg
	Sweet potatoes, boiled and mashed	1444 IU	8 mg
	Winter squash, baked	793 IU	7 mg
White Vegetables	Cabbage, boiled	60 IU	28 mg
	Cauliflower	7 IU	27 mg
	Celery	226 IU	1.5 mg
	Rutabaga	1.5 IU	16 mg
	Turnips	0 IU	10 mg

Source: U.S. Department of Agriculture—National Nutrient Database for Standard Reference

[a.] Vegetables are often the foods that clients will have an aversion to. Remember that substitutions have to be equivalent in nutritional value, so choose another vegetable(s) that is roughly equivalent to the content of the leader nutrients, vitamin A and vitamin C.

On a selective menu, there may also be items a client writes in as a special request. How this is handled depends on the facility policy. In general, health facilities attempt to honor write-in requests when practical. Many facilities develop a standardized list of write-in options to provide greater choice for clients.

Non-Selective Menus

A **non-selective menu** is one in which clients do not have the opportunity to make choices. Instead, they receive a standard, predefined menu. This is more common in a group dining experience such as a nursing home or assisted living. Even with a non-select format, you can focus on the clients by following their individualized food preferences with appropriate substitutions.

Glossary

Non-Selective Menu
A menu with no defined alternatives—a predefined menu plan

In a non-selective menu system, it is also important to review and modify standard choices to accommodate specific diet orders. You still want to follow individual food preferences, which may mean changing a food item. Substitutions must be of equal nutritional value. For instance, if someone doesn't like cabbage, the replacement should be a food that has similar Vitamin C, such as tomatoes. Since menus are planned to incorporate color, try to replace a food with a similar or a complementary color. Your facility should have a list of approved substitutes for your menu cycle. When making adjustments, always document the change and keep a record. This helps to prove during surveys that you are meeting client needs and preferences. See Figure 1.11 for food substitution choices.

Late Trays

In a healthcare setting, it is essential to have a system for providing meals to clients who have just been admitted, whose diet orders have changed, or who have missed a meal due to testing or special procedures. Trays delivered between meal times are called **late trays**. Particularly in an acute care environment, diet-related information can change quickly.

In many situations, late trays are cumbersome and expensive to produce and deliver. Obtaining required adjustments just before tray assembly can sometimes reduce the volume of added trays. Many healthcare operations strive to reduce out of sequence requests through their meal system design. Room service is an example of a service model that can virtually eliminate late trays, because all meals are provided on demand.

Summary

Whatever menu or service style you use in your foodservice process, make sure there are adequate policies, staff training, and oversight to be able to provide the quality of service expected. You also need to establish policies for working with clients who choose foods that are contrary to the therapeutic diet that was ordered for them. In addition, a facility needs to devise procedures and provide adequate staffing to assist with person-centered dining.

Now that you know what Style of Meal Delivery Service you have and what Style of Menu you provide to your clients, you can consider your options for a culture change in your dining services.

Glossary

Late Trays
Trays delivered between meal times

Menus—The Foundation of the Department

Overview and Objectives

The menu is the starting point for many decisions involving purchasing, production, and service of food. You will examine the basics of menu planning and utilize techniques to provide satisfying meals for your clients. You will identify standard food weights and measures related to the meal service and portioning. You will also review both your legal and moral responsibilities for providing nutritious food to your clients. After completing this chapter, you should be able to:

✓ Identify how the menu impacts the dining services department
✓ List resources available for menu planning and development
✓ Identify how cultures can impact the menu
✓ Define how the menu affects the department budget
✓ Describe how management decisions affect the menu
✓ Evaluate the quality and accuracy of each meal service

By now, it is clear that a menu is a strong force in achieving client satisfaction. It has been said that the menu drives everything in the kitchen. It is also a means of communicating with clients—and even marketing your fare to future clientele. However, it's more than that; a menu governs the series of events that define the department's overall workflow. Figure 2.1 identifies this process in a simplified format.

As you can see, recipe specifications, the products you need to carry in inventory, production information for the prep staff, and the final food presentation all hinge on the menu plan. In addition, the menu may define the requirements for staffing, equipment, physical layout and design of the department. Figure 2.1 displays the basic steps in the workflow, starting with menu planning through to meal delivery.

Ultimately, the financial performance of your operation rests heavily on your menu. What it costs to produce and serve meals impacts your expenses. What you sell in cafeterias and retail venues impacts your revenues. In short, the menu is a critical and dominant force in your operation. As such, it merits special attention and careful planning.

As you learned in Chapter 1 there are several styles and types of menus used in Dining Services. Each one is designed to meet the needs of the individual facility. In this chapter, the process of writing and revising menus will be covered. This will include the steps to track and monitor the quality and approval of your dining service to the clients.

Figure 2.1 Simple Flow of Work in a Foodservice Operation

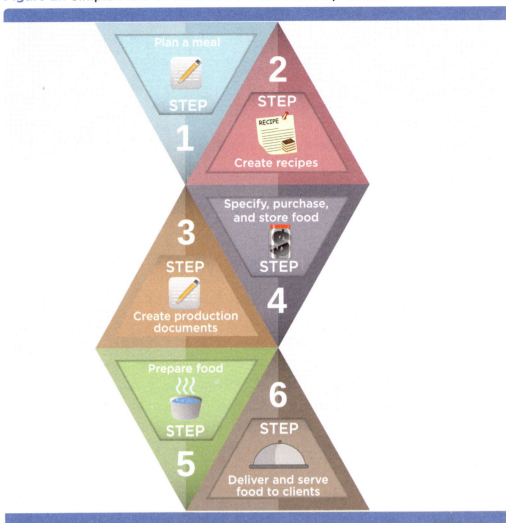

Menu Planning Considerations

Whether a menu is written in the facility or purchased from a third party, several points need to be considered to ensure a quality menu is offered to the clients.

Key Points

Customer/Client Satisfaction

The most important consideration in menu planning is satisfying your customers/clients. Chapter 7 will address the many ways to monitor and track customer satisfaction. Audits to evaluate "Plate Waste," client surveys or "Menu Score-Cards" help identify opportunities for menu edits.

In an effort to improve client satisfaction and meal consumption, many senior living facilities have moved to a more liberalized menu, allowing more options for all modified diets. However, it is still important to include special needs such as cultural factors, food habits, and especially food preferences and diets when planning your menus.

Facilities often use a menu developed by their corporate office or a third party. It is essential to adapt this menu to the needs, wants, and regional preferences of your clients.

Nutrition and Other Resources

Nutrition considerations should also be a primary goal of menu planning. It is important to maintain adequate nutritional status, to the highest extent possible. There are a number of resources to help; some of those include the **Dietary Guidelines for Americans**, (refer to the most updated at www.DietaryGuidelines.gov as these guidelines are updated every five years) the USDA DRI (Daily Reference Intakes), MyPlate (www.ChooseMyPlate.gov), facility diet manual, and Recommended Dietary Allowances (RDAs). Note that these resources are updated on a regular basis and the dietary manager should look periodically for the most current resources. Figure 2.2 on page 32 lists a number of standards that might be used to evaluate the nutritional content of your menus.

Modified or Restricted Diet Menus

Often in healthcare settings, menus need to be adjusted to meet the dietary restrictions ordered by medical staff. While many menu items will not need to be altered to meet the dietary restrictions, some items may require ingredient changes or elimination from the menu as planned.

Some managers have gone to a "one pot cooking" method for dealing with dietary restrictions. In essence, whatever the identified ingredient is that requires restriction is eliminated from all or most recipes making the recipe work across all diets. Many dining services have adopted a salt-free, fat-free and even sugar-free menu to allow for a single gravy, vegetable and entrée to be served to all clients. While this is a quick and simple answer to the problem it effectively penalizes all clients to the most restrictive of diets.

Most clients do not need to follow all of these restrictions and find the limited palate of meal options unsatisfactory. Keep in mind that client satisfaction may be related to reimbursements and clientele retention. Often the access to liberalized diets in senior living facilites allows for the use of a more acceptable variety of foods on the menu.

When the nutrient analysis of a menu dictates an alternate is required for some clients, the use of a modified recipe or totally different item is in order. Planning a menu with alternate items that mix well with the primary base menu (sides or entrées as appropriate) helps control the number of different items that need to be prepared.

Specific information on Nutrition Therapy and food restrictions are covered in the *Nutrition Fundamentals and Medical Nutrition Therapy* textbook which accompanies this textbook in many Dietary Managers' Training programs.

Cultural, Regional, and Religious Considerations

Cultural heritage should be a consideration when planning menus. To understand this aspect of menu planning, try asking yourself some questions. What does turkey and dressing with cranberry sauce mean to you? Many people will answer: Thanksgiving. This food has become part of a cultural tradition. Now, think about a wedding celebration. What food will always be served? Most people will answer: a wedding cake. Or, in China, the answer may be: roasted pig. Now, try another question. What food has become a symbol of American heritage and pride? Many people will answer: apple pie. From these examples, you can see that we regard food choices as cultural symbols. The meaning of these foods is much deeper than a sum of protein, carbohydrate, fat, vitamins, and minerals—the sheer nutritional values.

Many food choices arise from what we learn through our own cultural experiences. Holidays, festivals, and important events each have associated foods. In addition, daily

Glossary

Dietary Guidelines for Americans
Dietary guidelines that encourage Americans to focus on eating a healthful diet that focuses on foods and beverages that contribute to achieving and maintaining a healthy weight, promote health, and prevent disease

Figure 2.2 Nutritional Guides or Standards for Menu Planning

Name of Guide	Source
Dietary Guidelines for Americans	Department of Health and Human Services and U.S. Department of Agriculture: http://health.gov/DietaryGuidelines/
MyPlate	U.S. Department of Agriculture: www.choosemyplate.gov
Recommended Dietary Allowances	Nutrition.gov: http://fnic.nal.usda.gov/dietary-guidance/dietary-reference-intake?
Exchange Lists for Diabetes or Renal Disease	Academy of Nutrition and Dietetics or American Diabetes Association www.americandiabetes.com/using-exchange-lists-diabetes- meal-planning/ National Kidney Foundation: www.kidney.org/atoz/atozTopic_Nutrition-Diet.cfm
Centers for Medicare & Medicaid Services	CMS: www.cms.gov/Regulations-and-Guidance/Guidance/Manuals/downloads/SOM107ap_pp_Guidelines_ltcf.pdf
National Dysphagia Diet	American Speech-Language Hearing Association: www.asha.org/SLP/clinical/dysphagia/Dysphagia-Diets Nutrition411.com: www.nutrition411.com/?s=National+Dysphagia+Diet
National School Lunch	USDA Food and Nutrition Service: www.fns.usda.gov/nslp/national-school-lunch-program-nslp School Nutrition Association: www.schoolnutrition.org
Facility Diet Manual	Check with facility dietitian or state regulations for a current diet manual or complete an online search for "healthcare diet manual" for additional resources
Corrections Food Guidelines	http://www.acfsa.org/fedRegs.php

food choices vary by culture. Traditional German cuisine, for example, is likely to include sausage, schnitzel, spätzle, beer, and other specialties. Japanese cuisine includes sushi, tempura, and rice. Swedish cuisine may include pancakes, even at meals other than breakfast. Mexican meals include staples such as tortillas, rice, and refried beans. Creole cooking, popular in New Orleans, represents a fusion of French cooking using locally available foods such as shrimp and intense spices, mixed with influences from local Caribbean and Spanish cultures.

As a land of immigrants, the U.S. enjoys a multi-faceted cultural diversity. Our menu choices are as rich and complex as our population itself. It is important to look at the populations in the facility to determine what menu items should be added to meet the cultural diversity. Below are some of the more commonly seen ethnic regions that have migrated into the United States. Please note that this is not the full list but a sampling.

Hispanic/Latinos. The United States Census Bureau defines Hispanics as those who indicate their origin to be Mexican, Puerto Rican, Cuban, Central or South American (e.g., Dominican, Nicaraguan, and Colombian) or other Hispanic origin. The largest of these is the Mexican-American population, which represents at least two-thirds of all Hispanics/Latinos. According to a national survey conducted by the U.S. Department of Agriculture,

"Hispanics tend to eat more rice but less pasta and ready-to-eat cereals than their non-Hispanic white counterparts. Hispanics are also likely to consume vegetables, especially tomatoes, although they have a slightly higher consumption of fruits. Compared to non-Hispanic whites, Hispanics are more than twice as likely to drink whole milk, but much less likely to drink low-fat or skim milk. Hispanics are also more likely to eat beef but less likely to eat processed meats such as hot dogs, sausage, and luncheon meats." Legumes and corn in combination are good and common sources of protein and, along with cheese, are frequent ingredients in Hispanic ethnic meals.

East Indian Americans. Staples of the Indian diet include rice, beans, lentils, and bread. Rice is usually served steamed and mixed with flavorings. Indian breads include chapattis, round flatbread made of whole wheat flour; and naan, a bread that uses yeast. India's religious beliefs have also influenced the diet of Indians (e.g., Hindus believe that cows are sacred so they do not eat beef.) Chicken or lamb, in moderation, is augmented with vegetables, dried beans, lentils and split peas. Curry powder, a mixture of spices, is often used to flavor Indian foods. The heart of Indian cooking is the combination of spices that gives each dish its unique flavor. Indian cuisine has become increasingly popular during the first decade of the 21st Century with over 1200 Indian food products now available in the U.S.

Chinese Americans. Vegetables, rice, noodles, fruits, and foods made from soybeans (such as tofu and soy milk) are very important foods in the Chinese-American diet. Plain rice is served at all meals. Sometimes fried rice is served. Pork, poultry, and fish are popular and used in small amounts to flavor the rice. Foods are often seasoned with soy sauce, which is high in sodium. (Low-sodium versions can be purchased). Corn oil, sesame oil, and peanut oil are used. Tea is the main beverage and it is almost always enjoyed black—without sugar, cream, or milk. Fruits are important and few sweets are eaten. Cow's milk and dairy products are not used often (lactose intolerance is comparatively common in the Asian population).

Japanese Americans. Some people are surprised to learn that Japanese food is quite different in appearance and taste from Chinese food. While Chinese food is often stir-fried, Japanese food is often simmered, boiled, steamed, or broiled. Also, Japanese foods are not as highly seasoned as Chinese dishes. Sushi, a rice wrapped in seaweed has become a popular food choice in the U.S. in the past decade. Rice is the staple of many Japanese-American diets, along with a variety of noodles. As in Chinese cooking, soybean products, such as soy sauce, are important. Seafood is generally more popular than meat and poultry. Vegetables, such as watercress and carrots, are an important part of most meals. Tea is the most popular beverage, especially green tea, an excellent source of antioxidants.

Middle Eastern Americans. Foods of choice in a traditional Middle Eastern diet include yogurt, cheeses (such as feta and goat cheese), lamb, poultry, chick peas, lentils, lemons, eggplant, pine nuts, olives, and olive oil. A Greek specialty is baklava, a baked dessert made with nuts, honey, and filo dough. Common cooking styles are grilling, frying, and stewing.

See Figure 2.3 for cultural food influences. Here are more examples of cultural and ethnic food influences.

Figure 2.3 Cultural Influences on Food Intake in the U.S.

FOOD GROUP	HISPANIC/ LATINO	ASIAN (China, Japan, Korea, Southwest Asia)	MIDDLE EASTERN	EAST INDIAN
Grains	Tortillas (some made with lard) and rice	Rice noodles	Couscous, tahini, pita bread, and filo dough	Rice and whole wheat flatbread (naan)
Vegetables	Cactus, cassava, chayote, jicama, peppers, pinto beans, and tomatoes (salsa)	Garlic, ginger, mung beans, sprouts, bamboo shoots, bok choy, cabbage, and carrots	Tomatoes, olives, lentils, hummus, grape leaves, and eggplant	Red lentils, pigeon peas, legumes, and curries
Fruits	Avocado, bananas, guava, mango, papaya, plantain, and citrus fruits	Mango, banana, citrus fruit, coconut, and pineapple	Dates, figs, and citrus fruits	Coconut, watermelon, and mango
Meat	Chorizo (sausage and other processed meat), goat, meat, tongue, and pork	Small amounts of meat especially fish, eggs, and tofu	Small amounts of lamb, fish, and chicken	Mostly vegetarian— some mutton chicken and fish
Dairy	Goat cheese, goat milk, and whole milk	Soy milk	Yogurt and feta cheese	Milk, butter, and yogurt

Note: This is not a complete list of foods. All of these cultures have diets that vary from one region/country to another.

Regional Trends

Part of the cultural heritage unique to the U.S. is the development of regional culinary trends. Often, these trends reflect a mix of native cultures, foods that are grown and harvested in the area, and ethnic traditions contributed by settlers and immigrants over time. For example, New England is known for maple syrup, Boston beans, brown bread, and cranberry muffins. Maine is recognized for lobster. Blueberries are important in New Jersey and in the Midwest, where many are grown. In Pennsylvania and parts of Ohio, the Pennsylvania Dutch heritage gives rise to scrapple (a loaf made from meat scraps, broth, and flour), homemade noodles, and shoofly (molasses) pie.

Vidalia onions are a hallmark of Georgia's cuisine and are the official state vegetable. Peanuts and peaches are also key crops in Georgia. Florida is known for key limes and key lime pie, coquina soup, and other specialties. Kuchen is the official state dessert in

South Dakota. Most people associate Idaho with potatoes and New Orleans with Creole cuisine, such as jambalaya, dirty rice, and gumbo. Barbecued meats and pickled okra have special significance in Texas. In the Southwest (Arizona, New Mexico, Oklahoma, Texas), Mexican-style foods such as burritos and tacos are popular. Garlic is so important in California that the town of Gilroy celebrates an annual garlic festival. In fact, food celebrations, such as strawberry harvest festivals, maple syrup festivals, and many others, are key events in all parts of the country.

Religious Practices

Religious beliefs, along with religious customs and rituals, can exert a strong influence on menu planning. Fasting is one practice that many religions observe. The length of time one fasts varies with his/her religion and can range from one day to a month. Some Muslims observe Ramadan, which lasts for one month and fasting occurs from sun up to sun down.

Religious laws will also affect menu planning. For example, the Jewish faith has their own religious beliefs including building kosher kitchens which separate the meat from dairy when cooking. The Islamic faith has guidelines for the sourcing and cooking of halal foods.

Some religious beliefs are specific to the time of child birth and the 6-8 weeks following birth. Many religions and cultures have specific food requirements for their dying loved ones.

Developing a menu has now become more complicated for the Certified Dietary Manager as they must think about how to include these practices into the process for the facility. Identification of the presence and cultures of various ethnic and religious groups in your local population may require additional research into the food preferences and dietary restriction of those groups. Ethnic populations may influence large areas of the country, state or local community.

For example, one-third of all Somalis living in the United States live in Minneapolis, Minnesota. Just 10 miles away in St Paul, you will find the largest single community of Hmong residents in the United States. Both of these cities also share a unique blend of Norwegian, Swedish and Danish heritage along with the significant presence of Native American tribal history. The Certified Dietary Manager is well-advised to verify the multiple cultures and religions present in their local community and to incorporate the dietary restrictions and food preferences into their menu planning.

Government Regulations

Government regulation is another type of resource that plays a major part in menu planning. These regulations govern the type and quantity of food served at a meal. The Centers for Medicare & Medicaid Services (CMS) is a branch of the U.S. Department of Health and Human Services. CMS is the federal agency that administers the Medicare system and monitors the Medicaid programs offered by each state.

All healthcare facilities have mandatory state licensing requirements. The facility is held to the strictest regulatory requirements, either state or federal. It is important to know and follow local and state regulations. These guidelines are dynamic, meaning they change constantly. Work with your facility administrator to make sure you have the most recent CMS guidelines that impact menu planning.

If you work in a federal or state funded school system, you will be expected to follow the USDA National School Lunch Program. Critical upgrades were made through the Healthy,

Hunger-Free Kids Act championed by the First Lady, Michelle Obama. More details on the Nutrition Standards for the National School Lunch Program can be found at http://www.fns.usda.gov/school-meals/nutrition-standards-school-meals. Also work with your school administrator to make sure you have the latest guidelines.

Color, Texture, and Shape

Think about this menu, unbreaded baked cod, cauliflower, scalloped potatoes and vanilla pudding. Everything is white, round and the meal has strong competing flavors in the fish and cauliflower. This meal is often seen on menus and not widely accepted by clients. While there are times when the flavors and traditions, such as Thanksgiving Dinner, warrant a meal of competing flavors, it should not be seen on a regular basis.

Well written menus not only look at the nutritional balance but also look at the color, texture, mix of strong and mild flavors and the shape of food on the plate. When the meal looks and tastes good, clients will be more apt to enjoy their food.

One tip would be to prepare the planned menu and take a photo of the plate. This will tell the story around the appearance of the plate and what adjustments may need to be made. Look for all of these characteristics:

- **Color**—Is there a variety and balance?
- **Shape**—Is everything round, linear, wedged?
- **Texture**—Is it diced, chopped, formed or mushy?
- **Plate Coverage**—Is there a good balance across the plate (too crowded or empty)?
- **Seasoning**—Is there a mix of mild and spicy?
- **Flavor**—Is there bland or mild foods to complement the stronger meats or vegetables?
- **Food Group Balance**—Is there a mix of protein, vegetables, and starches?
- **Consistency**—Is everything in a sauce or gravy?
- **Overall**—Look at the whole meal as served, not just the main plate.
  > The grilled chicken breast with herbed rice and mixed vegetables may look fine until you see the rest of the meal with coleslaw and fruited (fruit cocktail) lemon gelatin, and sugar cookie.
  > Suddenly the whole meal is one color of mostly chopped up food items.

Photos of the plates and meals assist you in identifying some simple-to-make menu errors. It also helps the staff to maintain a consistent plate presentation for the client.

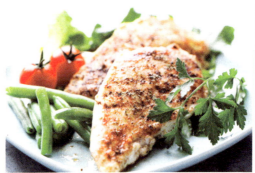 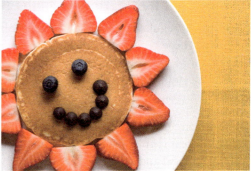

Sanitation regulations can also play a part in menu planning as they dictate the temperature to which foods must be cooked or reheated prior to service. A beautifully prepared roast beef may have perfect plate presentation when cooked for the time of service. However, the same roast in a cook-chill operation needs to be reheated to a rather well done 160° prior to service. How quickly food needs to be cooled, the appropriate storage time of cooked and raw foods and reheating guidelines all affect the safety and often the serving quality of foods.

More will be discussed related to sanitation in chapter 19. More details on the regulations can be obtained from federal, state, and local agencies.

Special or Single Use

Beyond the regular cycle menu that is planned for the clients of the facility, separate menus are often prepared to use for special events, theme meals or holidays. Many times these meals are designed to help break the monotony of a cycle menu. These menus may evolve out of a client food committee designed to incorporate their input into the meal planning process.

Retail cafeterias are typically located in schools, hospitals and other institutions that provide meal services that may be offered to the customer/student. This type of menu may provide a complete meal at a fixed price or al a carte pricing. A complete meal might include an appetizer, a salad, an entrée, a starch, a vegetable or fruit, a beverage, and possibly dessert. For example, a school lunch menu may offer a pre-defined list of foods that constitute a meal. Typically, these are planned in conjunction with USDA guidelines. See Figure 2.4 for an example.

Figure 2.4 Sample Special Menu 1 (St. Patrick's Day) for a Hospital Cafe

Appetizers

- Baked Spinach Artichoke Dip with Pita Chips
- Bruschetta with Edamame Pesto

Entrées

- Corned Beef
- Irish Stew

Accompaniments

- Baked Cabbage with Bacon
- Boiled Potatoes and Carrots

Bread

- Irish Soda Bread with Raisins

Desserts

- Crème de Menthe Pie
- Chocolate Zucchini Cake

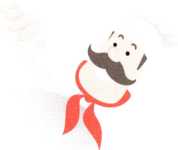

Reviewed 2015.

A la Carte

An a la carte menu allows clients to select each item they desire for a meal. In a retail setting, each menu item is priced individually. This may be used in campus dining or in schools. It is also common in many employee and visitor dining cafeterias.

Standard Weights and Measures

An essential part of menu planning is using standard food weights, measures, and recipes correctly. Within the menu planning process, consideration has to be given to the food being served in terms of quantity on the plate, nutritional value of the foods and cost controls. Serving sizes are specified in the menu design itself. If a cup of soup is planned as an appetizer, the quantity is significantly less than a bowl of the same soup served as the entrée of the meal.

The Purchasing Supervisor needs to know the serving sizes and number of servings so they order the appropriate amount of raw ingredients. The Production Team needs to know the serving sizes of items so they prepare the correct amount of food. The Serving Staff need to know the serving size of each menu item so they can plate the meal correctly. Registered Dietitian Nutritionist, Dietetic Technician, Registered/Nutrition and Dietetics Technician, Registered and /or Certified Dietary Manager need to know the serving sizes to evaluate the client meal intake for dietary intake tracking.

To plan a menu, you and your staff need to know how many servings in a full-size steam table pan, how many servings from a quart when using a disher/portion scoop, how many tablespoons in a cup, how many servings you can expect from a case of fresh broccoli, etc. One very helpful book that provides these charts for standard weights and measures is *Food for Fifty* by Mary Molt. This reference also contains many quantity recipes that may help you in revising menus to meet your facility/client needs. The need for accurate weights and measures in the recipe and production process are addressed in Chapters 3 and 4 of this textbook.

Menu Substitutions and Alternates/Standard Write-in Menu

Even with liberalization, another issue often arises—the need for substitutions on the menu. A substitution is a product that replaces a planned menu item when requested by a client or family member because he/she does not like or refuses to eat the food being served. Centers for Medicare & Medicaid Services (CMS) regulations specify that requests for substitutions should be permitted and honored, as long as they are reasonable and achievable. A substitution must be of similar nutritive value. On a selective menu, some Certified Dietary Managers use the term menu write-in to describe the same idea. A client may write an item on the menu that was not part of the planned cycle.

Providing substitutions upon request is part of the concept of giving clients control over their care; meal choice is considered a client right. Adjusting offerings to a client's requests helps to ensure optimal nutritional intake. In all, honoring substitution requests contributes to quality of life, especially for nursing facility clients.

What should a Certified Dietary Manager do with a substitution request? The answer is, honor it or provide an alternate choice. While some choices are not feasible, many options may exist. For a long-term client, a Certified Dietary Manager may be able to accommodate a special request. Sound management and practical realities dictate that the substitution process be planned and organized as part of the menu.

One way to provide substitutions is simply to offer alternate choices on a menu or in the service setting itself. This eliminates many of the challenges of providing substitutions at the last minute. It is one reason that some long-term care facilities have changed to selective menus. On a selective menu, clients can choose their substitutions or alternates in advance of service, and dining services staff can tally requirements in time for production.

With the goal of honoring client requests, a Certified Dietary Manager may also develop a list of "Always Available" write-in requests that can be accommodated in the kitchen. The manager can plan production of these items in conjunction with routine meal service or is at least prepared to honor these requests efficiently. Some write-in list offerings may cross over with items prepared daily for another service area, such as a cafeteria. Essentially, this write-in list becomes its own supplementary menu. Designated staff may refer to this menu to guide clients towards practical substitutions.

Management Considerations

Since the menu drives what you do in food production, it also drives your labor and food costs. Other management considerations are: delivery methods, timing, labor, equipment, and food availability.

- **Production, Service and Delivery Methods.** Your menu needs to coordinate with your type of service. For instance, if you are doing display cooking, a stir-fry would be a great menu item. However, for cafeteria service where food may be held on a steam table, stir-fried items may lose quality and prove a poor choice.

If you use cook-chill rethermalization methods for trays that are pre-assembled and chilled, it's important to examine what products stand up well to this process. Sometimes food thickness and the presence of liquids, gravies, sauces, and other aspects of the menu items you specify can influence quality achieved through various systems. Before adding items to a menu, test recipes through your own equipment and systems to find out how well they work.

- **Budget and Cost.** Next to labor, food cost is the second largest expense for your department and maybe even for the facility. This means managing food cost is a very important part of your job. Many facilities determine their food cost per client, per day and your budget is allocated accordingly. Whether your menu uses foods from raw ingredients or pre-prepared foods items, both will impact your budget and your menu planning process. Further discussion of this and other budget controls is in Chapter 26.

- **Timing and Labor.** How long it takes to prepare each menu item is an important consideration. Some menu items are more time-intensive than others. If you include a product that requires intensive preparation, you may need to pair it with a convenience or low-prep item to balance resources. The production schedule dictated by the menu must be realistic.

In addition, you must match your menu to the skills of employees responsible for producing the menu items. Culinary challenges presented to minimally trained employees can lead to increased costs through the loss of food or time. On the other hand, a facility that has a trained chef can use this resource to incorporate sophisticated techniques and preparation while holding food costs down. Through focused training, a Certified Dietary Manager can broaden the skills of food production employees so as to incorporate specific menu items that require specialized techniques.

Your foodservice department management team can help with menu planning by using their respective skills. For instance, the Certified Dietary Manager may provide input into the menu from the perspective of managing production. An Executive Chef can provide expertise on food items and preparation techniques. The Registered Dietitian Nutritionist can provide specific nutrition and therapeutic diet guidelines. The Diet Office Clerk or Serving Line Checker can identify the items that have frequent call backs for a second choice. The Dishroom Attendant can tell you what is returning on the plates uneaten. Each area of the department can contribute to the development of a better menu for the clients.

- **Equipment.** Menu items may require a broad variety of equipment. Consider each proposed menu item in terms of physical layout and equipment. You also have to consider what equipment will be in use at each time throughout the day. You may not have enough oven space if every menu item for a given meal requires the use of the oven. Storage equipment and transport/delivery requirements can be related concerns.

- **Availability of Food.** What ingredients are available for your menu may be impacted by where your facility is located. Consider a rural facility that is 100 miles from a metropolitan center. You won't be able to get an immediate delivery of a special menu item. With the current emphasis on purchasing locally, your menu may reflect the ingredients that are available in your geographic region, such as Idaho potatoes, Washington apples, or Wisconsin cranberries. Weather may also impact what menu items are available. If there is a freeze in Florida, oranges or orange juice might be available but at a price too high for your department budget. The availability of many of your produce items may be affected by weather and you may have to adjust your menu accordingly.

Monitoring the Menu and Meal Service

The best meal service starts with a well-planned menu and finishes with a well trained staff. No matter how well designed the menu is, staff competencies and performance determine the final presentation of the meal to the client. During the meal service there are several steps that require monitoring.

- Testing of the recipes for product performance and palatability is only the beginning.

- Training of the Production Team on the techniques required to make the menu items and the use of standardized recipes (discussed in detail in Chapter 3) starts the meal service.

- In addition to the standardized recipes, the use of Ingredient Pull Lists and Production Sheets with appropriate panning charts ensures the right items come to the serving line in the correct serving pans.

- Specification of portion sizes and serving utensils helps standardize the portion control.

- Pre-line meetings to taste the food and sample plate demonstrated the correct plating of the meal for consistency and presentation; and allows for any corrections to be made prior to the time of service.

- Documented pre-line temperature logs ensure that food is reaching the serving line at the appropriate temperature. It allows for any corrections to be made prior to the time of service; this is for both HOT and COLD food (milk sitting at room temperature during a one hour serving line will be close to room temp by the end of the line—yuck).

- Monitoring the start and stop times of the meal service, and the time needed to deliver the meals (longer delays cause greater temperature loss).

  > If the serving line is stopping for re-supply of items, either:

    - your production numbers were not correct—or they didn't make the amount specified;
    - the serving size on the line is over-portioned and they are running out;
    - the Production Team is not keeping up with the batch cooking; or
    - the Production Team is not focused on their primary task—Serving the Clients.

- Check random trays for accuracy to the items specified on the menu and compliance with all diet restrictions and allergies.

- Assess the trays for plate presentation, attractiveness and placement of the items on the tray or table setting.

Putting It Into Practice

2. How would you adjust the following menu so it doesn't overload the same equipment?
   - Baked Chicken
   - Scalloped Potatoes
   - Green Bean Casserole
   - Baked Apples

- The mid-line temperature of the food being served—are appropriate temperatures being maintained.

- Monitor the number and frequency of call-backs for a second meal selection.

- Record the Over Production and Run-Out/Shorts for the line.

  > Why were the production numbers wrong (over or short)?

  > What did you substitute for the products you were short?

- Observe the dishroom after the meal for what is coming back on the plate

- Conduct Meal Rounds in the dining rooms talking with the clients or in the patient/resident rooms during the meal service times

- Conduct Test Trays/Meals

  > Sample the food as a complete meal at the point of service in the dining room or in a patient/resident room

    - Take temperatures

    - Taste the food

    - Ask nursing and support staff to participate in the Test Trays

Information is your friend. Know what you expect and verify that it is the level of service you are providing.

Menu Revision

In the foodservice industry, most experts agree that a menu should not become static. For both ongoing and occasional clients, periodic revisions are a necessity. Here are some events that might signal a need for menu revision:

- **Client Feedback.** Client suggestions, along with information gathered through surveys, often begin to show patterns. A suggestion that arises repeatedly—or a complaint about a particular menu—can be triggers for revision.

- **Seasonal Change.** People choose different foods at different times of the year. Summer foods may include salads, chilled entrées, and produce in peak season. Winter foods (where winters are cold) may include more soups, stews, and seasonally available produce.

- **Trends and Fashions.** Ever-changing, the world of food experiences culinary innovations as well as trends. Keeping pace with these helps a facility compete in the industry. For instance: edamame was not well known 20 years ago; today it is a common restaurant menu option.

- **Special Requests.** A Certified Dietary Manager may monitor items that clients request or add to their own menus. If a request appears repeatedly, it may be time to add the item to the menu or increase its frequency.

- **Sales Records.** If you are monitoring sales records or selection data for the menu, you may discover that certain items are proving unpopular. One of the jobs of a Certified Dietary Manager is to identify menu "duds" and replace them with products clients prefer.

- **Quality Issues.** Similarly, a Certified Dietary Manager conducting routine quality checks may determine that a certain item is not holding up well on the menu. There may be a solution. Changing the procedure or the recipe, using different techniques or equipment, or training staff may make a difference. If not, the item may need to be replaced.

- **Changes in the Physical Facility.** Remodeling, renovations, or reallocation of space in a facility may impose changes on the foodservice department. Perhaps the opportunity exists to build an expanded cafeteria. A Certified Dietary Manager may explore a food court concept and its related menu implications. Or a facility may have an opportunity to build a group dining area, where buffet service is an option. The menu needs to change accordingly.

- **Service Revisions.** Sometimes a Certified Dietary Manager faces the need to develop new services or serve new clients. In addition, mergers and acquisitions may present new requirements to serve remote facilities. Integrating service changes with existing schemes may provide cause for re-evaluation of the menu as a whole and all related coordination issues.

A proposed menu revision should undergo evaluation for any nutrient standards that apply, as well as for costs. In addition, any menu revision creates ripple effects through the operational flow. To implement a change, systematically examine and plan related revisions required in staffing, service, delivery, inventory, purchasing, and food production.

In all, you can see that a menu has great impact on every aspect of the foodservice operation. Designing a menu that meets your clients' needs and expectations and uses your resources effectively is an enormous amount of work. However, the rewards are well worth the effort.

Tailoring Individual Menus—Honoring Legal and Moral Responsibiltiies

Every healthcare menu system must have a method for ensuring that every client receives a meal, even if selections have not been made. Clients who do not complete a selective menu receive a house diet or default selection. For a client whose preferences are known, a member of the clinical staff may complete a menu based on care plan or client preference record. This information may be tracked in a diet office software system.

Furthermore, every menu communications system must include control steps to ensure that foods planned for the individual menu meet the current diet order prescribed by the physician. Whether menus are selective or non-selective, spoken or paper-based, or implemented through trayline or buffet service, trained foodservice staff must assist with individual menu review before a client consumes the meal. Figure 2.5 on page 46 lists some of the criteria for menu review.

Reviewing menus can be time consuming. Certified Dietary Managers can structure menu systems to minimize this. For example, there are computer programs to review menu choices in order to check for compliance, calculate totals for restricted nutrients (such as sodium, protein, or fluid), eliminate allergenic foods, or automate routine food additions. This process requires that staff maintain a computerized set of care plans or client preference records.

When a foodservice staff member makes adjustments to a menu, communicating this with the client is important:

- If the client does not know the menu has been adjusted intentionally, the revisions may be perceived as an error.
- Menu review provides an opportunity for a dining services staff member to explain a meal pattern or other adjustment.
- Discussing adjustments opens a dialogue with the client about diet-related needs and preferences.

Putting It Into Practice

3. You decide to update your menu. What are three indicators of where to make changes?

Figure 2.5 Criteria for Individual Menu Review (Healthcare)

Before a client receives a tray and consumes a meal, trained foodservice staff must review individual menus and answer the following questions:

Q Do the selections provide a well-balanced meal, or has the client selected choices from nearly all categories (e.g., entrée, vegetable, starch, beverage, etc.)?

Q Are appropriate condiments included (e.g., margarine for bread, dressing for salad, etc.)?

Q If the client's diet order specifies combined modifications, such as sodium-restricted and carbohydrate-controlled, are selections compliant with these restrictions?

Q If texture modifications (e.g., mechanical soft diet or National Dysphagia Diet levels) are part of the diet order, does each menu selection comply with the order?

Q If the client has a meal pattern or a carbohydrate count, how do the totals compare to the plan?

Q Are portion sizes indicated on the menu appropriate for this particular diet order?

Q If the client has a fluid restriction, how do the figures add up?

Q If the client has requested a substitution, is the request honored?

Q If the diet order or kardex lists specific foods to avoid, (e.g., allergies or food intolerances) have these items been removed from the menu?

Q If the diet order or kardex lists specific additions for meals (e.g., nutrition supplements), are these items included?

It is the responsibility of the department director, dining services staff and Certified Dietary Manager to provide nutritionally adequate meals to clients. Sometimes there are specific requirements for patients, residents and school foodservice or one of customer choice. Planning a menu that meets the needs of both groups in a cost effective and efficient manner is the goal of every manager.

Putting It Into Practice

4. A client requests a menu item that is not allowed on their diet. What do you do?

Prepare Standardized Recipes for Food Production

Overview and Objectives

Even if you work in a corporate-owned facility where menus and recipes are pre-determined, it's important to be able to create and use standardized recipes. A standardized recipe is an essential tool in controlling costs in foodservice. It is a recipe for managing and controlling many aspects of the foodservice operation. After completing this chapter, you should be able to:

✓ Identify the different elements of a standardized recipe

✓ Calculate menus, recipes, diet census, tally sheets, and cafeteria needs to develop requisitions

✓ Compute proper portions using appropriate food charts/references

✓ Identify ways of calculating costs and nutrition content and a standardized recipe

✓ Define the steps in developing a standardized recipe

✓ Evaluate client acceptance of new recipes

A menu serves as a master plan for the food you serve. From the menu, a Certified Dietary Manager uses and develops recipes. A standardized recipe is the ultimate formula for the control of food. Each recipe has an effect on quality, cost control, and client satisfaction. A standardized recipe ensures consistency in quality, yield, nutritional value, the time required to prepare it, and staffing requirements. It is a fundamental and essential tool in the foodservice department.

A Standardized Recipe: The Ultimate Formula

A recipe is a formula for preparing a menu item. As such, it plays a strong role in control of your operation. It tells what ingredients to include and in what amounts. It tells how to prepare, portion, and present the food. It specifies what equipment and techniques to use. It controls what nutrients you will be serving clients.

Consider this scenario: You have just calculated the cost for a turkey casserole served every other week at lunch. It is coming out too high. To change this cost, one of your options is to go back to the recipe and adjust it. You can look at the cost and quantity of each ingredient. You may choose a different, less expensive form of turkey. Or, you may change the quantities you use for turkey, the most expensive ingredient. If your nutritional analysis tells you that scaling back the turkey will still allow the menu to meet nutritional standards, you may do just this. Alternately, you may see that you are using a cream soup base in the casserole. You may determine that you can accomplish a similar result with a small amount of milk, at a lower cost. This is just an example to demonstrate that a recipe indeed has clout, with financial impact.

Now, consider actual production procedures. One way to prepare a turkey casserole is to buy a frozen convenience food. In this case, the cook's task is to re-heat it according to directions. Another way to prepare it might involve using pre-cooked turkey cubes and a cream soup base as ingredients. Yet another might involve cooking raw turkey, chilling it, and cubing it. Again, it is evident that the recipe exerts control. The production methods specified in recipes control:

- how much time it will take to prepare an item (and how much lead time will be needed);
- what the labor cost of the recipe will be;
- what level of skill will be needed among preparation staff; and
- what requirements for equipment the recipe will impose.

What about final quality? A recipe capable of producing good results will contain the proper balance of ingredients. If you are making something as simple as gelatin, the amount of water added to the flavored powder makes all the difference in final quality. For a homemade minestrone soup, think about the seasonings included. Too much or too little can make the product unacceptable. Preparation procedures affect quality, too. For example, a prime fillet of fish will not turn out well if your procedure calls for baking it too long. Or, a stir-fry recipe will not turn out well if your procedure has you simmer the crisp vegetables in sauce for an extended period. In fact, the accuracy of a recipe, the procedures it defines, and even the ingredients it requires all affect final food quality. If you make changes to the recipe, you have to evaluate the quality of the final product, and exercise good judgment.

Standardized Recipes

Once you have selected or developed a recipe for a menu item, it's important to plan how you will consistently make products turn out every time you produce them. This is where standardization comes into play. A **standardized recipe** is a recipe that contains detailed specifications, and has been adapted and tested in your own operation. A standardized recipe tells exactly how much of each ingredient to use, how to add ingredients and in what sequence, and what procedures to use in producing the item.

By becoming very specific in a recipe, you can give instructions that can be repeated again and again by different staff members and still achieve the desired outcome. The use of standardized recipes helps all staff to maintain a consistent quality product regardless of who is cooking. This can be a great advantage, particularly in situations where a minimally trained employee may need to produce food or numerous employees may rotate through an assignment.

Quality. The result of using a standardized recipe is that you can produce a product that is consistent in quality, appearance and tastes the same. Clients notice this consistency, particularly if you have long-term clients, you can count on certain expectations. A client who enjoyed the banana bread last week expects to enjoy the same product again this week, and may be disappointed if it turns out differently.

Yield. A standardized recipe is consistent in **yield** and number of servings at a given portion size. A recipe for 100 servings always yields 100 servings. This is critical in ensuring you have enough food ready for service at any given time. You need to be able

Glossary

Standardized Recipe
A recipe that contains detailed specifications, and has been adapted and tested in your own operation

Yield
The number of servings a recipe will produce at a given portion size

to tell a cook how much food to make—and how much of each ingredient to include to ensure this happens.

Nutritional Value. A standardized recipe is also consistent in nutritional value. A serving that contains 8 grams of protein this week will contain 8 grams of protein again next week. In most non-commercial foodservice situations, you are responsible for assuring nutritional consistency. If you are complying with specific nutritional guidelines, standardized recipes become the formula for reliable nutrition. If you are not, you may still be marketing nutritional aspects of your products to clients. For example, the low-fat fare in a business dining setting needs to be reliably low in fat.

Time. In addition, a standardized recipe is consistent in time required for preparation. If it takes 75 minutes to prepare, you can generally count on that time and schedule the product to be ready for service. It is consistent in its labor requirements as well. This time-and-labor aspect of standardization is critical for devising effective employee schedules, and for assuring timeliness of service.

Cost. A standardized recipe is developed with specific amounts of ingredients and a given yield of servings. Because of this factor, you can use a standardized recipe to cost out your menus. What if employees choose not to follow a standardized recipe by increasing ingredient amounts or serving larger portion sizes and the cost has been figured into your department budget? You will be over budget, so making a standardized recipe work requires attention to the human factor as well.

It is important to note that a recipe out of a cookbook does not qualify as a standardized recipe. Why? Because the equipment may vary, cook's interpretation of "cook until done" or "add seasonings to taste" may vary, and the portion utensils and ingredients availability may vary. Each recipe needs to be standardized to your food preparation kitchen and staff.

The bottom line is that standardization allows you to manage the operation effectively. You want to be able to predict the inventory needed for food preparation, quantify purchasing needs and have ingredients on hand in time for production. You can predict and control expenses in your operation through standardized recipes. You can also predict staffing needs, and prepare an employee schedule far in advance. You need to plan exactly how much food to produce for each meal in order to feed all clients. For each of these tasks, standardization provides a useful planning tool. From the recipes, you know what you will need and can exercise strong management of the entire process.

Components of a Standardized Recipe

Now that you understand the concept of a standardized recipe, let's examine the details that define its consistency. An example of a standardized recipe appears in Figure 3.1. As you can see, the standardized recipe contains some key elements. These are described below.

Title. Each recipe must have its own unique title or name. The title in Figure 3.1 is *Alaska Cod Chowder with Black Beans and Corn*. While the need for recipe names may seem obvious, in operational practice, confusion actually can occur without attention to this detail. Let's say that you have two types of beef stew. One uses traditional carrots and potatoes, while another uses leeks and peas. You will need to distinguish these clearly from each other to avoid production errors. For clients, too, unique names make it easier to distinguish one menu item from another.

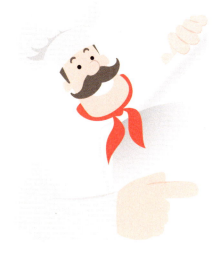

Figure 3.1 Example of a Standardized Recipe

1284: Alaska Cod Chowder with Black Beans and Corn

Category: Soups | **Yield:** 50 Servings | **Portion:** 1-1/2 cups | **Batch Qty:** 4.5 gal.

Ingredients

8 cups	onions, halved and sliced
1 (#10) can	diced tomatoes in juice
1 (#10) can	black beans, drained and rinsed
1 (#10) can	corn, drained
5 cups	chopped green chilies, canned or fresh/seeded
3 gal + 2 cups	chicken or fish broth
1/2 cup	fresh lime juice
1/4 cup	chili powder
1 Tbsp.	garlic powder
2 Tbsp	toasted cumin seeds, crushed
8 lbs., 4 oz.	Alaska Cod, thawed if necessary, cut in 1" pieces
1/2 cup	vegetable oil

Directions

1. In a large stockpot or steam-jacketed kettle, combine onions, tomatoes in juice, black beans, corn, and chilies.
2. Add broth, lime juice, chili powder, garlic powder, and cumin seeds. Bring to boil; reduce to simmer and cook 10 minutes.
3. Pan-sear cod in lightly oiled non-stick skillet about 3 minutes; add cod to chowder.
4. Simmer chowder an additional 20 minutes over medium-low heat. Verify that serving temperature is 155°F or higher.
5. For each serving, portion 1-1/2 cups soup into shallow bowl.

   Verify that serving temperature is 155°F or higher, held for a minimum of 15 seconds.

Source: Adapted from Alaska Seafood Marketing Institute

Category. Most facilities use a category designation to help keep recipes organized. Figure 3.2 provides some examples of category designations for recipes. Using categories helps you assign recipe production to the intended staff members. It also helps you group recipes for production on any given day. It helps you locate recipes for special menus as needed. If you use a computerized recipe system, categories help you use search features to find recipes. There is no right or wrong way to develop categories for your own operation. Categorization is simply a logical grouping that is useful to you.

Recipe Number. As you adopt recipes into your own facility, you will probably assign a recipe number to each as an additional way of identifying and controlling your bank of recipes. A computerized system typically requires a recipe number as a way of ensuring a unique identity for each recipe in the database. Some operations use numbering systems that relate to the categories. For example, a series of recipes beginning with 5000 may represent quick breads and muffins. A cinnamon muffin recipe may be number 5001. An apple walnut quick bread recipe may be number 5026 and so forth.

Figure 3.2 Sample Categories for Recipes

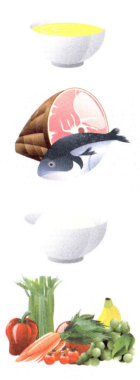

STARTERS
- Soups
- Appetizers

ENTRÉES
- Beef
- Pork
- Poultry
- Seafood
- Vegetarian
- Salads
- Pureed

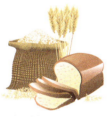

SIDES
- Side Salads
- Salad Dressings
- Rice and Pasta Sides

HOT VEGETABLES
- Potatoes
- Other

BREADS
- Quick Breads and Muffins
- Yeast Breads and Rolls

DESSERTS
- Cakes
- Cookies
- Pies
- Fruit
- Other

Yield. A yield is the number of servings a recipe will produce. Yield is closely related to portion size.

Batch Quantity. Sometimes yield is shown as the total volume of the batch, such as 4 gallons or 7.5 pounds.

Portion Size. This specifies what size each portion will be. It is expressed as a measurement. In the example shown in Figure 3.1 (adjacent), the recipe yields 50 servings of 1-1/2 cups each. Note that the same recipe would alternately yield 100 servings of ¾ cups each. Thus, it's important to specify portion size in every recipe. Otherwise, the yield becomes meaningless.

Portion sizes occasionally vary for use in different menus. This soup, for example, may be used as a 3/4 cup portion when the soup is an appetizer on a dinner menu. However, when it is featured as a main lunch entrée, the larger portion may be more appropriate. Traditionally, a "cup" of soup is ¾ cup and "bowl" of soup is 1 cup.

Sometimes, even at a single meal, portion sizes may vary for special diets. On a renal menu used for clients with limited kidney function, there is typically a restriction on meat, which contains protein. A standard portion of roast beef for a dinner meal may be 4 ounces. On a renal diet, though, it may be 2 ounces. In this case, each portion size must be specified on the recipe.

Ingredients. A standardized recipe specifies each ingredient. As with recipe naming, ingredient naming is a task that must always be tackled with precision. For instance, if you use flour in your operation, you need to be sure the names of various types are clearly distinguished. You may have all-purpose flour, self-rising flour, pre-sifted flour, whole wheat flour, cake flour, bread flour, and/or others. The success of a recipe for baked goods will depend on your cook selecting the proper ingredient. Very simply, a clear and precise name for the ingredient, used consistently, helps to make this happen. Computerized systems use ingredient numbers along with names to track, distinguish, and describe ingredients.

Typically, a recipe for quantity food production shows all ingredients in the order in which they are added. It is essential that every ingredient used in a recipe appear on the ingredient list. The list itself may serve as a tool for cooks in organizing their work. A common procedure is to measure each ingredient and have it ready before beginning production. The ingredient list in each recipe forms a basis for evaluating purchasing needs. An item that misses the list may not be purchased, and may not be available when needed. So, oversights in the ingredient list can lead to unnecessary work and error, and thoroughness is worth the effort.

Weights or Measures. An essential control in food production is measurement of ingredients. For most operations, three basic options present themselves. One is to measure ingredients by volume. Another is to measure by weight. Another, only feasible with certain ingredients, is to measure by count, or by the "each." Figure 3.3 gives examples of measurements. It is more accurate to weigh large amounts of dry ingredients and more cost effective.

Figure 3.3 Examples of Weights and Measures for Ingredients

BY WEIGHT	BY VOLUME	BY COUNT
• 3.5 lbs. of all-purpose flour	• 9 qts. of all-purpose flour	• 11 fresh, white onions
• 2 oz. iodized salt	• 3/4-cup baking powder	• 3 lemons
• 2.5 lbs. sugar	• 2 Tbsp. ground sage	• 45 bananas
• 12 lbs. turkey roast	• 1-3/4 cups skim milk	• 7 cloves of garlic
• 6.5 lbs. crushed pineapple	• 3 cups margarine	• 3, #10 cans of tomato sauce
• 1 oz. cinnamon	*Note: If accurate scales are available, dry ingredients should be weighed rather than measured.*	
• 12 lbs. raw apples		
• 5.5 lbs. chopped, fresh white onions		
• 8 lbs. margarine		

Food Safety Information. To support a food safety system, many Certified Dietary Managers also provide sanitation-related information on recipes. In a proactive system for managing food safety called HACCP (Hazard Analysis Critical Control Point), a particular step of the recipe may be identified as being critical for ensuring food safety. This step is called a **critical control point (CCP)**. The CCP may be noted on the recipe for reference and use by food preparation employees.

HACCP. The Hazard Analysis Critical Control Point system is also a component of the standardized recipe. Inclusion of safe food handling steps within the recipe helps ensure staff have appropriate guidelines on how to handle at risk ingredients and final cooking temperatures.

Some foodservice operations control ingredients by using an ingredient room. An ingredient room is a unique location where an assigned employee measures ingredients for all recipes, packages them, and labels them. Pre-measured ingredients are then distributed to assigned preparation staff. The ingredient room concept imposes several forms of control in the kitchen.

First of all, it ensures that ingredients are carefully measured by someone with specialized focus on measurement. This can support consistent yields and adherence to the measurements required for standardized recipes. Secondly, an ingredient room allows managers to limit access to food storage areas, which may be kept locked. This prevents pilferage or theft in a foodservice operation. Beyond these benefits, an ingredient room allows cooks to work very efficiently during the production process. In an ingredient room model, it is very common for all ingredients to be weighed.

Directions or Procedure. Detail and clarity in the directions for preparing a recipe help make it reproducible from one employee to the next. Steps for preparation must be presented in a logical sequence.

Pan Size. Many types of recipes include specifications for a pan size. A cake, for example, may use a 12" x 20" x 2" pan. Instructions for employees should indicate how to portion a pan (e.g., cut 8 x 10), or cut a pie (e.g., 6 slices). The pan specification may also relate to a layout for a steam table. Then, it is especially important that the cook use the right pan, so it will fit the layout. See Figure 3.4 for pan and portion sizes.

Batch Unit. Sometimes called unit of production, this figure tells what the batch size is for the recipe. Batch unit may not appear on all recipes, but is sometimes critical. Often, the quantity produced by a recipe does not match the yield you need. So, the recipe has to be scaled.

Scaling Adjusting the recipe ingredients upward or downward to generate specific yields. Other terms for this are extending or factoring the recipe. When you scale recipes, you often have to recognize batch units. Consider this example:

> You are making apple pies. Each pie yields 6 servings, with a portion of 1/6 of a pie. You need to serve pie to 211 people. To determine how many pies, divide 221 by 6.
>
> $211 \div 6 = 35.17$
>
> Since you cannot make a fraction of a pie, you have to round this up and make 36 pies. In portions, this is a yield of 216, or 5 more servings than what your estimated needs are.

Putting It Into Practice

1. Complete this question using Figure 3.4. Your lasagna recipe yields about 24 lbs.; you need 48, 6 oz. (1 cup) portions. What would be the best size pan to cook and serve it in? (Note: Assume that 1 lb. = 1 pint)

Figure 3.4 Pan and Portion Chart

PAN SIZE	PAN DEPTH	PAN CAPACITY		SIZE OF PORTION		# OF PORTIONS YIELDED*
		Quarts	Cups	Cup	Scoop #	
Full Size 12" x 20"	2-1/4"	7-1/2	30	1/4	18	120
				1/3	12	90
				3/8	10	80
				1/2	8	60
	4"	13	52	1/4	16	206
				1/3	12	156
				3/8	10	138
				1/2	8	104
	6"	19-1/2	78	1/4	16	312
				1/3	12	234
				3/8	10	208
				1/2	8	156
				1	6 oz. ladle	78
Half Size 12" x 10"	2-1/2"	3-3/4	15	1/4	16	60
				1/3	12	45
				3/8	10	40
				1/2	8	30
	4"	6-1/2	26	1/4	16	104
				1/3	12	78
				3/8	10	69
				1/2	8	52
	6"	9-3/4	39	1/4	16	156
				1/3	12	117
				3/8	10	104
				1/2	8	78
				1	8 oz. ladle	39
Third Size 12" x 6-7/8"	2-1/2"	2-2/5	9-3/5	1/8	2 Tbsp.	76
				1/4	16	38
				1/3	12	28
				3/8	10	25
	4"	3-7/8	15-1/2	1/8	2 Tbsp.	124
				1/4	16	62
				1/3	12	46
				3/8	10	41

Adapted from The Foodservice Tune Up by Wayne Toczek, Innovations Services, and Tim Bauman.
* Rounded down to lower portion

If your facility maintains vending machines, consider putting the five extra pieces in the vending machine or in the cafeteria/employee dining room.

A batch unit may be important for a meatloaf, cake, quick bread, roast, or other products that are conducive to be prepared in serving groups. When and how you round yields up depends on the batch unit. If you are preparing chili, stew, or soups, and you need 6.1 batches, consider rounding down. You would over-produce too much if you rounded up.

Seasonings (such as salt and sugar) do not always scale up and down as easily as flour or ground beef. Therefore, it's important to test scaled recipes prior to putting them into everyday production.

For some products, the batch unit is irrelevant, because you can scale the recipe into batches of single servings. Examples include sandwiches, individual cold plates, and most single serving entrée items such as chicken pieces and hamburgers.

Nutrition Information. This has become an expected component of a standardied recipe. Clients are asking for information about protein, calories, sodium and fat content. Identifying the nutritional benefits of menu items, such as "A good source of Vitamin A", helps clients make better choices in their food selections. Posting of nutritional content is being required for multi-unit chain restaurants, and as part of the "nutrition labeling" of pre-packaged and commercially packed food products.

There are a number of different sources available to calculate the nutritional value of a recipe. If the item is a ready-to-serve or a convenience product, then the nutrition labeling is printed on the packaging. Convenience items that require additional ingredients typically provide labeling both "as is" and as ready-to-serve based on their recipe.

When nutrition labeling is not readily available for a product, you may need to calculate the nutrition content based on the ingredients and scaling the quantity of each ingredient within a recipe. We used to rely on books available with tables of nutritional composition such as Bowes and Church's *Food Values of Portions Commonly Used* or the USDA National Nutrient Database. However, looking up individual ingredients, or even ready-to-eat foods, in a printed book format is cumbersome and time consuming.

Access to the internet or a computerized database of nutritional analysis can make the process much faster and more accurate. The USDA database is available online with thousands of items and detailed nutrient content. It is still a semi-manual process to collect the information for each ingredient and scale the values to match the quantities in the recipe.

A number of commercially available nutrition analysis software programs such as NutritionistPro®, NutriBase®, and The Food Processor® are used by clinical registered dietitian nutritionists to calculate the nutrient intake of their clients. Access to one of these nutrient analysis tools would make the calculations easier. Likewise, often food distributors offer recipes online that include the nutritional analysis.

The most effective means of determining the nutrient content of a recipe, or a complete menu, is to access the information via a computerized recipe program. In a full-service recipe module, you can edit the ingredients and add items to the recipe. The program will recalculate the nutritional content for the recipe, the meal, or even the entire day's menu based on your edits.

Recipe Sources. Generally, Certified Dietary Managers strive to find recipes specifically developed for quantity production. This is primarily a time-saver. Adapting a home recipe to large-scale production has some pitfalls and requires a fair amount of effort. A practical question to ask as you evaluate new recipes is: Has this been refined for quantity production? Even if you have a corporate office providing your recipes, you will want to address the following questions:

- What does this recipe cost per serving?
- What is the labor cost in producing this recipe?
- Do we have the proper equipment to produce it well?
- Do we have the match of skills required to produce a high-quality product?
- How does this recipe meet the nutritional requirements of our menus and recipes?
- How does this recipe fit the tastes, preferences and needs of our clients?

Computerized Menus and Recipe Management Systems

Computerized menu systems are designed to accomplish a wide variety of tasks from managing the patient/resident diet orders to standardizing the recipes used to meet those dietary restrictions. The interplay between the menu and the recipes is a little like which came first, the chicken or the egg.

A successful menu uses tested recipes that have high acceptance by the clientele for whom the menu is developed. Often the menu dictates the recipes to be used, but frequently variety is added by reviewing new recipes available. Computerized menu systems often provide a library of quantity foods tested recipes that may meet your needs.

Recipes in a computerized system use a standardized format for the recipes consistent with the points covered above. One of the options available with the computerized recipe is the ability to easily scale the recipes to any number of servings. This can be very handy if a recipe is designed for 50 servings and you need 215 portions.

The scaling of recipes in a computerized system is a simple math function, which may have some unusual side effects. By entering the number of portions needed the computer automatically divides or multiplies the base recipe to the level needed. However, the computer will not adjust the amount of seasoning in the recipe appropriately. The computer will also scale a recipe with unexpected quantities such as seven cups plus one tablespoon and one teaspoon of water. Remember, computers are very literal and do not round up or down well.

Steps in Adapting and Testing a Recipe

As you find recipes you wish to use in your operation, you are ready to begin adapting and standardizing them. When you obtain a recipe for foodservice that has already been standardized, you still need to test it in your own facility. Why? The standardization may change a little bit with the specific ingredients and equipment you use. Furthermore, variations occur with altitude. If a recipe for baked goods was tested at sea level, and you are at an altitude of 4,000 feet, you will need to make adjustments to create a similar product. In addition, a standardized recipe that meets one facility's standards may not meet another's. Thus, a safe practice is: *Don't believe it until you prove it in your own facility.* This ensures you know you have standards upon which you can depend.

Putting It Into Practice

2. Your new chef is anxious to introduce his new recipes to your clients. What would you suggest he do first?

The steps in adapting and standardizing a recipe are as follows.

Step 1: Verify that directions, techniques, ingredients and equipment specified all apply to your own facility. Edit them if necessary.

Step 2: Produce the original recipe in your own facility, using the equipment you expect to use for routine production. Portion out servings according to your portion and yield figures, and verify the numbers and acceptability.

Step 3: Name and categorize the recipes in a way that makes sense for your own facility.

Step 4: Specify the portion size you wish to use to comply with your own menu needs.

Step 5: Set the yield for which you wish to standardize the recipe. This should be the yield in which you expect to produce it most often.

Step 6: Scale and cost out the recipe accordingly (described under Recipe Math below).

Step 7: Assure that measurements are expressed in terms you always use for each ingredient and are easy to understand.

Step 8: Prepare the new recipe. Taste and evaluate the final product for quality. This is often done through a taste panel, a group of individuals who all taste and evaluate the food. A sample evaluation for members of a taste panel appears in Figure 3.5.

Step 9: Document any adjustments needed, and re-test if warranted. Some experts advise adjusting only one ingredient at time, so that you may fully evaluate the impact of each change.

Step 10: Prepare a finalized, clearly documented version of the recipe for reference. At this point, you may be entering it into a computer-based management system, or, you may be filing an original copy in a secure location.

Figure 3.5 Recipe Evaluation for Taste Panel

Date: _____ Menu Item: _Blueberry Muffins_____

Evaluator: _____ Recipe Number:_____

Instructions: Check (✓) your reaction to each of the following factors used to describe the menu item.

Evaluation Factor	Exceptional	Like Very Much	Acceptable	Like Slightly	Unacceptable
Evenly browned.					
Rounded, not peaked top.					
No tunnels.					
Blueberries evenly distributed.					
Cake-like texture.					

Comments:

In large facilities, recipe testing occurs in a test kitchen. A test kitchen is a designated location with proper equipment and staffing for trying out, verifying, adjusting, and standardizing recipes. Whether or not you have a test kitchen, the steps are similar.

In this process it is important to be precise and accurate so that you may be certain you have developed a meaningful, standardized recipe.

As you adapt recipes, you may make adjustments that affect both cost and nutrients. Many managers run both cost and nutrient analyses when the standardization is complete, and again verify that all figures are acceptable.

Recipe Math

Scaling a recipe to produce different yields calls for recipe math. First, you convert the yield from old to new. Then, you adjust all ingredient measurements accordingly. Let's take a closer look at the calculations.

The most common method is to determine a **conversion factor**. A conversion factor is the number by which you will (initially) adjust everything to arrive at a new yield. The steps for scaling a recipe are as follows.

Step 1: Divide the new yield by the original yield. This gives you a conversion factor. Note that when you are reducing a yield, the conversion factor will be less than 1.0. When you are increasing a yield, the conversion factor will be more than 1.0.

Example: Your original recipe yields 100 portions. You want a yield of 225 portions.

New yield ÷ original yield = 225 ÷ 100 = 2.25

2.25 is your conversion factor.

(*Tip:* Remember that *n* comes before *o* in the alphabet. To obtain a conversion factor, use *new* yield divided by *old* yield.)

Step 2: Multiply the measurement for each ingredient by the conversion factor.

Example: The original recipe calls for 3 oz. of sugar. The new measurement is:

3 oz. x conversion factor = 3 oz. x 2.25 = 6.75 oz.

Step 3: Consider additional adjustments that may be necessary. Some ingredients do not need to follow the conversion factor precisely. Spices and seasonings, for example, can appear in smaller quantities than you might calculate. Oil used for sautéing vegetables may not need to increase in proportion.

Step 4: Specify and verify the batch unit if applicable. For example, if you are adjusting a recipe for whole pies, be sure the final quantities you have determined will make some number of whole pies. Likewise, if you are working on a recipe that must be prepared in steam table pans, baking pans, or something similar, examine the batch unit.

Glossary

Conversion Factor
The number by which you adjust each recipe ingredient to arrive at a new yield.

In Step 2 of this process, many experts suggest you use only weight measurements (e.g., if measuring flour in cups, first change it to pounds and ounces). This is generally the most precise and easiest to convert. To do this, use a reference table of conversions from weights to measures, found in many quantity cookbooks, such as *Food for Fifty*, and built into many computer-based recipe management systems. When you are finished, you can use the same table to convert back to volume measurements if desired. Figure 3.6 shows an example of a set of weight and volume conversions for flour.

Converting a recipe to new yields requires careful attention to the proper calculations. Your final answer may come out as a unit of measure that is not usable in daily operation or, it may come out as a decimal, such as 2.79 teaspoons. In this case, you need to round the decimal to a usable fraction. Keep in mind how the recipe will be used, and strive to make it simple to understand. Finally, after scaling a recipe and converting measurements, be sure to retest the recipe for accuracy.

Figure 3.6 Example of Weight and Volume Conversions for Flour

BACKGROUND

You are scaling a recipe that contains all-purpose flour. Your original recipe calls for 5 cups of flour. You wish to scale this recipe to a higher yield using a conversion factor of 3.3.

1. Convert Cups to a Weight

1. Look up the volume-to-weight equivalent in a cookbook and find that 4 cups of all-purpose flour = 1 lb.
2. Create an equation to show the relationship: 4 cups/1 lb. = 5 cups/? lbs.

   Tip: *When you are setting up an equation like this one, always put the volume measurement on the top of each side, and the weight measurement on the bottom of each side (or vice versa). This assures that you have set up the equation correctly.*

3. To solve this, you cross multiply the top number (numerator) of one side by the bottom (denominator) of the other to create a new equation:

$$\frac{4}{16} = \frac{5}{x} \quad \text{Cross multiply and then divide}$$

$$4x = (5 \times 16)$$
$$4x = 80 \qquad \text{Now divide both sides by 4}$$
$$\frac{4x}{4} = \frac{80}{4} \qquad x = 20 \text{ oz.}$$
$$\frac{x = 20}{16 \text{ oz. or 1 lb.}} \qquad x = 1.25 \text{ lbs.}$$

4. Divide each side by 4.
   $$5 \div 4 = x \quad x = 1.25 \text{ lbs.}$$

2. Scale the Measurement

Scale the measurement for the new yield. Multiply the original measurement in weight by the conversion factor: 1.25 lbs. x 3.5 = 4.125 lbs.

3. Convert to Volume

This is an optional step. If you measure flour by volume, it is important. If you measure flour by weight, you can stop here. You create an equation to show the relationship.

$$\frac{x}{4.125} = \frac{4}{1}$$

To solve this, you cross multiply the top (numerator) of one side by the bottom (denominator) of the other to create a new equation.

$$4 \times 4.125 = 1 \times (x) \quad or \quad 4 \times 4.125 = 16. \, 5 \text{ cups}$$

To make this measurement easier, convert this final volume measurement to a manageable unit. From a cookbook, you can also learn that 4 cups = 1 quart. So you may change this figure to: 4 pt. + 1/2 cup.

Food production references such as *Food for Fifty* by Mary Molt provide direct reading tables so you don't have to calculate.

Using Standardized Recipes to Determine Standard Portion Costs

Additional math used with a standardized recipe is costing. A standardized recipe helps you with cost control because recipe amounts and portions are predetermined. Costing a recipe without using a computer program can be time consuming. As the Certified Dietary Manager, you should decide whether to include ingredient costs on the standardized recipe. Perhaps you could begin with the recipes that are most expensive, such as your meat items and your supplements.

Regardless of whether you use ingredient costs on your standardized recipes, you need to know how to calculate the cost of a recipe. Here's how to calculate the cost of a recipe.

Step 1: Create a standard recipe costing form such as the one in Figure 3.7 and fill in the ingredient and amount columns.

Step 2: Calculate unit cost and determine the total cost of the ingredient.

Total cost of the ingredient item = unit cost x the quantity/amount of the ingredient.

Unit Cost = Total cost ÷ by number of servings per package

Example of calculating unit cost: You have a 2 lb. package of bacon @ $7.78/pkg. A salad recipe calls for 12 pieces of bacon. Bacon is about 1 oz./piece. Two lbs. = 32 pieces. Determine unit price by dividing the total cost of the package by 32: $7.78 ÷ 32 = $.243 per piece/unit. This becomes the unit price on the recipe. The total cost of that ingredient is then $.243 x 12 pieces called for on the recipe or $2.92.

Step 3: Determine if any recipe ingredients have a different yield from the amount purchased. (See section on Understanding Product Yields.) Calculate the Edible Portion cost.

Step 4: Total all ingredient costs.

Step 5: Divide by the total number of portions for the recipe to determine cost per portion.

Understanding Product Yields

When you purchase fresh produce, you will clean it, peel it, core it, etc. before you use it. This preprocessing reduces the final amount available for a recipe. You might also remove skin from chicken pieces, trim fat from pork chops or remove bone from a ham steak. You are changing the amount purchased (aka **As Purchased [AP]**) to an **Edible Portion (EP)** amount. For costing purposes, you must calculate the cost of the Edible Portion of an ingredient. Thus, the ingredient information in recipes must be adjusted or converted to reflect the cost of what is actually consumed. Use the Yield Factor to determine the As Purchased amount of product needed.

Cooking may also change the amount purchased to an Edible Portion amount. You know when cooking a roast, turkey, or ground beef that the amount you end up with is less than the amount you started with.

How do you know what the Edible Portion (EP) is for any produce you use? You can weigh the product in its As Purchased (AP) form, and then weigh it again after you have completed the preparation or cooking. There are many reliable resources available that provide you with tables showing the **yield percentage** of an as purchased amount to an Edible Portion. One such reference is *Food For Fifty* by Mary Molt. This book includes many food production tables and quantity recipes and would be a valuable resource for any foodservice department.

Glossary

As Purchased (AP)
The raw weight, without any pre-production

Edible Portion (EP)
The final quantity produced after all preparation is done

Putting It Into Practice

3. Your chef wants to standardize a new recipe. The old recipe yield is 20 servings and she wants the new yield to be 75 servings. What is the conversion factor? Use that conversion factor to determine how much chicken is needed in the recipe if the old amount was 4 lbs.

Calculating Edible Portions from As Purchased Amounts. Most facilities use a yield percentage to determine the ingredient amount from the raw purchased or AP amount. The yield percentage is the percentage available after preproduction, portioning, or cooking has been completed.

Edible portion (EP) cost = AP cost ÷ yield percentage

Example of determining the Edible Portion cost of a recipe ingredient: The yield percentage table (from a reference book) indicates that each pound of 85% lean ground beef yields 0.80 lbs. of cooked, drained ground beef. 10 lbs. x 0.80 = 8 lbs. of cooked ground beef. The AP price of 85% lean ground beef is $13.90 for 10 lbs. The EP cost = $13.90 ÷ .80 or $17.38 for 10 lbs. To determine the price per pound, divide the total EP cost of $17.38 by 10 =$1.74 (round up) per EP pound.

Example of determining ingredient cost using yield percentage: Recipe calls for 15 lbs. of fresh green beans. The unit cost of the green beans is $.69 per pound. The yield percentage on fresh green beans is 88% or .88. The EP cost of one pound of green beans then is $.69 ÷ .88 = $.78/pound

Figure 3.7 shows ingredient costing where the AP and the EP are the same and an example of calculating an ingredient cost where the AP and EP are different.

Note: This process is also very important when determining the nutrient value of a recipe ingredient. The nutrient content should be determined based on the Edible Portion, not on the amount purchased.

Figure 3.7 Standardized Recipe Cost Sheet Sample

Menu Item: French Dip Sandwich					
Total Yield: 50 Sandwiches	Portion Sizes: 3 oz. meat, 1/4 cup au jus					
Ingredients			**Ingredient Cost**		
Item	AP Amt.	Yield %	EP Amt.	AP $	Total Cost
Roast Beef**	15 lbs.	66% or .66	10 lbs.	$2.39/lbs.	$35.85
	50 servings x 3 oz. = 150 oz. 150 oz. ÷ 16 oz./lbs. = 9.9 lbs. (round up to 10 lbs.) 10 lbs. x 66 100 (10 x 100) ÷ 66 = x 1000 ÷ 66 = 15.1 lbs.				
Au Jus, Canned Item	12.5 cups or 2, 51 oz. cans			$5.38/can	$10.76
Kaiser Roll	50 each			$0.17 ea.	$8.50
				Total Recipe Cost:	$55.11
	Roast Beef purchased raw and then cooked.			# of Portions:	50
				Cost per Portion:	$1.10

Computerized Recipe System

Scaling and costing recipes on a daily basis requires a great deal of time. Many Certified Dietary Managers scale a single recipe to several common quantities, and simply use these. With chicken soup, one manager may maintain a reference recipe scaled to 200, 250, and 300 servings. When a recipe calls for 215 servings one day and 235 for another day, the facility may produce 250 servings.

This is practical and expedient, but also results in over-production of food. When amplified by dozens of food items in a single day, this over-production incurs significant unnecessary expense and food waste. In dollars, some managers have described this over-production as representing 5-10 percent of the food budget.

This is one reason that many managers choose to use a computer-based system for recipe management. Software can scale and re-scale recipes at any time. So, if a core recipe is in the computer, the system may produce scaled recipes for each day of production, based on projected usage figures the manager specifies (or the system calculates). In the above example, this would mean the system produces a recipe for chicken soup scaled to 215 servings on one day, and 235 on another. Thus, it reduces food waste.

Calculating recipe costs using computer software expedites the process of calculating food costs. If the software is linked to your electronic inventory program, your recipe costs can be updated as prices change, thereby providing more current information. The more current your recipe costs are, the more accurately you can stay within budget.

Recipe Costing versus Meal Costing

Recipe costing assumes that you have perfect preparation and portioning of the recipe with no leftovers or waste. With single serve items such as a grilled chicken breast the number produced and the number consumed can be tracked and the waste factor calculated. With menu items that are not single serve, the number of portions and the actual portioning become a consideration in the cost of the meal.

If you are serving baked fish for lunch, the case of product may cost you $48.75 for 40 – 4 oz. portions.

> The recipe costing would be $48.75 \div 40 = \$1.22$ per portion
>
> You plan to serve 60 portions of fish so your cost would be 60 x $1.22 = \$73.13$
>
> However, you only served 47 portions and had 13 pieces of fish leftover
>
> Your true Meal Cost for the fish is the total cost divided by the actual number of servings used. (There is no "popular" use for leftover baked fish so the remaining portions are going to be thrown out) or $73.13 \div 47 = \$1.56$

Recipe costing is a valuable step in the recipe standardization process. It provides you with the beginning calculations for your food cost by meal or patient/resident day. Just keep in mind that the recipe cost is not the same as your food cost.

Encouraging the Use of Standardized Recipes

Making standardized recipes work requires communication. Remind staff of the importance of standardized recipes by holding short in-services annually to review how and why to use them. Make sure that your department standards (such as standardized recipes) are part of new employee orientation. If you notice over or under production problems, follow up on them immediately with the cooking staff.

Putting It Into Practice

4. Calculate the yield percentage of ground beef if the AP weight is 10 lbs. and the EP weight is 7.5 lbs. Using the yield percentage, calculate the ingredient cost of 2 lbs. of ground beef if the AP price is $1.69 per lb.

Conducting pre-line taste testing panels daily will establish a pattern of evaluating the food items being prepared. This allows you and the entire team to assess the quality of the food being served and ensure a consistent use of the recipes. In addition, there are several ways to make a standardized recipe user-friendly and improve compliance:

Sequence of Ingredients. As you list ingredients on a recipe, verify the sequence of ingredients matches the sequence in which they are used. This helps to prevent oversights and errors.

Consistent Units of Measure. Recognize that there are many ways to measure any given ingredient, and standardize your units of measure for each one you use in your operation. For example, if you decide that flour will be measured by volume, then be sure it is always done this way on every recipe. There may be a few exceptions, where ingredients are used differently in one recipe than another. In a computer-based system, a user may actually specify two different ingredients that can appear on recipes, such as: margarine, measured in 1-lb. blocks; and margarine, measured by volume. Make sure that for whatever measurements you specify, measuring utensils are available. For example, if you use quart measurements, have a quart measure on hand.

Consistent Abbreviations. There are variations in abbreviations used to describe common measurements. For example, teaspoons may be: tsp or t. Tablespoons may be: Tbsp. TB or T. Pounds may be: lbs. or #. There is no right or wrong to any of these designations. However, the use of abbreviations must be standardized and consistent on all recipes to minimize confusion.

Consolidated Measures. When scaling a recipe, you may arrive at measurements such as: 18 cups or 24 teaspoons. If you ask staff to make these kinds of measurements, you lengthen the time required for production and increase the opportunity for error. When possible, consolidate smaller measurements to larger units, using a chart of equivalents. For example, 18 cups becomes 4.5 quarts, and 24 teaspoons becomes 1/2 cup. See Figure 3.8 for common equivalents.

Figure 3.8 Common Equivalents

Volume Measurements	Fluid Measurements	Weight Measurements
• 1 bushel = 4 pecks	• 1 gallon = 4 quarts	• 1 lb. = 16 oz.
• 1 peck = 8 quarts	• 1 quart = 4 cups	• 1 oz. = 30 grams
• 1 gallon = 4 quarts	• 4 cups = 2 pints	
• 1 quart = 2 pints	• 1 cup = 8 fluid oz.	
• 1 pint = 2 cups	• 1 fluid oz. = 2 Tbsp.	
• 1 cup = 16 Tbsp.		
• 1/2 cup = 8 Tbsp.		
• 1/3 cup = 5-1/3 Tbsp.		
• 1/4 cup = 4 Tbsp.		
• 1 Tbsp. = 3 tsp.		

Consistent Temperature Standards. It is also helpful to standardize all temperature measurements to one system, such as degrees F (Fahrenheit) or degrees C (Celsius). Generally, this has to match available readings on actual equipment, and many operations use Fahrenheit.

Proofread Recipes. As you finalize tested recipes, take the time to proofread them carefully. Small errors can magnify in the food production kitchen. Imagine the results that could occur if you omitted baking powder from the cornbread recipe, or accidentally noted teaspoons instead of tablespoons, or specified a baking temperature as 425° instead of 325°F. Check final amounts carefully. In addition, ensure that every ingredient in the ingredient list is used in the text of the procedure—and that every ingredient called for in the procedure appears on the ingredient list. Finally, make sure the procedure is clear and cannot be misunderstood. Attention to detail helps ensure the recipe will be carried out as it is intended it to be.

To ensure the ongoing success of standardized recipes, it's also important to encourage feedback from production employees. Tell employees that if they encounter suspected errors in recipes or believe that a standardized recipe is producing unacceptable results, you would like to hear about it. Encouraging communication allows you to pinpoint areas for correction and involve production staff in tweaking recipes that are then updated with the new information.

Employees who feel they cannot talk to the Certified Dietary Manager about recipe problems are much more likely to make their own adjustments to "fix" a recipe. In this way, a flawed recipe can slip through the system for a long time. When a new employee comes in and prepares the same recipe, it can flop. It's always better to edit the recipe and create a document that can generate reproducible results.

Using Standardized Recipes

Standardized recipes are useful for more than just production needs. Use them to determine your requisition needs and to improve portion control.

Requisitions

In large facilities, there may be one staff member whose job is to retrieve items from the storeroom for production needs. That person will work from a requisition that lists all of the items needed for the day's production. If your standardized recipes are computerized, your computer software can generate the requisition from those recipes.

If your recipes are not computerized, you can still generate a requisition from the standardized recipes. When starting a new menu cycle write down, or better yet, open a computer file such as Excel, Lotus 1-2-3 or Macintosh Numbers, and enter each ingredient used and the quantity needed in all of the recipes used during the day. If you have the same ingredient used in multiple recipes in the same production area, you could pull it all at one time. For example, if you are making Turkey a la King you might need:

15 lbs.	of turkey breast is needed for the regular entrée
+	
1 lb.	for the chopped and ground turkey PLUS
+	
2 lbs.	for the carb controlled recipe
+	
15 lbs.	for the cafeteria
33 lbs.	**TOTAL**

The requisition list would show a total of 33 lbs. needed.

Putting It Into Practice

5. Your facility is researching the need to expand their computer system and have asked for your input. Currently all you have is a computerized inventory system. How would you justify expanding the computerized inventory system by adding a computerized recipe system?

A requisition sheet helps with inventory control, purchasing and storeroom management. This will improve the storeroom process and staff efficiency by reducing trips to the storeroom for forgotten items.

Portion Control

Ensuring that food served matches portions specified in standardized recipes and on menus is critical because portion control is intertwined with recipe yields. **Portion control** is essential for managing the value of a standardized recipe, such as predictable costs, predictable nutrient content of menu items, and predictable number of servings for each product. Portion control also builds client satisfaction, as the portion sizes of foods are predictable and consistent.

Responsibility for portion control may be shared among various employees, from production staff to trayline employees to servers. For example, portion control for applesauce pre-portioned into dishes in the cold food production area becomes the responsibility of a cold food production employee. Meanwhile, portion control for hot mashed potatoes served on a buffet becomes the responsibility of the server. As the Certified Dietary Manager, you need to explain and reinforce the importance of portion control to all involved employees, provide training, and allow employees to practice the techniques. For example, have them practice using a common big spoon, a spoodle and a disher to portion a set number of portions of mashed potatoes. Usually, these portion sizes will vary and will demonstrate the need for a standard portion utensil.

Carrying through portion control often requires some tools for measurement. For example, when you specify 1/2 cup as a portion size, how do you know it will be served that way? Common measurement tools used in foodservice facilities include portion/dishers, scoops, and ladles. Portion scoops/dishers, and ladles designed for non-commercial foodservice have standardized sizes and are an aid in portion control. Portion scoops/dishers have designated numbers. For example, a #8 disher equals 1/2 cup, and a #16 equals 1/4 cup. This number is equivalent to the number of servings in a quart or 32 oz. So a #8 **disher** means 8 servings in a quart. (Note: a disher is frequently called a scoop or an ice cream scoop. The proper term is disher or **portion scoop** so it is not confused with another utensil called a scoop and used for dry ingredients such as flour.)

For some foods, portioning is achieved by weighing on a scale. For example, the 2-ounce serving of beef for a renal diet may be weighed to ensure compliance with the diet order. However, it is not always practical or cost-effective to weigh every portion of a food. In portioning the roast beef for a trayline service, a cook may weigh several portions in order to establish the thickness and dimensions of a 4-ounce serving and use this as a visual guide for the remaining portions. Finally, managers have many pre-portioned foods available to them today. These eliminate many of the challenges related to portion control. For example, you may purchase pre-portioned chicken breasts or fish filets for service. Figure 3.9 provides examples of how portions may be measured.

Glossary

Portion Control
Control of the serving sizes so they are standardized

Disher/Portion Scoop/Spoodle
A portion control serving utensil used for dishing vegetables, fruits, desserts, or starchy items like rice and potatoes

Figure 3.9 How Portions are Measured

PRODUCT	PORTION	METHOD
Diced peaches	1/2 cup	Use a #8 disher/portion scoop to portion individual servings into bowls.
Individual chicken fillets	5 oz. cooked weight	Portion each as one serving.
Vanilla cake	1/24 of pan	Slice cake as a 6x4 equal portions.
Apple pie	1/8 pie	Slice pie into eight equal pieces/portion.
Hearty chicken stew	1 cup	Use 8 oz. ladle to portion into bowls at the time of service.
Mashed potatoes	1/2 cup	Use #8 disher/portion scoop to portion individual servings onto plates.
Whole banana	1 each	Offer one banana each.

As you have seen, one advantage of standardized recipes is that you can specify standard portion sizes. But how do you know what the portion size should be? There are many references that describe standard portion sizes such as the Academy of Nutrition and Dietetics (Academy) Exchange Lists [formerly known as The American Dietetic Academy (ADA)].

Standardized Recipes and Food Allergies

The use of standardized recipes is of particular importance to people with food allergies. Food allergies and sensitivities are a potentially life-threatening concern for millions of people. Allergic reactions to the presence of an allergen can vary from an itchy or tingling feeling of the skin, nose or mouth to anaphylaxis (ana-fil-lax-is).

Anaphylaxis can cause difficulty in breathing, reduced blood pressure and gastrointestinal symptoms such as vomiting and diarrhea. If untreated, a severe anaphylactic reaction can lead to death. According to the Food and Drug Administration website:

> Each year in the U.S., it is estimated that anaphylaxis to food results in:
> - 30,000 emergency room visits
> - 2,000 hospitalizations
> - 150 deaths
>
> http://www.fda.gov/Food/ResourcesForYou/Consumers/ucm079311.htm

The most common "Big Eight" food allergens are:

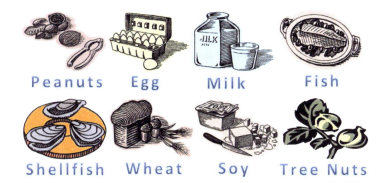

Peanuts   Egg   Milk   Fish

Shellfish   Wheat   Soy   Tree Nuts

Your clients rely on you to follow your recipes. At home, they can manage the ingredients of the meal items they prepare. However, when they are in your dining room, or when they are living in your care center, residence hall or detention center, they cannot control the ingredients in their foods.

When asked what is in the apple crisp, standardized recipes provide the staff with the list of ingredients that can be reviewed with clients. The consistent use of standardized recipes ensures that the baker did not add some chopped walnuts (a tree nut) to the apple crisp topping today.

For more information on Food Allergies and Anaphylaxis, refer to websites such as FDA. gov, WebMD, or FoodAllergy.org.

Recipe Acceptance

Recipes are planned and edited to provide our clients with meals and menus they will enjoy and that meet their dietary restrictions, if any. Developing a standardized recipe also has to include how well the dining clientele accept the item. Talking with diners during the meal, circulating Menu Surveys or Scorecards, and observing plate waste are all part of the feedback loop as you trial or present new recipes. Sometimes new items are not well accepted just because they are different. Oftentimes though, you may have a great item but the clientele prefers more oregano and less onion. You will not know unless you ask.

Standards and Procedures for Preparing Food

Overview and Objectives

This unit is all about managing production. Standardized recipes are one way to manage production; specifying standards and procedures for preparing food is another important consideration in managing production. The Certified Dietary Manager needs to establish the standards for food and production as part of the quality management initiatives. This chapter will address the production steps involved in the preparation of food. As with all standards, follow-up and continuous coaching of employees will ensure that standards are met. After completing this chapter, you should be able to:

✓ Develop food quality control standards; e.g., appearance, temperature, acceptance

✓ Implement procedures to monitor food production

✓ Develop procedures for monitoring food waste control

✓ Identify appropriate HACCP steps for food preparation

The development of standards for the preparation of food begins with identifying quality standards for raw and prepared foods in your facility. Specifically, you want to identify purchasing, preparation, and storage standards for foods served in your facility. Storage standards are covered in Chapter 18 and 19.

Section A   Purchasing Standards

First a little history. Having written specifications for each ingredient in your storeroom is an essential and practical matter. Prior to national food distribution companies and government oversight of food manufacturers, more items were produced and purchased locally. Standard definitions for what could be included in ground beef or white bread were far less structured and specific. Organizations purchased more raw ingredients to make their spaghetti sauce from scratch or bake their own homemade dinner rolls.

In today's marketplace, government oversight of healthcare and school foodservice, in particular, requires that food products be purchased from approved vendors only. Rarely do facilities make or purchase homemade tomato sauce to use in their "home-style" spaghetti sauce. They use a commercially prepared and marketed tomato sauce from their vendor (local grocery store or nationwide distributor).

Most items purchased today in any foodservice organization are prepared, packaged and processed under some level of government monitoring. Grading of meats, canned goods and dairy products are provided by the **USDA** (United Stated Department of Agriculture) and stamped on the labels of the products or cases.

Federal guidelines also dictate what labeling is required from the manufacturers: the list of ingredients, nutrition labeling, expiration or use by date, contact information and pack or lot numbers for tracking purposes. The pack or lot numbers become critically important information in the event of a product recall.

Before you purchase foods or write your specifications, you want to identify general information and guidelines about the food you procure. That information can be used to document standards for your facility.

Eggs and Dairy Products

Eggs

Eggs have many uses in most foodservice facilities. You and the chef/cook need to consider what type of eggs best fit the production needs. The type of eggs used will depend upon the number of clients served and the menu. (i.e. Do you have an on-site bakery?) There are three different egg products you might use: fresh, processed (frozen and liquid eggs), or dried eggs.

Fresh Eggs. The USDA provides the following information about shell eggs. There are three consumer grades: U.S. Grade AA, A, and B. The grade is determined by the interior quality of the egg and the appearance and condition of the shell. Eggs of any quality grade may differ in weight (size).

U.S. Grade AA eggs have whites that are thick and firm; yolks that are high, round, and practically free from defects; and clean, unbroken shells. Grade AA and Grade A eggs are best for frying and poaching where appearance is important. U.S. Grade A eggs have characteristics of Grade AA except that the whites are "reasonably" firm. This is the quality most often sold in stores. U.S. Grade B eggs have whites that may be thinner and yolks that may be wider and flatter than eggs of higher grades. The shells must be unbroken, but may show slight stains. This quality is seldom found in retail stores because they are usually used to make liquid, frozen, and dried egg products.

For more than 10 years the FDA and USDA guideline for the use of shell eggs has been to use pasteurized eggs. **Pasteurization of eggs** is a process, using a combination of time and temperature, that heats eggs in the shell, destroying bacteria and eliminating salmonella contamination. After pasteurization, a food-grade wax is added to the shell to prevent recontamination and maintain freshness. Pasteurized eggs are approved for whole egg products such as "sunny-side up", poached, or the making of egg based sauces such as fresh Hollandaise. Non-pasteurized eggs are intended for use in baking, quiches or other products where the egg will be *fully* cooked, which eliminates any *Salmonella* contamination. Pasteurized liquid eggs are recommended for most baking, egg bakes and scrambled products.

Healthcare and school surveyors have cited some facilities for having both pasteurized and un-pasteurized shell eggs in the same cooler. It may be wise to have only pasteurized eggs in the facility. Refer to the Food Code, CMS, USDA and state regulations for information pertinent to the specific operation.

Putting It Into Practice

1. Coffee is available in your cafeteria throughout the day. You want to make creamers available that don't need refrigeration and can be displayed next to the coffee. What type of creamer should you purchase?

Frozen, Liquid, and Dried Eggs. Processed eggs save time when used for baking or cooking omelets and scrambled eggs in large quantities. Processed eggs help meet the food safety regulation that prohibits pooling eggs (breaking raw shell eggs into a container and storing them for later). All processed products are processed under sanitary conditions and must display the USDA inspection mark. Processed eggs are broken and separated into yolks and whites and then pasteurized before processing into dried, frozen or refrigerated liquid products. There are several different processed liquid and dried egg products. Figure 4.1 shows both liquid and dried egg products, how they are packaged for purchase, their uses, and storage and handling guidelines. Pasteurized dried egg white powder should be used for meringues or desserts that are not cooked. Note: "Egg Substitutes" are comprised of egg whites, food coloring and some seasoning. They should be handled like liquid egg products.

Figure 4.1 Egg Products

REFRIGERATED LIQUID EGG PRODUCTS

- Whole eggs, whites or yolks
- Sugared egg yolks
- Salted whole eggs or yolks
- Scrambled egg mix
- Extended shelf life whole eggs, whites, yolks or scrambled egg mix

Usage	Foodservice and the commercial food processing industry.
Availability	Bulk tank trucks, totes, metal or plastic containers, polyethylene coated fiber or laminated foil and paper cartons and hermetically sealed polyethylene bags. Container size from small bags to cartons (8-oz. to 5-lbs.), intermediate size bag in boxes and pails (20- to 40-lbs.) and larger drums and totes (200- to 3,500-lbs.).
Advantages	Pasteurized, quick and easy to use.
Storage/ Handling	Refrigerated egg products should be kept at 40°F (4°C) or below, but do not freeze. Use well within expiration dates.

DRIED EGG PRODUCTS

- Whole eggs, white or yolk solids
- Dried egg or scrambled egg mix
- Egg whites
- Free-flowing whole eggs or yolk solids
- Blends of whole eggs and/or yolk carbohydrates

Usage	Ingredient especially for the commercial food processing industry.
Availability	Foodservice: 6-oz. pouches, 3- and 25-lb. poly packs Commercial: 25- and 50-lb. boxes, 150-, 175-, and 200-lb. drums
Advantages	Pasteurized, long shelf life, stable and mixable.
Storage/ Handling	Keep cool at less than 50°F (10°C) to maintain quality. Once containers have been opened, reseal tightly to prevent contamination and absorption of moisture. Dried egg products should flow freely and not be clumped or hardened. Use well within expiration dates.

Source: American Egg Board. Used with permission.

Cheese

Cheese is important because it can add calcium and protein to menu items. With the wide variety of cheeses available, it can also add unique flavors. There are processed cheeses and natural cheeses.

Processed Cheeses. When you are selecting cheese for use in hot items, such as heated sandwiches, casseroles, or sauces, select a cheese with a suitable flavor and texture that will melt consistently and easily. Processed cheeses are a combination of natural cheeses that have undergone a heat process. They melt more easily and smoothly but provide less of the variety of unique flavors because they are a combination of cheeses. They work well in casseroles and sauces. If you have a signature hot sandwich, you might have a higher client satisfaction with a natural cheese slice because of the more pronounced cheese flavor. Processed cheeses come in a variety of forms such as sliced, block, or spreads.

Natural Cheeses. The flavor of the natural cheese depends upon the type of milk (cow, goat, or sheep) and the length of time the cheese is aged.

There are several varieties of natural cheeses:

- Fresh cheese such as ricotta, mozzarella, or feta
- Soft cheese such as Brie
- Semisoft such as blue or Monterey Jack
- Firm cheese such as Cheddar, provolone
- Hard grating cheese such as Parmesan

Aging does decrease the lactose content so if you have lactose intolerant clients who prefer cheese, they might be able to tolerate an aged natural cheese. Natural cheeses come in a variety of forms such as grated, sliced, and cubed.

There are hundreds of varieties of cheeses and you can determine which type and form to purchase by reviewing your recipes and consulting the chef/cook. There are many websites that can help you determine the characteristics and purchasing information of cheeses or use a food production book such as *Food for Fifty* by Mary Molt.

Milk

Milk is another staple in the foodservice department and is commonly used in recipes as well as for a beverage.

Fluid Milk. Generally, there are four different types of fluid milk used for beverages:

- Whole milk—contains 8 g of fat per 8 oz. cup and the federal standard requires that whole milk be at least 3.25% fat
- Reduced fat milk—2% fat and contains 4.7 g total fat per cup
- Low-fat milk—1% fat and contains 2.6 g total fat per cup
- Nonfat or skim milk—0.5% fat and contains 0.5 g total fat per cup

The availability of goat milk is increasing and for Certified Dietary Managers who work in hospitals, you may need to establish a source for it. Goat milk has a higher concentration of medium chain fatty acids (MCFA) and research has shown that clients with various medical conditions, such as malabsorption syndrome are more tolerant of goat milk. For infants who are allergic to cow's milk, goat milk may be an acceptable alternative.

Sensitivity or intolerance to fluid cow's milk has led to the development of lactose-free dairy products. Alternative "milk" products such as soy, almond, and rice have become easily accessible in grocery stores for customers with intolerance or wanting to decrease their intake of animal-based foods.

Fluid milk products must be **pasteurized** to be served in commercial facilities. Pasteurization means heating fluid milk or cream to a specific temperature for a specified amount of time. Both fluid milk and cream products may also be **ultra-pasteurized**. Ultra-pasteurization takes the pasteurization process to higher temperatures for a shorter period of time. Finally, these products can also be **ultra-high-temperature processed**. The products are heated at a high enough temperature to kill all of the bacteria. Ultra-high-temperature products can be held without refrigeration for up to three months. Once they are opened, they must be treated like all fluid milk or cream products, refrigerated and used within a few days.

Yogurt. Yogurt is a product cultured with lactic acid-producing bacteria. It is available with whole milk, low-fat, or skim milk. Some Greek yogurts have much higher protein content (i.e. 11-14 gm as compared to 7 gm for the traditional yogurt). For cancer clients or those needing increased protein and calories, consider purchasing a whole milk, Greek yogurt. There are many flavorings, sweeteners, and fruits added to increase client acceptance.

Butter

Butter is considered a dairy product because it is made with pasteurized cream and has 80% milkfat content. Butter is usually graded according to federal standards with Grades A or AA. Grade B butter is made from sour cream. When butter is churned, salt or a salty brine is added. Unsalted butter is available as well as whipped butter.

Unsalted butter is called for in some baking recipes because the butter flavor is more pronounced. Whipped butter doesn't convert well in baking recipes; it is used more as a spread.

Grains

Grains are the seeds or kernel of cereal grasses. Grains come in many different forms depending upon the amount of milling:

- Whole grains—contain the bran (outer shell providing fiber, B vitamins, trace minerals), the endosperm (provides energy—carbohydrate and protein), and the germ (provides antioxidants, Vitamin E, B-vitamins). Whole grains that are cracked, crushed, or flaked during milling but still retain the same proportion of bran, germ, and endosperm as the original grain are also considered whole grains.

- Pearled grains—bran and germ layers are removed resulting in less fiber but faster cooking times; also known as polished grain.

- Grits—corn or oat kernels cut into smaller pieces so they cook more quickly; they are still considered whole grains. Steel-cut oats is one example.

- Flakes—whole grains that are rolled into a flattened kernel.

- Meal—whole grains that are finely ground; corn meal and graham flour are examples.

- Bran—the outer part of the grain kernel that can be flakes or fibers. Oat bran, wheat bran, and rice bran are examples.

- Germ—the bottom of the grain kernel that contains the fat and fat soluble vitamins; because of the fat content, it has a shorter shelf life.

• Flour—kernels that are ground and sifted; not considered a whole grain if the bran and germ are removed.

Cooking with whole grains and serving whole grains should be encouraged in your facility because of the added nutrient content. There are some new grains on the market that will enhance the nutrient content of your menus if used: Amaranth seeds are higher in protein content and can be used with flour in breads or pancakes. Quinoa (pronounced KEEN-wah) is higher in protein, calcium, and iron than any of the other grains. It is a small seed from South America and is used like rice.

The interest in gluten-free products has skyrocketed in the past few years. Gluten is a type of protein found in many grains. As the Certified Dietary Manager, you need to know which products are gluten-free to meet the increased demand from your clients. See Figure 4.2 for a table of grains that are considered whole grains, not whole grains, and gluten-free grains.

Flours

Flours can be made from almost any grain. Besides fiber, one of the characteristics that differentiate flour is the amount of gluten it contains. All-purpose flour is blended wheat flour with a lower protein content than bread flour. It serves dual purpose for baking, breading, and general cooking needs. Bread flour, being higher in protein, is also higher in gluten. Gluten helps give yeast breads a higher volume. For pastries such as biscuits and cookies where high gluten content is less desirable, large commercial bakeries use pastry flour that is low-protein flour made from soft wheat. Self-rising flour contains leavening agents and added salt and should be avoided with low-sodium diets.

Figure 4.2 Whole Grains Guide

WHOLE GRAINS	NOT WHOLE GRAINS	GLUTEN-FREE GRAINS
Look for these terms on the label:	Not whole grain if the label reads:	
• Cracked wheat	• Flour, white flour, wheat flour	• Quinoa
• Crushed wheat	• All-purpose flour	• Rice
• Whole wheat flour	• Unbleached flour	• Sorghum
• Graham flour	• Bromated flour	• Teff
• Bromated whole wheat flour	• Instantized flour	• Amaranth
• Whole (wheat or corn)	• Self-rising flour	• Buckwheat
• Wheat berries	• Any grain product labeled "enriched"	• Corn
• Oat groats	• Bread flour	• Hominy
• Rolled oats	• Cake flour	• Millet
• Brown rice	• Durum flour	
• Brown rice flour	• Corn or hominy grits	
• Wild rice	• Farina	
• Amaranth	• Semolina	
• Whole barley	• White rice	
• Quinoa	• Couscous	
• Kasha/buckwheat groats	• Pearled barley	
• Whole millet		
• Wild rice		
• Whole rye flour and flakes		

Corn starch is similar to flour in that it is finely ground endosperm, the starchy part of the kernel. It is used as a thickener in place of flour because the final cooked product is translucent rather than opaque. A substitute for corn starch as a thickener is arrowroot or tapioca.

Pasta

Pasta is made from high-protein wheat flour or durum semolina flour. Pasta comes in a large variety of shapes, most of which can be used with sauces or in casseroles. Your menu, your recipes, and the chef/cook can help decide which pasta shapes to purchase. Ask your foodservice vendor for a poster with the various pasta shapes or do a quick Web search for a guide to pasta shapes and sauces. Another consideration besides the shape is whether the pasta will be made with an egg product, such as egg noodles, and whether you will purchase fresh or dry pasta. Fresh pasta is highly perishable. Some pasta is available frozen.

Some Asian recipes call for other types of noodles such as rice noodles, made from rice, or chow mein noodles made from wheat. Bean starch noodles or cellophane noodles are made from mung bean starch. Both rice noodles and cellophane noodles can be fried very quickly and added to dishes as a garnish. Asian noodles are usually stir-fried or used as a base or garnish rather than served with a sauce.

Meats

Beef, Pork, Lamb and Veal. Meat will obviously be the high dollar item in your food budget. Therefore, knowing about meat quality, how it is handled after delivery, and cooking methods are extremely important. Fortunately, there is help from the **National Association of Meat Purveyors (NAMP)**. They publish a *Meat Buyer's Guide* based on the USDA's **Institutional Meat Purchasing Specifications (IMPS)**. The guide is available for purchase at this URL: www.namp.com/namp/Default.asp

Most of the meat today is purchased portioned or a retail, ready-to-use cut rather than in wholesale large cuts such as a hind-quarter. All meat that crosses state lines is required to be inspected by the federal government; if it is processed and sold within a given state, the inspection must be equivalent to the federal standards. Grading of meat, such as prime and choice for beef, is not mandatory. However, the grading process helps to identify for consumers the relative eating quality of the product. If you are responsible for procuring meat in your facility or department, use the *Meat Buyer's Guide* to help you understand the purchasing language and process.

Poultry

The past ten years has seen an explosion in the selection of cooked and processed poultry products available to Certified Dietary Managers. As with the other products, examine your menu and recipes. Together with the chef/cook, decide which poultry products would be the best buy for your facility and clientele. If the chef is skilled at making homemade soups, purchasing whole poultry or cut-up pieces that will yield bones for stock might be a good investment. Would portioned cuts be the best for the skills of the staff? Pulled chicken, rather than uniform diced pieces of chicken, might be needed for salads or casseroles. Before finalizing the purchase order, know what your needs are in terms of the types of poultry cuts.

Glossary

NAMP
National Association of Meat Purveyors. They publish the industry standard *Meat Buyer's Guide* based on the USDA's Institutional Meat Purchasing Specifications (IMPS)

Poultry has a mandatory inspection for wholesomeness and optional grading. Grade A poultry is most commonly sold to commercial facilities. The grading relates to the fat covering, discolorations, feathers, thickness of flesh and other overall quality criteria.

Irradiated Stamp

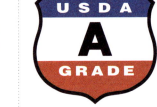

Grade Stamp

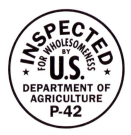

Inspection Stamp

Today, both raw meat and raw poultry products may be irradiated to increase product safety and extend the shelf life. The **FDA** requires that irradiated meat and poultry be labeled as such.

Fish and Shellfish

When it comes to purchasing fish and shellfish, fresh is not always the best choice. As soon as fish is caught, it loses its ability to fight off bacteria. Most fish today is quickly frozen within hours of being caught and this fresh-frozen choice may be the best option depending upon your geographic location. If fish are intended for raw or undercooked consumption (such as sushi or cold-smoked salmon), it must be properly frozen before being served to kill worms deeply imbedded inside fish muscle. Look for labeling or other information to assure that the fish was properly frozen.

The U.S. Department of Commerce does voluntary inspection of fish and shellfish. Look for the **Packed Under Federal Inspection (PUFI)** mark on packages to assure that the fish is safe, wholesome, and properly labeled. There is also grading for fish similar to other meats. The Grade A stamp assures that the product is free from blemishes and defects, and is of high quality with good flavor and aroma. The **FDA Food Code** recommends that fish be purchased from a state-approved vendor and that it be commercially or legally harvested.

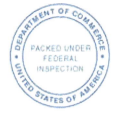

Fish can be purchased in many sizes and shapes. The following are common examples of what you might purchase:

- Fish fillet—product is cut the length of the fish parallel to the backbone; it can be an irregular shape and size
- Portioned cuts—square or rectangular cuts from a block of frozen fish; fish sticks are one example
- Steaks—product is cut across the fish into slices

See Figure 4.3 for a Seafood Buying Guide. The buying guide only addresses commonly served fish and shellfish. If your facility serves high-cost shellfish, be sure you investigate the proper storage and purchasing information for products such as fresh lobster, oysters, clams, and mussels. Make sure that you are purchasing from an approved seafood vendor and that the seafood is "commercially or legally harvested" per the FDA Food Code guidelines.

Figure 4.3 Seafood Buying Guide

FISH OR SEAFOOD TYPE	CHARACTERISTICS TO LOOK FOR
Fresh or Thawed Fillets and Steaks	Mild odor; firm, elastic flesh; no bruising, blood spots or browning
Fresh or Thawed Shrimp—sold by the count per pound (e.g., extra large shrimp are 26-30 shrimp per pound)	Flesh completely fills the shell; no strong odors; no black edges or spots; moist but not slimy feel
Surimi	Firm and moist; possess an off-white color; no strong odors; flesh should have a light pink tint
Frozen Seafood	No signs of frost on seafood or package interior; no signs of drying as in white patches; no strong odors; should be solidly frozen
Smoked Fish	Clean, smoky odor; firm texture; no signs of mold or salt crystals

Fresh and Canned Produce

Fresh or canned produce is most likely part of every meal served so having purchasing standards will be critical to serving quality meals.

Fresh Produce

There are changes occurring in the fresh produce industry: 1) purchasing fresh produce at farmer's markets is gaining in popularity; 2) pre-cleaned and cut produce is widely available today and in some case may be less expensive than the whole product.

Farmers' Markets. Fresh produce is best at peak harvest and you will have the highest quality and nutritional value if you purchase from local farmers. Farmers' markets rarely sell graded products as the USDA grading program is voluntary. They may sell their products under a different name for a grade such as firsts and seconds. Check your menu and recipe needs to determine what level of quality is needed. If exterior appearance is important (i.e. when you are serving whole or pieces of fresh fruit or vegetables), then pay for the top-quality product. If the product is going to be mashed, chopped, or pureed, then choosing the lower quality grade will be your best buy. Check state and local regulations regarding the use of local suppliers and compliance with the "approved vendor" status. Get to know your vendors and how they keep the product fresh between harvesting and market. They might also be willing to deliver products to your facility.

Pre-Cleaned and Cut Produce. Again, you have to know your menu and recipes and what staff time and skill level is available to determine the best produce to purchase. If the pre-cleaned or cut produce is cheaper and meets the needs of the facility, go one step

Putting It Into Practice

3. Your university foodservice has decided to offer Sushi at least once during each menu cycle. What purchasing standard should you consider for Sushi?

further and make sure vendors have HACCP (Hazard Analysis Critical Control Point) plans in place. Pre-cleaned and cut produce should be processed in clean, cold facilities and delivered in refrigerated trucks.

Canned and Frozen Fruits and Vegetables

Processing slightly reduces nutritional content of canned and frozen products but not enough to abandon the use of them. Frozen products have a higher quality appearance because freezing doesn't cause color and texture changes as much as canning. This is especially true for the **IQF (Individually Quick Frozen)** products. Frozen products can contain more nutrients than fresh because they are processed soon after harvesting. Many fresh products sit in store rooms or produce counters for a long time after harvesting, thus losing nutritional value.

The USDA has voluntary grading of quality for many canned and frozen vegetables and fruits. The most common are U.S. Grade A (Fancy), U.S. Grade B (Extra-select or Choice), and U.S. Grade C (Standard). Grading is paid for by the packer and packers may use different terminology. Grades are based on appearance criteria: color, uniformity of size, shape, lack of blemishes, or lack of stems/leaves. Like fresh produce, purchase only the grade that you need. If you are using canned tomatoes for pasta sauce, you don't need to purchase Grade A or Fancy.

Section B   Preparation and Quality Standards

Preparation tips indicated below are not meant to be cooking or production instructions. Consider purchasing a book like *Food for Fifty* by Mary Molt to find recipes and full cooking instructions. When preparing standardized recipes, consider adding a quality standard to the recipe. Some organizations maintain a notebook of photographs of the final plate presentation for their different menu items. That way, production and serving staff will be reminded what the product should look like, down to the garnishing, when it is completed. You will find more detailed quality standards in *Food for Fifty*.

Eggs, Cheese, and Milk

Eggs

Preparation. The two most important principles for preparing egg products are to use low temperatures and minimize cooking time. It is also helpful to review grades and sizes of shell egg products discussed earlier in this chapter. Pasteurized Grade A or AA is a good choice for eggs that will be prepared whole, such as poached or fried, because the yolks are firm and high. For other uses, Grade B is fine. Eggs are also sized. You will want to match shell egg sizes to sizes specified in any of your standardized recipes.

Menu items featuring eggs can range from scrambled eggs to omelets to frittatas to soufflés. With modified diets, you can use egg whites or egg substitute products that have been modified to reduce cholesterol and saturated fat. Figure 4.4 lists some common egg preparation problems and solutions.

Quality Standards. Quality standards for egg products should include the following:

- Fresh egg products, such as scrambled, omelets and custards, should have a soft, semisolid structure with no water separating from the cooked eggs.
- The color should be a soft yellow with no greening.

Glossary

Individually Quick Frozen (IQF)
A process of rapid freezing that yields smaller ice crystals and maintains the individual units of fruits, berries, vegetables, and meat items

Figure 4.4 Egg Preparation Problems and Solutions

GREENING

PROBLEM: Cooked eggs may turn green (a natural chemical reaction) if held over heat for an extended period of time.

SOLUTION:

Omelets and Scrambled Eggs

- Use fresh eggs (Grade AA or A). Greening is more likely in older eggs.
- Cook eggs in small batches, no larger than three quarts.
- Substitute a medium white sauce for the liquid in the egg mixture. (One part white sauce to five parts egg.)
- Use temperatures of 135°F and above for steam table holding.
- Do not hold hot foods on buffet line for longer than 1 hour.
- Use only stainless steel equipment and utensils.
- Try a liquid egg product if greening is frequent. (Many of these contain citric acid which slows greening.)
- Beat in 1/4 teaspoon lemon juice for every 18 large eggs, or 1/4 teaspoon citric acid crystals for every dozen large eggs.

Hard-Cooked Eggs

- Simmer eggs (185-190°F) in water. Don't boil.
- Cool immediately in cold water. Peel when cool.

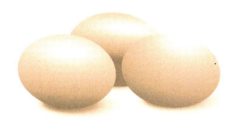

WEEPING

PROBLEM: Water separating from cooked eggs is caused by overcooking or by cooking and holding at high heat or from the addition of watery ingredients.

SOLUTION:

Scrambled Eggs

- Prepare eggs in small batches, no larger than three quarts.
- Substitute a medium white sauce for the liquid in the egg mixture. (One part white sauce to five parts egg.)
- Use temperatures 135°F and above for steam table holding.
- Use egg products with stabilizers (i.e. gums) added.
- Limit the amount of added ingredients and make sure they are well-drained.

Meringues

- Lack of volume of the foam during beating or cooking:
  > Beat whites until frothy before adding sugar.
  > Add sugar slowly.
  > Stop frequently and lift whites from bottom of bowl to ensure thorough and even beating.
  > Use a clean metal or glass (not plastic) bowl.
  > Beat until sugar is dissolved, the peaks barely fold over and whites do not slip from sides when bowl is tilted.
- If the meringue is to be used on a pie, place it on a hot (160°F or above) filling, and brown immediately at 350°F for approximately 15 minutes.
- For pie meringues containing a larger number of egg whites, reduce baking temperature and increase baking time to achieve temperature of 160°F and mixture tests done (knife inserted near center removes cleanly).

RUBBERY AND DRY EGGS

PROBLEM: The problem is the result of overcooking and high heat. It generally follows weeping.

SOLUTION:

Omelets and Scrambled Eggs

- Cook at medium heat until no visible liquid egg remains.
- Cook in small batches, no larger than three quarts.
- Use a medium white sauce as liquid in egg mixture. (One part white sauce to five parts egg.)
- Use temperatures 135°F and above for steam table holding.

Fried Eggs

- Cook over medium heat on preheated grill or pan.
- Use the right amount of fat to avoid toughening, about one teaspoon per egg.
- Baste with fat or steam-baste by adding small amounts of water and covering.

Cheese

Preparation. Cheese can add calcium, protein, and unique flavor to menu items. When you are selecting cheese for use in hot items, such as heated sandwiches, casseroles, or sauces, select a cheese with a suitable flavor and texture. Generally, it should be sliced (for sandwiches), shredded, or cubed. Low temperatures, generally no higher than 350°F, help prevent curdling, toughness, and stringiness. For food safety, a foodservice operation should select only pasteurized cheeses.

Quality Standards. A quality product containing cheese will have the cheese evenly distributed and melted with little or no browning the on top. The cheese flavor will blend with the other flavors and not be overpowering.

Milk

Preparation. Your menu and recipes will drive what milk products to purchase for cooking. See Figure 4.5 for descriptions of milk products used in cooking.

Figure 4.5 Milk Products Used in Cooking

PRODUCT	CHARACTERISTICS
Evaporated Milk	Comes as whole milk, low-fat, or fat free. Fluid milk with about 60% of the water removed.
Sweetened Condensed Milk	Comes as whole or fat free. It is evaporated milk with added sugar and processed to one-third its original volume.
Dry Milk	Comes as whole or low-fat. Dissolves in cold water; whole dry milk has a shorter shelf life because of the fat content.
Buttermilk	Can be purchased as fluid or dry product. The fluid product has a bacteria added to make it thick and tart. Dry buttermilk is dried from the liquid produced when making butter.
Half-and-Half	A mixture of whole milk and cream with 10.5-17% fat. May be used in place of light cream or table cream.
Light Cream, Table Cream	A lower-milkfat cream; cannot be used for whipping.
Light Whipping Cream	Contains a minimum of 30-36% fat and does work for whipping.
Heavy Whipping Cream	Contains a minimum of 36% fat and is preferred for whipped cream because it whips easily and holds it shape.
Sour Cream	A cultured product like yogurt except it is cultured cream. It contains 18-22% fat.

Glossary

Coagulate
To cause transformation of a liquid into a soft, semisolid, or solid mass

When cooking or reheating products containing milk or cream, use a low heat setting. Like cheese, milk is high in protein. When heated to too rapidly, protein **coagulates** causing the milk product to potentially curdle. The film on the top of cooked milk or custards is another example of coagulated protein.

Quality Standards. Products containing milk or cream such as cream soups, sauces, and desserts will appear smooth with a uniform texture and no film. The color will be light and opaque. Products containing cream will also have a rich mouth feel and texture.

Grains

This section will address products made with grains such as yeast and quick breads, pasta, rice and dessert products.

Yeast Bread

Preparation. Yeast breads are leavened with yeast and may be a lean dough (using little or no sugar and margarine) or a sweet dough (using sugar, margarine, and/or eggs). Lean dough is appropriate for French bread, sandwich rolls, and similar products; while sweet dough makes good caramel rolls or raisin bread. See Figure 4.6 for preparation problems and solutions.

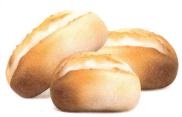

Quality Standard: Uniform golden brown color, sounds hollow when tapped; crisp, tender crust; uniform grain, moist texture.

Figure 4.6 Yeast Bread Preparation Problems and Solutions

PROBLEM	SOLUTION
Coarse, Heavy Texture	Be sure yeast is not killed by water that is too hot in initial stages or excessive equipment-generated heat in processing [use a thermometer; extend kneading time; check proofing time (may be too long or too short)]; check to be sure excessive salt was not used.
Loaf is Cracked	Avoid adding excessive flour when forming the loaf; shape loaf with care, not forcing it.
Loaf is too Big and Light	Check flour ingredient (may be too much gluten); check oven temperature (may be too low); check yeast measurement (may be too much).
Loaf Collapses	Re-check and limit proofing time; make sure oven temperature is not too low.

Quick Bread

Preparation. Quick breads include biscuits, muffins, and loaves such as banana bread or nut bread. Quick breads can be made from batter (as with muffins) or soft dough (as with biscuits that are rolled and cut).

For any baked product, it is important to measure flour correctly. Be sure to match the product to the recipe, as presifted flour does not have the same volume as unsifted flour.

Some ingredients require packing. An example is brown sugar. Failure to pack the sugar when specified could reduce the sugar in the recipe by as much as 50 percent and affect the final product significantly.

Note that unlike yeast breads, quick breads do not rely on developing the gluten in flour, so mixing should be limited. Too much mixing causes the gluten proteins to develop, resulting in tunnels in the product.

Biscuits contain similar ingredients, but the proportion of flour is higher. A muffin dough has 2 parts flour to one part liquid, whereas a biscuit dough has three parts flour to one part liquid.

Figure 4.7 lists quick bread problems and solutions.

Quality Standard. Muffins and biscuits should be uniform size and shape; have a tender crumb, even cell structure, rounded, not peaked top, pleasing flavor, moist texture, no tunnels and a uniform golden brown color.

Figure 4.7 Quick Bread Preparation Problems and Solutions

PROBLEM	SOLUTION
Coarse Texture with Tunnels	Avoid over mixing; re-check measurements of ingredients.
Dry Product	Avoid over baking; also check flour measurement (may be too much).
Quick Breads Become Soggy	Remove from pans after about 5 minutes; do not let sit in pans too long.
Muffin or Biscuit Texture is Tough or Rubbery	Limit mixing; only moisten dry ingredients.
Biscuits are Dense and Don't "Rise" Much	Mix and handle the dough less.

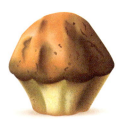

Pasta and Rice

Preparation. When preparing rice, macaroni, noodles, spaghetti, or similar products, general cooking principles are:

- Cook quickly in boiling water until tender. Salt the water if specified in the recipe.
  - > It is not recommended to totally eliminate salt in the cooking of Pasta, Rice or Grains as the lack of salt changes the final product to a flat hollow taste.
- Drain quickly and stir in fat, if specified. Do not rinse.
- Avoid washing rice before cooking or rinsing pasta after cooking, as these procedures wash away valuable nutrients such as B-vitamins.

Quality Standard. Pasta should have some resistance to the bite (called al dente or tender to the tooth); not too soft or mushy. Rice grains should also be tender, not too soft, and separate easily.

Meat, Poultry, and Fish Products

The quality of meat products will depend upon the quality of the ingredients, the equipment in place, and the skill level of the cooking staff. Endpoint cooking standards for meat products are extremely important and are located in Chapter 19.

Beef, Pork, Lamb, and Veal

Preparation. When cooking meats, choose a *dry* or *moist heat* method. For example, tender cuts that contain little connective tissue, such as steaks and roasts, do well with dry heat methods. These include roasting, baking, broiling (for individual portions that are 1-2" thick), and frying. Less tender cuts of meat with more connective tissue require moist heat to develop tenderness and flavor.

You can use meat timetables as a general guide for cooking meat. Timetables, available in most cookbooks, are useful in determining production scheduling requirements, i.e. when to start the cooking process so that products will be done in time for service. You can measure doneness with a thermometer placed in the center of the product, not touching bone. The temperature of a roast may continue to rise after it is removed from the oven.

Quality Standards. Meat products should be evenly browned, not burned, tender, and moist. To ensure food safety, meat products are cooked to the appropriate time and internal temperature recommendations. (See Chapter 19 for a more detailed discussion on food safety and internal temperature controls of cooked food items.)

Figure 4.8 Cooking Time and Temperature Guide (Suggested Minimums)

FOOD ITEM	TEMP.	TIME	COMMENTS
All whole cuts of meat such as pork, steaks, roasts and chops	145°F	15 sec.	Allow the meat to rest for 3 minutes before consuming.
Poultry, game, stuffed fish, stuffed meat, stuffed pasta	165°F	15 sec.	
Chopped or ground seafood or meat (includes ground beef, ground pork, veal, lamb and mechanically tenderized meat)	155°F	15 sec.	
Fish, seafood, meats not listed above	145°F	15 sec.	
Eggs on steam table	155°F	15 sec.	Cooked to hold
Egg, single-serving	145°F	15 sec.	Cooked to order
Fruits and vegetables	135°F	N/A	
Food cooked in microwave	165°F	2 min.	Hold time after cooking
Reheating leftovers	165°F	15 sec.	

Note: These are standards recommended in the FDA Food Code. Please consult your local standards, which may be different. Also review manufacturers' instructions for processed foods.

Poultry

Preparation. Poultry is available in various cuts, from whole birds to cut pieces. Generally, poultry should be cooked at a low temperature (325°-350°F) to produce a tender, juicy product. Preparation options include roasting, broiling, grilling, oven frying, and other frying methods; as well as moist-heat methods such as braising, stewing, or steaming.

As with meats, you can use timetables as a general guide for cooking poultry. It is important to verify end-point cooking temperatures with a thermometer.

Putting It Into Practice

4. Your menu calls for a Blushing Pear salad that uses canned pear halves. What grade should you consider purchasing for this salad?

Quality Standards. Poultry products should be lightly browned, tender, and moist. To ensure food safety, poultry products are cooked to the appropriate time and internal temperature recommendations.

Fish

Preparation. Fish should generally be cooked at a moderately high temperature, rapidly enough to retain juices and moisture, but slowly enough to ensure thorough cooking. You can match preparation techniques to the product. For example, fatty fish such as salmon lend themselves to baking and broiling. In general, consider ten minutes cooking time per one inch thickness at 400-425°F.

Quality Standards. Fish products should be juicy, flavorful, and tender. Breaded products should be a uniform golden brown color. To ensure food safety, fish products are cooked to the appropriate time and internal temperature recommendations.

Fresh Produce

Fresh produce should be prepared as close to serving time as practical to preserve the fresh appearance and nutritional value.

Fresh Vegetables

Preparation. Careful attention to preparation techniques can help preserve nutrient values in produce, as well as flavor, appearance, and overall quality. It's important to consider the needs of the clients served, ensuring that vegetables are tender enough for any clients with chewing limitations. Sometimes chopping or grating vegetables (as in a coleslaw, for example) is an option for serving fresh vegetables. Cook vegetables in small amounts of water or steam them until they are tender but firm. If possible, schedule prep work as close to final service time to maintain quality and minimize nutrient losses.

In the past, some chefs have used baking soda to brighten the color of cooked vegetables. Not only does this make the vegetable mushy, it also decreases the nutrient quantity of the vegetable. When cooking fresh vegetables, pre-cook only until color brightens and the vegetable is still crisp. Plunge into ice cold water, drain, and store in the refrigerator until ready to complete cooking immediately prior to service. This helps to preserve the color and texture. Do not over-blanch the vegetables as it can increases the nutrient loss, particularly anti-oxidants.

Quality Standards (this is also appropriate for canned vegetables). Vegetables are cut into bite-sized pieces as appropriate for the clientele. They are cooked to a tender but firm consistency. Color is pleasing and appropriate for the vegetable.

Fruit

Preparation. Fresh fruits may be served whole, halved, or in pieces. Wash fresh fruits thoroughly before serving. Some, such as peaches and bananas, can turn brown after slicing. To prevent this, you can dip slices in ascorbic acid or diluted lemon juice after peeling or cutting. As with vegetables, you should cut or prepare fresh fruits as close to service time as practical.

Dried fruits may be served as stewed fruit or in pies, cobblers, crisps, whips, and salads. Frozen fruit should be served as soon as it has thawed (preferably before all the ice crystals have melted).

Putting It Into Practice

5. The chicken breasts for dinner were dry and tough. They don't meet the standard. What might have happened to cause this?

Quality Standards (this is also appropriate for canned fruits). Fruits are cut into bite sized pieces as appropriate for the clientele or the fruit recipe. Color is pleasing and appropriate for the fruit. Frozen fruit is not watery and has some ice crystals. Flavor is mildly sweet and appropriate for the fruit.

Sauce

Preparation. There are several basic sauces; not all of them are thickened with a grain or starch based process:

- **Simple sauces:** A simple sauce is the au jus made from the drippings of roasted meat. The caramelized drippings are dissolved in water by stirring over heat with no thickening added. Concentrated canned soups may be used as a sauce (with no or minimal dilution); simply heat and serve hot.

- **Butter sauces:** Butter or margarine adds richness and flavor as a sauce and holds additional seasonings well. To make a butter sauce, stir seasonings into melted butter or margarine.

- **Bread sauces:** To prepare dry bread sauce, stir and brown breadcrumbs in a hot skillet with melted butter. For moist bread sauce, use two ounces of dry breadcrumbs to thicken one quart of stock.

- **Sauces thickened with egg:** These include mayonnaise and cooked sauces such as Hollandaise. The principles involved in the preparation of these sauces include the absorption of fat into the egg yolk and the ability of the egg yolk to act as an emulsifying agent and hold oil in suspension, as is the case in mayonnaise. Select pasteurized egg products for these recipes.

- **Tart or savory sauces:** Examples are barbecue sauce or teriyaki sauce. These sauces are often used on baked, broiled, and grilled meat, poultry, and fish. Marinades can be used to flavor and tenderize meats. Some include acid ingredients to help tenderize meat. If meat is marinated, do it under refrigeration. Discard the excess marinade before cooking.

- **Starch-thickened sauces:** These products use starch ingredients such as flour, cornstarch, tapioca, or others to thicken the product while heating. Cereal starch requires a boiling temperature to complete gelatinization, or the swelling of the starch granules which causes thickening to take place. Boiling must continue for five minutes to ensure complete swelling. Root starch begins to gelatinize when heated to 150°-160°F, and complete swelling is accomplished before boiling. If boiling continues, the starch granules will break down; the sauce will lose its thick appearance and become sticky. When preparing a starch-thickened sauce, it's important to stir continuously to prevent lumps.

A basic method for preparing a starch-based sauce begins by mixing the starch with fat. This is called a **roux**. To make a roux, blend an equal weight of melted fat and flour, and cook together three to five minutes for a white roux, five to seven minutes for a blond roux, and ten minutes for a brown roux. Next, remove roux from the heat and add to the hot liquid, whipping with a wire whip. Return to heat while stirring until it reaches a boil. Cooking thickens the sauce and removes the starchy flavor.

Quality Standards. Quality standards for gravies and sauces should include: smooth texture; not too thick; lightly salted. The appearance and texture depends upon the type of sauce or gravy:

Glossary

Roux
Is made from equal parts fat and flour and used to thicken sauces and gravies

- White sauce (made with milk): White, opaque color
- Cream sauce (made with cream): Light yellow, rich mouth-feel
- Béchamel (made with part milk or cream and chicken or fish stock): Light yellow, rich mouth-feel
- Veloute (made only with chicken or fish stock): Light yellow
- Brown sauce (made with browned roux): Rich brown color, lightly toasted flavor, have a slight sheen.

Section C — Other Food Preparation Standards

Purchasing and preparation are only two of the standards needed for quality control. Chapter 3 discussed two others, standardized recipes and portion control. What about special diets? What happens if you need to make a substitution? Can these be controlled?

Ingredient Substitutions and Monitoring Food Waste

During food production, sometimes things go wrong. An ingredient may be unavailable due to a delayed delivery, a shortage from the supplier, or an error. Or a recipe may fail due to errors in standardization, changes in ingredients, or errors made by a cook. In each of these situations, a Certified Dietary Manager is likely to be called upon to solve the problem.

Substitutions

When ingredients are not available, the Certified Dietary Manager needs to make a decision about substituting ingredients. A reasonable policy is to have substitutions routinely approved by a manager, rather than left to the cook's discretion. This policy ensures that the manager will become aware of supply problems. This allows the manager to further investigate the problems and take steps to ensure against repeated shortages.

Work with the staff to develop a standard ingredient substitution list. Some ingredients do not substitute well. However, many common ingredients can be changed. Figure 4.9 lists examples of common ingredient substitutions that may be acceptable in many recipes.

Occasionally, it may also be necessary to substitute entire products in a menu, due to shortages. To make these decisions, look for the most similar product you can identify. For example, a substitution for breaded chicken strips might be breaded chicken breasts. A substitution for meatloaf might be Salisbury steak or a ground beef patty. A substitution for cooked oatmeal might be cream of wheat. In each of these decisions, double check the intended substitution for each special diet served. Key nutritional components, such as calories, protein, fat, and carbohydrates, should remain about the same. Also give special consideration to any client with unique restrictions, such as food allergies or intolerances.

Beyond the substitution issue, sometimes there is an error in production leading to unacceptable products or recipe flops. Figure 4.10 lists ideas for dealing with common production problems.

Figure 4.9 Common Ingredient Substitutions

These substitutions work in some recipes, but not all. Substitution decisions require culinary experience and sound judgment.

FOR...	SUBSTITUTE...
1 lb. butter	1 lb. margarine
1 cup milk	1/4 cup dry milk plus 1 cup water
1 cup buttermilk	1 cup plain yogurt or 7/8 cup milk plus 1 Tbsp. vinegar or lemon juice
1 tsp. baking powder	1/3 tsp. Baking soda plus 1/2 tsp. cream of tartar
1 cup cracker crumbs	1 cup bread crumbs
1 Tbsp. cornstarch (for thickening)	2 Tbsp. flour
1 clove garlic, minced	1/8 tsp. garlic powder
1 tsp. lemon juice	1/2 tsp. vinegar or 1 tsp. lime juice
1 lb. dried beans	Approx. 5 cups cooked beans (adjust liquids)
1 cup packed brown sugar	1 cup granulated sugar (may add 1 Tbsp. molasses)

Figure 4.10 Solutions for Common Production Problems

PROBLEM	SOLUTION
Soup or sauce curdles	Add milk and beat rapidly
Chips are stale	Heat in oven at 350°F for 10 minutes
Soup is under yield	Add broth, tomato juice, or other liquid as appropriate
Baked product is overly browned	Cut off dark edges
Product is too salty	Add a small amount of sugar (if not for special diets) or if it is a soup
Product is too dry	Add a small amount of sauce or gravy

Source: Adapted from F&N Training Paks, © 1998, The Grossbauer Group

Putting It Into Practice

6. The cream of broccoli soup curdled and there isn't time to make another batch before the meal service. Is there a way to solve this problem?

Monitoring Food Waste

There is an old management adage in foodservice: "You can't control what you don't measure." When it comes to controlling food costs and food production, you also need controls for what food is wasted. Implement a waste log and ask employees to record what was wasted and why. This waste is then calculated as part of the food cost. See Figure 4.11 for a Food Waste Standard Policy and Procedure.

Figure 4.11 Leftover Food Usage

Date Effective: _____

Date Revised: _____

Date Reviewed: _____

Approved By: _____

Issuing Department: _____

Policy

It is the Dietary Department's goal to maximize food usage in order to avoid waste. To this end, certain leftover foods are reused, with restrictions.

Procedures

- Cool foods to 71° F within 2 hours and then to 41°F within the next 4 hours. Ice baths, vigorous stirring, and transfer to shallow dishes are options for ensuring a quick cool down.
- Store all ready-to-eat food that are prepped in-house for a maximum of 7 days at 41° or lower. After 7 days you must throw the food out to prevent bacteria from growing to unsafe levels.
- Label foods prepared in-house that are made with previously cooked food with the discard date of the previously cooked item, not the newly prepared item. For example, if you make soup with previously cooked chicken, you must label it with the discard date of the chicken (7 days after it was originally cooked).
- Place leftover foods in containers with tight-fitting lids. If food is stored in a zip-top plastic bag, push the air out of the bag before sealing.
- Label all containers clearly with the date and time that the food was first prepared.
- Reheat food to a minimum of 165°F for a minimum of 15 seconds.
- When in doubt, throw it out. Smelling food is not a reliable means of determining whether or not it is still usable. Never taste food as a means of judging freshness.

Review Date 4/12 | G-0615

References and recommended readings: National Restaurant Association. Serve Safe Essentials. 5th ed. Chicago IL: National Restaurant Association, 2008. US Food and Drug Administration. FDA Food Code. Available at: www.fda.gov/Food/FoodSafety/RetailFoodProtection/FoodCode/default.htm. Accessed April 16, 2012.

It is also important to occasionally monitor items that are discarded daily. There have been incidents where employees have hidden food in trash bags and then transferred it to their vehicle.

Another control is using food waste that is edible (such as leftovers) that can't be used for another meal, as donations to hunger relief charities.

As follow-up to any problem that arises during food production, investigate the causes and seek to make improvements. Whether the situation relates to inventory management, reliability of suppliers, errors in standardized recipes, or skills of employees, it is up to the Certified Dietary Manager to implement improvements.

Nutrient Control and Special Diets

If you are serving special diets, you may have the responsibility to supervise the amounts of certain nutrients during food production. Foods served to clients following sodium (salt) limitations, for example, need to provide consistent and reliable amounts of sodium. The same is true for fats, as well as many other nutrients.

Meanwhile, many clients who have no special diet orders may still follow special nutritional guidelines, through personal choice and attention to healthful practices. For these clients, you also have a responsibility to standardize and control nutrient content of menu items. Furthermore, if you label foods served by nutritional content, you have an obligation to ensure the labeling is truthful on an ongoing basis.

To ensure this control, specify salt, fats, and other ingredients in standardized recipes. Avoid using phrases like, "salt and pepper to taste" or "add butter as desired" or "pour olive oil liberally over all." Instead, test and standardize quantities for these ingredients. It is also important to standardize amounts of salt to add to water for pasta, rice, and vegetables.

Vegetables, stir-fries, hamburgers, and many other foods can be produced on a batch basis throughout service. Often, cooking in small, continuous batches minimizes holding times, preserves nutrients, and boosts final quality of products at the time of service. This is called **batch cooking.**

It is also essential to practice meticulous portion control. Not only does portion control affect the success of standardized recipe yields and food costing plans, it also affects nutrient control. Over-portioning a product by 10 percent increases calories, fat, sodium, protein, and other nutrients by 10 percent. An accumulation of portion control errors through a one-day menu can seriously violate the controls intended by a special diet.

In producing food, also pay special attention to texture and consistency, especially for products served to clients with swallowing disorders. Variations from standards established for product consistency can make meal time difficult, or even dangerous, for a client with a swallowing disorder.

Making special diets appealing sometimes requires culinary creativity and a flair for presentation. Particularly in a healthcare or a correctional facility, you may be serving clients whose appetites are compromised due to illness, disability, side effects from medications, psychological stress, or even depression. Extra attention to presentation, attractive garnishes, and other visual details can play a strong therapeutic role.

Dysphagia/Purèed diets in particular require planning. In a skilled nursing facility, a quarter of clients (or more) may be eating from a texture modified menu containing plain purèed foods. These foods typically offer little visual appeal (such as pale brown for purèed meat).

Experienced Certified Dietary Managers use food processors to blend casseroles, rather than serving plain foods. They also emphasize using seasonings, thickening ordinary foods, serving slurries, and adding milk or other ingredients to bring entrées up to required protein and calorie needs.

Today, healthcare foodservice managers use specially developed recipes, color combinations, flavor combinations, and safe garnishes to make puréed menu items interesting, attractive, and appealing. Puréed meat products can also be molded to look more like their source foods.

Garnishing

Garnishing foods is a small touch that goes a long way. A simple garnish provides a polished appearance with professional zest and can entice appetites. Garnishes can be part of many standardized recipes and foodservice staff can benefit from training in presenting food. An appropriate garnish is always edible and safe to eat. Often, it complements the color and flavor of the food, such as a lemon wedge on fish or minced parsley on soup. Remember to calculate the cost of garnishes. While there are many possibilities for garnishing, here are a few ideas:

- Lemon or orange wedge (on fish, chicken, salads)
- Fruit sliced in a fan shape
- Melon balls (with cold plates)
- Cucumber and/or carrot curls; cherry tomatoes (with sandwiches)
- Croutons (on soups or salads)
- Grated cheese (on soups, salads, or hot vegetables)
- Parsley, dill, or rosemary sprig (with meat, poultry, or fish entrées)
- Minced herbs (on soups or casseroles)
- Whipped cream (on desserts or beverages)
- Maraschino cherry (on desserts)
- Flavored syrup (drizzled on cakes in a zigzag pattern)
- Carved vegetables (with entrées or cold items)
- Paprika and/or minced chives (on potato products)
- Grated summer squash on salads
- Hard candy on clear-liquid diet trays

Glossary

Garnish
Enhance food appearance by adding edible decorations

Food Production Systems

Overview and Objectives

There are many factors that go into the production and distribution of food. The difference between quality foodservice and poor foodservice is the Certified Dietary Manager who compares the key standards to current practice and takes necessary action to ensure quality production. After completing this chapter, you should be able to:

✓ Check quality/quantity of food served

✓ Check adherence to delivery schedules and procedures

✓ Keep records for monitoring and accountability

Chapters 3 and 4 have already addressed production controls and standards such as standardized recipes, purchasing, preparation standards, and portioning. Other controls in the production and distribution process that affect the quality of food are time and temperature controls, production planning tools, staff training, and managing energy usage. Each of these controls produces records for monitoring and accountability.

Quality Control is built on the premise that monitoring, testing and documenting time after time, will detect an impending problem before any damage is done, for example Temperature Logs for the walk-ins. **Quality improvement (QI)** or **continuous quality improvement (CQI)** is the implementation of a plan developed to improve the quality performance of some aspect of your department, e.g., reducing tray errors and missing items. This may also be referred to as a Performance Improvement Plan.

There are many different quality documentation and tracking systems available through websites like Nutrition411.com, Becky Dorner and others that provide forms commonly used in foodservice operations, either as part of their service or built into their digital policy and procedure manuals. Your organization may have defined formats for CQI that they require. You could also find out who has spreadsheet skills in your organization and can help you develop your own forms. You can create your own using spreadsheet programs like Microsoft Excel, Lotus 1-2-3, or Macintosh Numbers.

Time and Temperature Controls

One of the greatest influences on the quality and quantity of food served is controlling time and temperature. So far, examples of quality standards for preparation addressed criteria such as purchasing the appropriate quality of product, using low heat when

Glossary

Quality Control
Monitoring existing systems for consistent performance

Quality Improvement (QI)
Managing the change in a process for better outcome

Continuous Quality Improvement (CQI)
The philosophy that most processes can be improved—not just those that are broken

preparing high protein foods, and comparing end products to expectations prior to service. Time and temperature controls should be added to your standardized recipes so that foods are cooked to the proper temperature, within a given amount of time, and then cooled and stored properly. These standards combined with the sanitation guidelines from the **Food and Drug Administration (FDA Food Code)** help ensure food safety for your clients. They also help to improve the quality of food.

How do you supervise time and temperature to ensure food quality and quantity? Let's assume that you have procedures in place to take the temperature of foods at the time of delivery and before, during, and after service. As the Certified Dietary Manager, your job is to make sure that those procedures are in place, they are working, and you take any necessary corrective action. In this instance, you can do that by checking the temperature documentation and taking the temperature yourself occasionally to compare to the documentation.

What if food is being served at an improper temperature? What is the corrective action? The immediate action is to adjust the food temperature. For instance, if the food is too cold, reheat the food to 165°F for 15 seconds and return it to service which addresses the temperature issue but may create a food quality problem. The second action is to address the performance problem with the staff member responsible.

Deal with the performance issue as early as possible. If the problem occurred due to lack of training, arrange for one-on-one training right away. If the problem occurred due to lack of equipment (thermometers weren't readily available), fix it. If the person can do the job properly and just didn't do it, review the standard and hold the person accountable.

You should also have a policy that foods are tasted prior to service at each meal. Pre-meal test plates allow you to evaluate the meal to be served for consistency with the recipes as they were standardized. This step can assist in defining the plating of the meal for presentation to the client and taking temperatures of the food as it is coming off the serving line. While pre-meal test plates seem unnecessary for an established menu (after all, everyone should know how to plate and serve this meal) it becomes even more important to ensure a quality product, that you not assume compliance.

Production Planning Tools

Supervising the production and distribution of food requires using production planning tools. These tools include forecasting, food production scheduling, supervision of quality, and training for production staff.

Forecasting

Have you ever wondered how Certified Dietary Managers know the amount of food to prepare for any given meal or event? **Forecasting** is the process of estimating future needs for food. It identifies both how much food to produce and how much food to order. Based on your own facility, you will determine how far in advance you need to forecast. About a week ahead is not uncommon. Based on the menu, purchasing systems, and inventory management system, a timetable or schedule for forecasting becomes a routine part of the daily operation. To create a forecast, there are several types of information typically used.

Many Certified Dietary Managers keep records of the quantity of food served in the past. Maintain a **production history** of your past production numbers and usage. Using a menu cycle, along with past production sheets, allows you to track how much was produced the last time the item was on the menu and how much was actually used. Knowing if you were over by 50 servings or short by 10 servings helps refine the number of servings to be produced next time. If a computerized menu system is being used, the production history is automatically tracked for future reference.

Census Figures. Depending on the facility, this may be available in one or more forms. In a healthcare environment, the manager may use the overall daily census, or more specifically, the client count of patients/residents receiving each of a variety of menus or diet types on corresponding days of the menu cycle. Keeping track of census can be as simple as writing the count on a wall calendar every day.

In this process, the manager then checks the current census to estimate adjustments. Figure 5.1 shows an example of this process. A census may also be available in a school, a university, and corrections environment. Many complex formulas and options exist for using census data. One facility may average the figures for the past five menu cycles. Another may examine figures from one year ago.

Figure 5.1 Using a Census to Create a Forecast

BACKGROUND

You serve clients in a skilled nursing facility based on a three-week cycle menu. You are currently forecasting needs for day 15 of the cycle, coming up in about a week.

PROCESS

1. You examine the census for Day 15 of the previous menu cycle. You see that you served 152 clients on the regular menu, 34 clients on a pureed menu, and 51 clients on a modified fat and sugar menu. The total client count was 237.

2. You check today's census, and see that the client count is 235, with a very similar distribution among diets.

3. You carry over the numbers from the last Day 15 to the future Day 15.

Tally Figures. In a computerized menu system, the program may tally each item selected or served on a menu. These tallies become valuable detail for the next forecast. In this system, a Certified Dietary Manager essentially transfers the tally figures on the computer from a past menu cycle day to the next one, making any manual adjustments desired.

If you are conducting a manual tally of items for production, keep in mind that the only recipes that really need to be tallied are those for items that are made by the each at the time of service. A tally counted at 10:00 for Beef Stew to be served at 11:45 is of no value to the production team. You have already thawed the beef and made the stew in enough quantity to meet the needs based on prior history (forecasting). However, an accurate count of how many of the made to order Roasted Turkey on a Croissant Cold Plates you will need is very important.

Using historical data such as census and tallies, a Certified Dietary Manager also has to evaluate whether the predictions were accurate the last time around. For example, did the service line run out of food before the service ended? Or, did the cook report large quantities of leftovers of any item? These must be taken into account for the next estimate. A standard procedure is to provide a form for documenting **shortages** and **leftovers**. Managers may include an over/short column on the Production Sheets (Figure 5.2 below) that the cooks use, or on the Panning Charts that the serving line uses.

Glossary

Census Figures
The count of clients and customers present or available to access your services

Tally Figures
The actual count of individual items needed for a meal service

Shortage
The number of additional servings needed, but not available, for a meal

Leftovers
The number of servings remaining after a meal has been served

Figure 5.2 Sample of a Simple Production Sheet with Over/Short

MONDAY	WHO PREPARES	AMOUNT	INSTRUCTIONS	OVER/SHORT
Lunch				
Vegetable Soup				
Vegetable Egg Roll				
Chicken Chow Mein				
Turkey Avocado Sandwich on a Ciabata				
Steamed Rice				
Oriental Blend Vegetable				
Relish Plate				
Mandarin Oranges				
Dinner				
Tossed Salad				
Beef Pot Roast				
Tabouli Salad				
Pargiot Chicken				
Israeli Grilled Chicken				
Parsleyed Potatoes				
Steamed Baby Carrots				
Frosted White Cake				

Keep these records for at least 2 or 3 times through the menu cycle and review them frequently. If there are excessive leftovers, this can be a sign that the forecast needs to be decreased. However, if a particular product consistently runs out before service ends, this is a sign that more should be produced. It is particularly important to encourage employees to complete production records accurately when service ends, and to monitor overproduction and underproduction for continued planning.

Weather plays a big part in how many meals are served for different facilities. Attendance at K-12 schools, a college or university, and a retirement center or senior housing may all be dramatically affected by the weather. Along with your census figures, make a note about the weather. If you have a record of how many were served on a rainy day, you can use this information for future rainy days. Even though forecasting figures might be pre-set in your electronic software, the system can be overridden to adjust the forecast on days when weather or campus events are likely to affect the count.

Catering can significantly impact your forecasted and tallied numbers. Typically, you ask for advance notice of catering events so you can plan appropriately for production and staffing needs. Many meetings and activities are on a regular schedule such as the third Thursday of the month. Maintaining a calendar of known catering events helps to better forecast the impact of those events on the daily production schedule.

For a catered event, you generally have an advance client count that can be used in forecasting. The last minute notice of catering needs, while not desired but are often unavoidable, can be disruptive to production planning.

Point of Sale (POS) Records. Another source for historical figures is a point of sale (POS) system or computer-based cash register system that tabulates menu items sold. This is useful in a cafeteria setting. The data may be available as a printout tape from the POS system, and/or the system may include software for forecasting that electronically accepts sales records.

Sales reports can provide a record of service problems. For example, the production sheets show that 150 servings of macaroni and cheese were prepared for lunch on Day 12. However, the cash register tapes document that the last 2 times macaroni and cheese was on the menu, the cafeteria ran out of macaroni and cheese at 11:45 AM. In this case, the production quantity needs to be boosted for the next time on the menu.

Known Changes. There may be certain changes you can predict for the future. In a hospital, for example, what if the upcoming Day 4 of the menu cycle is also a holiday? You can likely predict that the census will go down, as clients are discharged for the holiday. Likewise, in a campus or business dining environment, known scheduled activities can help predict times when fewer (or more) clients are likely to arrive.

These are just a few examples of records that may be used for determining a forecast. In addition, an alternate practice is to **pad** or increase forecast figures by a small increment, such as three to ten percent. In the Figure 5.1 example, if the forecast is for 235 residents, what happens if five more are admitted to the facility before the next Day 15? You never want to cut the forecast so closely that you cannot serve a few more clients. The amount of padding needed depends on how much variation is normal for client count. On the other hand, you do not want to pad excessively, as this may generate food waste and lost dollars.

To determine a forecasting methodology, ask the following questions:

- How can I best capture historical figures about the amount of food served?
- How can I verify whether these figures will carry through to the future?
- How can I capture and incorporate notes about food shortages or leftovers?
- How much variation is typical for my facility, and how much do I need to pad the figures?

A forecast is expressed in the number of servings for each menu item. Products served on multiple menus are totaled for a final count. Figure 5.3 provides a partial example of a forecast.

Glossary

Point of Sale (POS)
Refers to the computer-based cash register systems menu item counts

Pad
The amount added to a forecasted menu item to ensure adequate quantities available

Putting It Into Practice

1. Your school celebrates the return of spring with a week-long celebration that culminates in a large outdoor picnic. You normally serve 450 students and their guests. The day of the picnic arrives and it is cold and rainy. What steps would you take to adjust the meals for the forecast?

Figure 5.3 Partial Forecast for Day 15 Lunch

PRODUCT	PREDICTED COUNT (No. of Servings)
Multigatawny soup	124
Macaroni and cheese	78
Turkey salad sandwich on wheat bun	54
Pureed macaroni and cheese	17
Tossed salad	67
French dressing	22
Cottage cheese	2
Fresh banana	81

A forecast is more than number-crunching. It requires a willingness to make judgment calls. It is not an exact science. Effective methods for predicting needs are not universal, but vary from one facility to another. Client groups, menus, and service models all affect the forecast. Starting with standard approaches, most Certified Dietary Managers learn from experience, and refine their forecasting methods to the individual facility. In addition, foodservice facilities with very stable client counts on a cycle menu often devise a standard forecast that is used routinely, with only minor adjustments from cycle to cycle.

The results of effective forecasting include:

- Smooth operations, as products are available when they are needed
- Satisfaction, as clients receive the foods they expect
- Cost control, as accuracy minimizes food waste

Production Scheduling

With quantities of food to deliver at single points in time, a Certified Dietary Manager needs to give special attention to **advance preparation** practices. Advance preparation is a general term that describes any tasks that can or must be completed before main production takes place. To determine what steps of advanced production should be completed, ask questions such as these about each recipe:

- What ingredients need to be thawed before a cook will be able to use them in this recipe (and how long will it take to thaw them following safe techniques)?
- What sub-recipes have to be produced in order to make the main recipe?
  - > A sub-recipe is a distinct recipe routine that must be completed before production of a main recipe is possible. An example of a sub-recipe is the tomato sauce that will be used in lasagna, the pie crust that will be used in chicken pot pie, or the cooked shrimp that will be used in shrimp salad.
- What pre-preparation processing is required to bring an inventory product into the form required by the recipe?
  - > Examples of advance processing include washing lettuce, peeling and slicing apples or potatoes, trimming fat from meat, dicing meat, crushing garlic, chopping onions, soaking dry beans, and many others.
- What products need to be pre-portioned before production can begin?

Glossary

Advanced Preparation
Any tasks that can be completed prior to the time of recipe production such as thawing meats, chopping vegetables, or making sauces

It is not always necessary to perform all possible advance preparation as a separate group of tasks. However, doing work in advance when possible often eases the workload in the few hours before service and makes it easier to meet service requirements.

Once the tasks are identified that can be performed in advance, it is helpful to establish timetables. For example, thawing frozen meat in the refrigerator may take several days. So, the **production schedule** or **daily production sheets** should indicate the need to transfer it in time. This may be referred to as the **pull list** and included at the bottom of the Daily Production Sheets. Figure 5.4 lists tips for thawing foods.

Figure 5.4 Thawing Tips and Times

TIPS	THAWING TIMES
• Schedule thawing so that meat will be cooked soon after thawing is complete.	• Timing for large meat roasts: 4-7 hrs. per pound of meat
• Do not thaw at room temperature. Use one of the approved thawing methods.	• Timing for small meat roasts: 3-5 hrs. per pound of meat.
• Withdraw from freezer only the amount of meat/poultry needed for one-day use.	• Timing for chops, steaks: 12-14 hrs.
• Remove from carton and thaw in original wrappings in the refrigerator.	• Timing for chicken, whole: 1 day
	• Timing for chicken pieces: 12-14 hrs.
	• Timing for whole turkey—18 lbs. or larger: 4-5 days
• Space packages on refrigerator shelves so that air can circulate around them.	• Timing for whole turkey—under 18 lbs.: 2-3 days
	• Timing for seafood in blocks: 1-2 days

Sub-recipes can sometimes be prepared in advance and then held under proper storage conditions until needed. Often, the decision to separate sub-recipes as advance preparation tasks depends on a judgment of quality and food safety. A tomato sauce for lasagna, for example, can readily be made in advance, chilled rapidly, and held for a day. However, a traditional hollandaise sauce cannot be held. As with the Pull List, pre-prep recipes are often included on the Daily Production Sheets as assigned tasks.

Advance processing of vegetables can be batched for greater efficiency. Consider this example:

• Cook A needs a total of 4 quarts of chopped onions for beef stew plus 2 quarts of chopped onions for homemade bean soup for the same production period.

• Cook B needs 1 quart of chopped onions for a chicken salad plate and 3 cups of chopped onions for guacamole.

• The employee responsible for the salad bar needs another 4 quarts of chopped onions.

In this example, each of three employees would obtain onions for preparation. Each cook would wash and peel the onions, set up a food processor, chop the onions, and then clean up. This would generate a lot of work. Alternately, one person could go through the process one time and prepare all the chopped onions needed for all three areas. Then, the employee could portion and distribute the chopped onions. Even in a very small operation, consolidation such as this is labor efficient and cost-beneficial.

Glossary

Production Schedule/Daily Production Sheet
A document that outlines what to produce, how much to make, and who is responsible

Pull List
Typically included on the Daily Production Sheet for items to be pulled from the freezer for future use

Putting It Into Practice

2. What are the production steps for the recipe below? Indicate with a star the steps that are advance preparation.

Chicken Wrap:
• 96 (6-inch) tortillas
• 9 lbs. grilled chicken breast, cubed
• 1 #10 can cooked black beans, drained
• 8 lbs. pre-chopped mixed lettuce (romaine and iceberg)—purchased pre-chopped
• 3 lbs. crumbled feta cheese
• 3 lbs. roasted red peppers, chopped
• 1-1/2 qts. commercial Caesar Dressing

Some facilities have utilized an **ingredient control room** concept where the storerooms and walk-ins are closed to the staff and all inventory is managed through **requisitions**. An employee responsible for issuing inventory would process the requisitions, typically starting with the consolidated pre-processing of the ingredients, and then distributing all of the needed ingredients to the respective cooks.

While consolidation provides greater economy and convenience, the disadvantage of this approach is the burden of predicting exact needs. In some systems, a cook reviews the upcoming schedule and assigns advance preparation needs. In others, the Certified Dietary Manager establishes a schedule for pre-preparation in conjunction with the forecast.

Here is a situation in which computerized systems can offer support. A well-designed food management software package may:

- Handle pre-processed ingredients as a type of inventory item and requisition them automatically according to established lead times and forecasts.
- Consolidate needs for pre-preparation and generate a distribution list for each product.
- Generate labels for products undergoing ingredient room processing or pre-processing.
- Review upcoming needs for thawed products and generate advance thawing schedules that tell a storage clerk when to transfer products to refrigeration.

Use of an automated system makes it more practical to consolidate and manage production schedules without risking oversights and emergencies.

Production Schedule Resource Management. As you build your production schedule around standardized recipes with controlled inventory and trained staff, the equipment that is available must also be considered. A production schedule that requires oven space for 10 hotel pans may not work in a kitchen with only one oven. While fryer space may be no problem to meet the production needs, you may not have the staff to assign to each of the fryers.

Designing a Production Schedule requires you to think backwards. Not everything can come out of the oven at the same time. Scheduling when items are made is like a big jigsaw puzzle based on their equipment needs, cooking time, finishing time and if the item can be prepped and then held in a hot box until the time of service.

- Start with the defined meal service time:
- To meet that schedule how much time do you need for final handwork on the menu item such as slicing of the meat or panning up of the soups?
- What is the cooking time needed to get to the finishing handwork?
- Add how much prep time is needed prior to the cooking time?
- This is the recipe production time.
  - > Can you cook and hold it (even a day in advance) or is this a cook and serve item?

During the menu planning process, discussed in Chapter 2, consideration has to be made for the needed recipe production time, equipment available and staffing coverage. A fabulous menu that exceeds your production resources, equipment, labor or time will frustrate the staff and fail to meet client expectations.

Production Schedule Communication. As you forecast production, plan staffing, and schedule activities, it becomes clear there is another critical piece in the flow of food production. This is communication. Scheduling production is an excellent example of a task that requires clear and precise communications for assigned staff. The main production activities require direction, too. A cook needs to know what to make, how many servings to make, when to have items ready, and where to deliver the finished products.

How this is communicated varies by facility. In some small facilities, actual food tallies or counts reach the cooks before preparation. For example, in a healthcare environment, automated menu counts may be handed to the cooks on a daily production sheet with an instruction to add a pad of several servings per item. A sample production sheet appears in Figure 5.5.

The daily production sheet identifies meal, product, number of servings, and distribution instructions. Details like the number of servings needed for patient/resident meals, with a separate count for a cafeteria and yet another count for the doctor's dining room or the administrator's board meeting is all included on the production sheets. As explained above, daily production sheets can also include the items to be pulled from the freezer (pull list) and **pre-preparation recipes** of products that will be used tomorrow or the next day.

In a manual system, a Certified Dietary Manager should maintain a set of production sheet forms for cooks based on a cycle menu. This is a project to get set up, but once established it defines the daily flow of activity in the kitchen. Specific production numbers of products to be produced must be manually edited and adjusted from cycle to cycle.

In any large, multi-site facility, it is virtually essential that a computerized production system be used to manage the paperwork and communications involved with food production. A set of computer-generated production sheets can provide a daily, detailed schedule for each cook, along with standardized recipes scaled for the number of servings forecasted.

After production, it is also important to document leftovers and shortages of each product. This information helps with future forecasting, and careful attention to this process can both improve service (supply) and reduce food waste. In some facilities, this documentation is the responsibility of cooks. In others, it is the responsibility of trayline or service personnel. Figure 5.6 illustrates another format for a food production planning and leftover report form.

At the end of each work day, production records such as these should go back to the Certified Dietary Manager or person in charge of forecasting. In a computerized system, this data may be entered into the system for use in automated forecasting for future menus.

Supervision of Quality

Another aspect of ongoing food production management is the supervision of quality. A Certified Dietary Manager should look at foods during both production and service. In addition, some facilities set up small taste panels of foods produced, either daily or at periodic intervals. Production and management personnel join together to taste samples of all products, evaluate for quality of appearance, flavor and texture (especially for texture-modified products), and make suggestions for improvement.

Another point to monitor is to observe plate waste. Spend some time in the room where plates are being returned or in the dining room. What is on the plate? Are you seeing servings of the same food item uneaten? What is the appropriate corrective action? The initial response is to test the food still on the serving line and assess the item for current problems, over-salting or even salting, when it should have been sugar, are mistakes that happens.

Figure 5.5 Sample Production Sheet

CYCLE		1		DAY: MONDAY		POS.		EC COOK/CA			
				Amount to Prepare				Amount to Send			
RECIPE #	BREAKFAST	Portion Size	Total Amount		Temp. at Finish	SS	CY	OE	RS	Cafe
1052	Oatmeal	6 oz.	3	gal	165	2	1			
1266	Scrambled Egg	#16 disher	90	ea	145	60	30			
1149	Bacon	2 slices	120	ea	165	70	50			
4955	Pureed Eggs	#16 disher	5			5				
4867	Pureed Bacon	#16 disher	5			5				
RECIPE #	LUNCH									
3975	Roast Turkey	3 oz.	130	prtn	165	50	20	6	4	50
2648	Stuffing	1/2 c. (#8 scp.)	130	prtn	165	50	20	6	4	50
8422	Gravy			3 gbs	165					
3387	Hamburger on Bun	4 oz./1	100	ea	160	25	15	5	5	50
7521	Steak Fries	1/2 c. (#8 scp.)	116	prtn	165	40	20	5	6	45
7501	Mashed Potatoes		103	prtn	165	35	15	5	3	45
6982	Glazed Carrots	1/2 c. (#8 scp.)	164	prtn 20 bgs	165	65	35	10	4	50
6257	Lettuce/Tomato/Pickle/Cheese		0							
5164	Chicken Noodle Soup	4 oz./6 oz.	75	prtn	165	15	7	4	4	45
4381	Purée Turkey	#16 disher	4		165	4				
4254	Purée Hamburger	#16 disher	1		165	1				
4266	Purée Rice	#16 disher	4		165	4				
4457	Purée Carrots	#16 disher	5		165	5				
4316	Ground Turkey	#16 disher	4		165	4				
4356	Ground Hamburger	#16 disher	0		165					
	Cafe									
			0							
	Sandwiches (variety)		14	ea						14
	Thaw:		Prepare for Next Day:							
	Ribs for Thursday menu		Add to Week 5 Sun—tear bread for stuffing on Monday (1, 3-4 inch long pans)							

Figure 5.6 Food Production Planning and Leftover Report

Date: _____   Meal: _____

SERVICE START TIME:			**SERVICE END TIME:**					
Item	**Portion Size**	**Qty. of Portions to Prepare**	**Employee Assigned**	**Comments**	**Qty. of Portions Left Over**	**Actual Qty. Served**	**Leftover Disposition**	**Shortage: Ran Out at _____ (time)**

Determine if the problem is an issue with the recipe itself, the ingredients used, the cook who did or did not follow the recipe, the visual presentation of the item, or does the product not meet local food preferences. When you understand what caused the issue, you can take the right steps to fix it.

Throughout the food production process, a manager should be highly visible and accessible to cooks, trayline or plating staff, and the servers. A manager needs to monitor activities and observe practices related to culinary technique, food, and employee safety. A manager should be a coach to employees who are learning new skills. In addition, a manager should be ready to intervene when it appears that production is behind schedule and make decisions when problems or substitution needs arise.

Finally, a manager needs to listen to the concerns and suggestions raised by preparation staff, servers and the clients. For example, a staff member may suggest an improvement to a standardized recipe, an alternate production method, or an idea for presenting food more attractively. An effective manager continually seeks feedback and input from their team members in order to improve quality.

Staff Training for Production Employees

As production employees perform their work, technique becomes critical. Many aspects of final quality rest with the cooks, including measuring, preparation techniques, presentation and garnishing. Not every cook enters a facility with special training. However, someone in the facility should have a high level of culinary expertise.

This may be the Certified Dietary Manager, an executive chef, or an experienced production manager. In turn, this person should coach other members of the staff to develop skills and talents. Some facilities have a short production meeting each day to make sure production questions are answered.

Putting It Into Practice

3. At the end of each day, your cooks document production results. What items should they document?

Each cook needs some special training about food production. For example, a cook needs to know:

- The purpose of standardized recipes
- Standard terms used on each recipe, such as yield, portion size, etc.
- Ingredient descriptions and the distinctions among products (e.g., the difference between kosher salt and iodized salt; all-purpose flour and self-rising flour, sifted or unsifted flour, etc.)
- Utensils and methods for measuring ingredients
- Abbreviation system for measurements
- Food safety and/or HACCP standards in place for each recipe
- Procedures for requisitioning ingredients
- Cooking terms used throughout the recipe, such as sauté, simmer, bake, broil, roux, etc. A list of common cooking terms appears in Figure 5.7
- Employee safety and ergonomic practices that protect the cook and others from injury
- Proper methods for using all required equipment
- Methods for portioning and/or panning food
- Methods for holding food and/or transporting it to service
- Established timetables for production
- Procedures for addressing questions and problems

As a basic work process, a cook can follow several steps to ensure an efficient work flow:

- Read through the production sheet and be sure all assignments are clear
  > Question anything that is unclear
- Read through each recipe, and be sure all instructions are clear
- Assemble all needed ingredients
- Verify that all needed equipment, bowls, knives, and utensils are available and ready for use
- Follow the recipe procedure exactly, taking each step in sequence
- Clean up between tasks and keep the work area orderly
- Follow established sanitation guidelines
- Group errands (such as trips to the storeroom, dishroom, or trash area) and work as efficiently as possible

Beyond basic orientation, many foodservice employees enjoy further culinary training. You may ask your most skilled culinary employee to present cooking classes, featuring basic techniques, garnishing tips, and more. When a culinary expert is not available on staff, consider inviting a local talent to present a special in-service session or series of classes.

Another option for training is to use culinary instructional videos, which are readily available from many sources. Culinary reference information, slide shows, and even video clips illustrating culinary techniques are available free on several websites. When feasible, schedule production employees to attend food and trade shows. Finally, if your facility offers a continuing education program, you may encourage employees to attend seminars or classes in preparation and culinary techniques.

Putting It Into Practice

4. What would you monitor to assure production staff training has been effective? What do you do if you find the training was not effective?

Figure 5.7 Common Cooking Terms

Al dente	An Italian term literally meaning "to the tooth"; refers to food that is cooked just enough to have a little resistance to the bite.
Bain-marie	A water bath used to warm or cook food. A container of food is placed in another container of water, either in the oven or on the stove.
Baste	To put stock or other liquid over meat while it is cooking (usually roasting) in order to keep it moist.
Beat	To briskly mix ingredients, usually with a whisk, electric mixer, or fork.
Bard	To cover or wrap raw meat with some type of solid fat before cooking.
Blanch	To pour boiling water over food (often fruit, vegetables, or nuts) in order to soften it or to remove the hulls or skins. Other methods include simmering the food and then placing it quickly in cold water, or steaming the food for a short period of time. Often confused with parboiling; see definition below.
Braise	To prepare food by browning it, covering it, and then slowly cooking it in the oven or on the stove with as much as 1/2 inch of liquid.
Brown	To cook food, usually in a small amount of fat, until it is brown; often a first step in another cooking process.
Broil	To cook food by exposing it to direct high heat, usually in the broiler of an oven or on a grill.
Butterfly	To cut a food directly through the center, splitting it almost in half.
Clarify	To remove food particles from grease used for frying, or to remove the top fat from melted butter, by heating and straining and/or skimming.
Coddle	To slowly cook a food (usually eggs) in liquid at a low heat. Usually done by placing it in boiling water and then immediately covering the pot and removing it from the stove.
Cream	To bring solid fat and dry ingredients (usually sugar and butter, margarine, or shortening) to a smooth, creamy consistency with a mixer or large spoon. The fat is creamed first; then the sugar is added gradually.
Cut in	To combine a dry ingredient and a solid fat with a fork, two knives, or a pastry blender (curved wires or thin, dull blades attached to a handle). They are mixed in a gliding cutting motion until they form small, separate pieces.
Dice	To cut a food into tiny chunks or cubes.
Deglaze	To make a sauce or sauce base using the juices and food bits remaining in a pan after cooking (broiling, sautéing, etc.) meat or fish. After some or all of the fat is removed from the pan and liquid is added, the mixture is heated and stirred and the pan is scraped until all of the food particles and juices are mixed.
Dredge	To coat food with a flour mixture or bread crumbs, usually before frying.
Dust	To sprinkle food with a dry ingredient by hand with a sifter or a can made for dusting.
Fold	To gently blend two ingredients or mixtures, such as whipped egg whites and cake batter. They are layered on top of one another, the bowl is tilted, and the mixing is done with a sweeping top-to-bottom motion.
Fry	To cook food quickly in fat that is usually at a high temperature. If a small amount of fat is used, it is called stir frying, sautéing, or pan frying. If the food is immersed in fat, it is called deep fat frying.

(Continued)

Figure 5.7 Common Cooking Terms *(Continued)*

Garnish	An edible item used to decorate a dish or the process of decorating it. A garnish can be as small and simple as a sprig of parsley, as ornate as a small vegetable sculpture, or as substantial as the starch and vegetables on the plate used to garnish the meat.
Grate	To produce small bits or shavings of a food by rubbing on a grater or using a food processor.
Julienne	Used to describe food that has been cut into matchstick-like pieces 1/8 of an inch thick and 1½ to 3 inches long.
Knead	To develop the gluten in dough by hand or with a kneading attachment on a mixer. When done by hand, it is folded, pressed down, and turned ¼ turn repeatedly until it becomes smooth and pliable.
Macerate	To soak fruit or vegetables in liquid.
Marinate	To soak meat in a seasoned liquid.
Mince	To finely chop food.
Pare	To cut the skin from fruit or vegetables.
Pan-broil	To cook meat on the stovetop using an uncovered skillet and very little or no fat. Each side of the meat is browned and fat is poured off during cooking.
Parboil	To partially cook food in water that is already at a rolling boil. A large quantity of water is used so that the food does not interrupt the boiling.
Poach	To completely cook a food in liquid just below boiling, usually in a covered pot.
Purée	To process cooked food or soft raw food in a blender.
Reduce	To cook a liquid food over high heat, allowing the water to evaporate.
Render	One process is to melt fat off of meat during cooking, with the cooked meat being the product. Another is to separate pieces of tissue from meat fat by heating and then straining it. This prepares the fat as well as the crisped tissue for other uses.
Roast	To cook food, usually meat, in the oven without it sitting in liquid.
Roux	A thickening agent using equal weights of fat and flour.
Sauté	To cook food in a small amount of fat at a temperature high enough to quickly sear it. This is done in an open skillet with constant stirring motion.
Scald	To cook food (usually milk) just below boiling, usually at about 185°F.
Scallop	To cook food in a cream sauce in the oven.
Shred	To process food into long bits and pieces, either by hand or with a grater.
Sear	To quickly brown food (usually meat) and seal in the juices by placing it on a very hot cooking surface. The surface of the food should be relatively dry, and depending on its natural fat content, little or no fat is used.
Simmer	To cook food or have food immersed in liquid below boiling usually between 130° and 185°F.
Steam	To cook food in direct contact with steam, either over boiling water or in a pressure cooker.
Whip	To process food rapidly with a spoon, whisk, or mixer. The utensil is swept up and down to incorporate air. This is the same as beating when the object is to thoroughly blend ingredients. Depending on the recipe, whipping may refer to lengthening the process and greatly increasing the volume of the food by incorporating a large quantity of air, as in whipped cream.

It is important to encourage, acknowledge, and reward advances in knowledge and skill. Follow up to ensure the training is implemented. Often, the simple availability of training is enough to motivate employees to challenge themselves and tap into their own talents. Skillful food production brings on the immediate rewards of seeing a product that looks good, tastes good, and generates positive satisfaction ratings.

Controlling Energy Usage

You might wonder how controlling energy usage fits into this chapter on supervising the production and distribution of food. If you think about it, very little can be produced in foodservice without the use of energy. The next decade will be an exciting, and probably challenging time as we become more efficient. All types of foodservice industries are being encouraged to try new methods for becoming more "green" by utilizing or re-directing food waste for energy, reducing consumption through energy efficient equipment, and turning off equipment and lights when not in use. Can you think of other ways to conserve in your department?

Figure 5.8 Commercial Building Energy Cost Per Square Foot (Dollars)

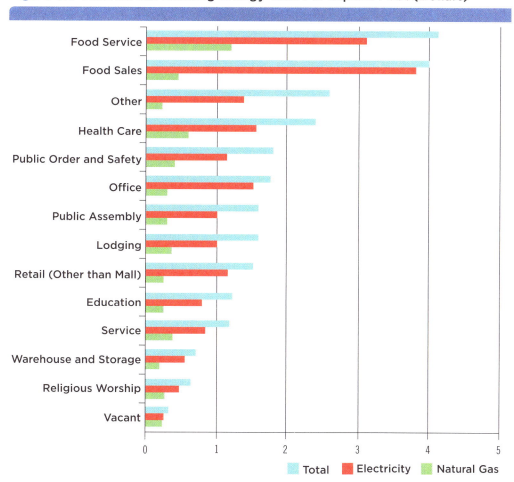

Source: Sustainablefoodservice.com and Energy Information Administration, www.eia.doe.gov. Used with permission.

Foodservice departments utilize significantly more energy than other departments and this may be a controllable expense worth investigating. Figure 5.8 shows the Commercial Building Energy Cost per Square Foot and Figure 5.9 shows how this energy use is divided in a restaurant.

Figure 5.9 Restaurant Energy Use

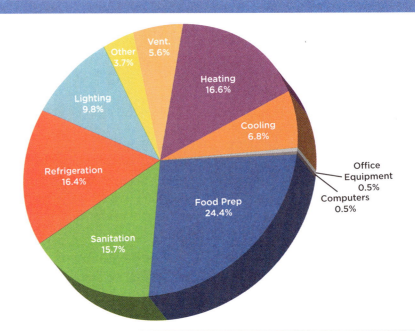

Source: Sustainablefoodservice.com and Energy Information Administration, www.eia.doe.gov. Used with permission.

How do you begin controlling energy costs?

- Start with contacting your local energy companies.
  - > They may offer design consulting services to help you design and order equipment for maximum efficiency.
- A local energy company may also conduct kitchen equipment test reports giving you specific information about the energy usage of cooking and food preparation equipment.
  - > A local college or university may also have a program where students could provide this service as part of their learning activities.
- Your energy company may also conduct an on-site survey resulting in a list of recommended actions to cut energy use and costs.

Figure 5.10 shows energy conservation tips to consider for your facility.

Like the other supervision activities in this chapter, control of energy costs mean keeping records of utility costs and monitoring equipment use.

- Track your energy/utility costs monthly and look for dramatic changes or trends.
- Total your water usage each month and ask your staff to help you find ways to conserve water.
- Use training to get your staff on board with energy conservation and how controlling energy use affects operational costs.
  - > Since your staff are the ones using the equipment, they can be the keys to success in monitoring equipment use.

Controlling energy costs may well be wiser in the long run than trying to meet your budget by reducing the quality of food.

Figure 5.10 Energy Saving Tips

1	Switch from incandescent EXIT lights to LED EXIT lighting. They last ten times longer with an average annual savings of $40, excluding maintenance costs.
2	Switch from Incandescent Light Bulbs in exhaust hoods and walk-ins to Energy Star® Light Emitting Diode (LED) lamps. Replacing a single 60 watt incandescent lamp, operated 12 hours per day over 365 days with a 12 watt LED lamp will save approximately $20 in annual operating cost at a utility rate of $0.10/kWh.
3	Turn off door heaters on reach-in refrigerators and freezers. Commercial reach-in refrigerators and freezers have door heaters to help prevent condensation build up around the door frame, however, in dry climates condensate may not be an issue and many refrigerators and freezers have door heaters which can be manually turned off. A single door heater has an approximate annual operating cost of $50 at a utility rate of $0.10/kWh.
4	Use Strip Curtains or plastic doors on walk-in coolers and freezers to prevent warm air infiltration and reduce compressor runtime. Utility studies have shown an annual savings of $100 for a typical 10 x 10 walk-in freezer equipped with a strip curtain assuming a utility rate of $0.10/kWh.
5	Fix all water leaks. A seemingly innocent hot water leak with a flow rate of half a gallon per hour can have an annual cost of $90 if left unabated. Cost assumes a natural gas cost of $1.00/therm and a water/sewer utility cost of $8.00/CCF.
6	Clean dirty refrigeration system—evaporator and condenser coils. They should be inspected monthly for dust, lint, and other obstructions and cleaned if necessary.
7	Set Water Heater to Proper Temperature. Only heat water to the temperature required for specific tasks in your operation. Facilities with high temperature dish machine typically require 140° F supply hot water and those with a low temperature machine can require supply hot water as low as 125° F. A water heater set 10°F too high in a typical casual dining restaurant using 2,000 gallons of hot water per day will cost an extra $900/year, assuming a natural gas utility cost of $1.00/therm.
8	Replace high flow pre-rinse sprayers with high performing, low flow sprayers that have a flow rate no higher than 1.6 gallon per minute. Retrofitting a high flow nozzle rated at 5.0 gpm with a low flow unit rated at 1.2 gpm in a dish room where operated one hour per day over 365 days will save approximately $1,700 in natural gas and water costs.
9	Implement a strict start up and shut down schedule for all cooking appliances. Fryers, ovens, griddles and charbroilers require no more then 20-30 minutes to pre-heat. Pay special attention to charbroiler and manually controlled griddles—shut them entirely off, partially off or down during slow service periods.
10	Install and/or maintain programmable thermostats to manage heating and air conditioning systems. Properly program the thermostat so that during unoccupied periods, cooling is set to 85° F and heating to 55° F. During occupied hours set the cooling set point as high as possible and heating set point as low as possible, but still being mindful to maintain staff and customer comfort. As a rule of thumb, for every cooling degree set point increase and heating degree set point decrease, system operating cost lowers by 3% - 4%.

Source: Fisher-Nickel Inc., Food Service Technology Center-fishnick.com. Costs are based on average National rates.

Preparation and Delivery of Between Meal Snacks Supplements

Overview and Objectives

A large percentage of clients receive some type of between-meal supplements. Certified Dietary Managers have to be prepared to manage the preparation and service of these supplements as well as manage the burgeoning cost of supplements. After completing this chapter, you should be able to:

✓ Identify clients who need nourishments or supplemental feeding

✓ Define schedules/needs for special food preparation/foodservice

✓ Monitor implementation of special foodservices

✓ Identify appropriate supplemental products

✓ Monitor cost of supplements

✓ Monitor the passing of nourishments and supplements

✓ Use a system to audit the passing of nourishments or supplements

The dual role of meeting nutritional needs and satisfying the personal menu requests of your clients is a challenge. Protein and calorie malnutrition is fairly prevalent today, and you will have clients who need specialized nutrition support. The diet order will be the primary tool used to identify clients who need nourishments or supplemental feedings. You may also gather information for the Registered Dietitian (RD) on clients in poor nutritional status or with high nutrient needs. These clients are often in need of concentrated sources of nutrition. **Nutrition support** is a general term for providing foods and liquids to improve nutrition status and support good medicine.

Generally there are two approaches to providing added protein, specific nutrients and/or calories. One is to use conventional foods selecting those that are particularly nutrient-dense. Another is to add commercial **nutritional supplements** to menus of individual clients. Each has its pros and cons. Conventional foods have the advantage of familiarity and are often readily accepted by clients. The decision to provide nutrition support of any kind beyond what the normal diet provides has clinical and financial impacts that must be considered.

Not all clients benefit from more food in general, and often require less food overall, but more of specific nutrients. Starting with the addition of "regular food" to the existing menu can be highly effective, particularly for seniors. Nutrition support can start with simply adding margarine or sweeteners to the menu items of the day. Adding half a sandwich as a bedtime snack can boost the daily intake for protein and calories.

Glossary

Nutrition Support
General term for providing foods and liquids to improve nutrition status

Nutritional Supplements
A food or commercial product intended to enhance the nutritional intake

To effectively impact the nutritional status of a client, it is important to start the dietary recommendations with a complete diet history and discuss food tastes, preferences, and tolerances with a client. This helps to identify good candidates for "regular food" menu enhancements or those who will be better served through a commercially prepared supplement. See Figure 6.1 for menu planning techniques for nutrition support.

Figure 6.1 Menu Planning Techniques for Nutrition Support

- Use margarine liberally on bread, toast, vegetables, rice, pasta, and in sandwiches.
- Add gravies or sauces to entrées and side dishes.
- Add sour cream to potatoes, casseroles, and fruits.
- Use real whipped cream on top of desserts and fruits.
- Add 2 tablespoons dried milk powder to each cup of whole milk. Use for drinking and when making cream soups, hot cereal, pudding, custard, hot chocolate, mashed potatoes, casseroles, milkshakes, and creamed dishes.
- Add dried milk powder to scrambled eggs, gravies, casseroles, meatloaf, and meatballs.
- Spread peanut butter or other nut butters on toast, English muffins, crackers, cookies, apple slices, and celery sticks.
- Add cheese to sandwiches, scrambled eggs, casseroles, vegetables, and sauces.
- Add chopped eggs and diced or ground meat to salads, sauces, casseroles, and sandwiches.
- Use mayonnaise liberally on sandwiches.
- Choose desserts such as custard, bread pudding, rice pudding, and fruited yogurt. Serve with real whipped cream or ice cream.
- Offer whole milk products or cream in place of skim milk, or, offer milkshakes as beverages.
- Cook cream soups or hot cereal with whole milk; add margarine or butter.
- Serve six small meals rather than three large ones.
- Add ice cream to enteral products as a milkshake.
- Use enteral pudding supplements as a topping for cake desserts.
- Add olive oil or flavored oils to potatoes and vegetables.

Use food first as a supplement. Providing foods at meals that the client likes will encourage them to eat better. In some cases this may not be the menu of the day. If a resident wants a sandwich at every meal and they eat it, that is better than giving the meal of the day and only having a 25-percent meal completion.

The use of commercially prepared nutritional supplements and tube feedings often requires medical staff approval. Nutrition formulas are available to supplement what a client is already consuming or may provide 100% of a resident/patients' nutritional needs in a liquid form. There are literally hundreds of different products from several different manufacturers, each designed to meet a specific need.

Glossary

Enteral Nutrition
Supplemental feeding, by mouth or by tube, of liquid formulas that contain essential nutrients

Enteral nutrition refers to the feeding, by mouth or by tube, of liquid formulas that contain essential nutrients. It requires that the gastrointestinal tract be functioning. Specialized commercial products exist for providing nutrition support. A standard enteral formula provides one calorie per milliliter (ml). (About 240 ml equals one cup.) Other enteral formulas may provide 1.2, 1.5 or 2 cal/ml. A complete enteral product contains a nutritional balance of protein, carbohydrates, fat, vitamins, and minerals. Some are flavored so they can be taken orally.

Incomplete nutritional supplements offer another way to boost nutritional intake. For example, a product of carbohydrate powder with minimal flavor can be stirred into beverages, soups, applesauce, and other foods to add almost invisible calories. Another commercial product is protein powder used to boost protein content when added to mashed potatoes, hot cereal, soup, or other products.

A third type of nutrition support product you might be purchasing are the formulas for parenteral nutrition. **Parenteral nutrition** is the administration of simple essential nutrients into a vein. Parenteral solutions may contain dextrose, lipids, amino acids, electrolytes, vitamins, and trace elements. They may be used in cases where the client's gastrointestinal tract is no longer able to digest and absorb food properly; to maintain fluid and electrolyte balance both before and after surgery; or when a client is not receiving enough nourishment by other feeding methods.

> **Clinical Note:** The Registered Dietitian Nutritionist should work with the clinical staff and medical provider in establishing the use of medically appropriate nutrition support (from basic supplements to parenteral nutrition) to meet the needs of the client. Likewise, the clinical team should regularly assess the effectiveness and impact on the clinical outcomes of the nutrition support and implement changes as needed.

Implementation of Special Nourishments and Supplemental Feedings

Work with your Registered Dietitian to select special nourishments and supplemental feedings. In selecting an enteral product for oral or tube feeding, a nutrition caregiver should consider the following:

- Taste, texture, and individual client acceptance in an oral supplement
- Tolerance of lactose
- Product concentration of specific nutrients
- The need for nutritionally complete formulation
- Needs for modification in carbohydrate, fat, or protein composition
- Location of the feeding tube if tube fed
- Whether or not to include fiber
- Cost

Many of the commercial manufacturers have developed a "decision tree" to assist clinicians in the selection of the most appropriate product. Work with registered dietitians, pharmacists, nursing managers and purchasing to define a **formulary** of products that will be stocked in your organization and define the criteria for each product's use. Approval and support from the Medical Staff Director is usually required and will help "ease" the transition by all medical staff to a defined number of products. Nutrition411 (also known as Nutrition411.com) has a good sample policy defining the scope of the Enteral Feeding Formulary.

Advantages and Disadvantages to Commercial Supplements for Your Own Facility

Does the staff have the expertise and/or the time to prepare your own supplements and nourishments? Perhaps you can combine commercial products with conventional foods. For example, a client who does not enjoy a liquid supplement may enjoy a milkshake made from the supplement plus ice cream. Instead of purchasing protein powder, consider adding Nonfat Dried Milk (NFDM) to mashed potatoes, soups, and desserts.

For your clients who prefer it—or for certain dysphagia diets—specialized nutritional pudding products represent another choice. Pudding supplements that are nutritionally similar to the liquid products that are available. A garnish of real whipped cream, chocolate shavings, or fruits may also make these products more appealing.

Some disadvantages to commercial supplements include acceptance and cost. Client acceptance may vary, as clients may perceive a flavor described as "medicinal" or tasting "like vitamin supplements." On the other hand, these products are available in a variety of flavors and textures that may help to overcome this drawback.

When offering commercial supplements, it is important to allow a client to taste several products and choose what seems most enjoyable. Some facilities have a client taste panel to help determine what supplements the dining services department will purchase.

The cost of nutrition supplements can range from less than the cost of a typical snack to being outrageously expensive. As the Certified Dietary Manager, you may be expected to manage these expenses as part of your food costs. Some facilities purchase their supplements through the pharmacy and the cost is not allocated to dietary. In some cases tube feedings are paid for by nursing and oral feedings by dining services. Whatever purchasing policy your facility has, it is important to remember cost cannot be the only consideration; it is just one of them.

Keep in mind that the cost of the items used should be directly related to the beneficial clinical outcome. If the client does not consume the mid-afternoon strawberry flavored supplement because "I told her that I like strawberries but now I am sick of it" means that the supplement is not being consumed. The medical care provider and the clinical staff all believe the client is receiving added calories and protein when, in reality, the cost is being thrown away and the client never received the added nutrients. This is where a rotation of different snacks can reduce the flavor fatigue and increase supplement intakes.

Nourishment Delivery Systems

Many of the liquid supplements are better accepted when served very cold. If your delivery system isn't efficient, those supplements may arrive too warm and therefore may not be consumed. When managing nutrition supplements it is important to consider when and how they are delivered to clients.

Nearly all healthcare facilities offer snacks to clients. Not all snacks are supplements. A snack may be a simple cookie offered midmorning or birthday cake in the afternoon. Snacks may be part of the daily routine or may be scheduled only for clients with specified dietary needs, such as a diet order for six small feedings each day or a snack coordinated with insulin injection for a client with diabetes. An evening snack is generally standard for senior living residents and most clients with diabetes.

To make it even more confusing, not all supplements are commercially made or come in a can. Many of the items available today are "nutritionally enhanced" food items, not pharmaceutically produced supplements. Some commonly used items include:

- A packet of Instant Breakfast and 8 ounces of milk
- Individual cartons of frozen enriched milkshakes
- High protein power drinks
- Many of the "sport drinks" are high in electrolytes

Snacks and nourishments must comply with the diet order and may be pre-assembled by an assigned staff member or team. These may be delivered as a group to each nursing station for delivery by nursing staff or delivered directly to clients' rooms by dining services staff. In some settings the supplements are included on the **MAR (Medical Administration Record)** which requires the nursing staff to verify the consumption of the item.

While prescribed supplements are prepared and delivered to specific clients, between-meal and evening snacks are often provided through nursing unit pantries from which nursing staff withdraw items requested by clients. In some locations, dining services employees travel from room to room with a rolling cart and offer diet-appropriate snacks.

Both options allow clients to choose what they want at the time of service and receive personal attention to their requests. In many cases they improve turnaround time for processing requests and may also streamline labor requirements. Dining services and nursing staff providing snacks on demand must be familiar with dietary restrictions and must assure that foods offered meet the diet order.

Part of your supplement system should be to give supplements between meals and not with meals unless the supplement is part of a fortified liquid diet. This is to encourage the client to eat the meal and not just drink the supplement. Be careful that the nutrition supplement does not become a meal replacement. Consider this scenario:

> It is 11:15 and lunch is served at 11:30. The dining room tables are set for the residents. The assigned location for Mrs. Jones includes the place-setting, a glass of water, a glass of juice, a cup of coffee and a glass with a chocolate flavored supplement. Mrs. Jones chats some with her table mates and is sipping on the beverages. By the time the lunch plate is served, Mrs. Jones has half a glass of water left and has drunk the other fluids.
>
> At the end of lunch, a nurse asks Mrs. Jones why she did not eat the baked chicken and mashed potatoes. Mrs. Jones replies that she just wasn't all that hungry. The nurse notes that Mrs. Jones only ate 25% of her meal—maybe, given her recent weight loss, she needs a between meal supplement to boost her nutritional intake.
>
> Did you see that Mrs. Jones drank the 6 oz. of juice PLUS the 6 oz. of coffee PLUS the 8 oz. of supplement PLUS 3 oz. of water? She had 25 ounces of fluid in her stomach by the time lunch was served at her table and you wonder why she did not eat much of her lunch.

Every facility will have a different variation on their nourishment delivery systems. It will be important to meet with your **Interdisciplinary Team** to discuss the best process for your facility. Then develop a policy and procedure that outlines what part the dining services department plays in this process. See Figure 6.2 for a sample policy and procedure for delivery of between-meal snacks.

Between Meal Snack and Supplement Cost Implications

While the cost of between meal snacks and supplements seems minor it can become a black-hole of expenses. The labor to make the items and deliver them to the unit or the client directly can add up. The cost of the products themselves quickly move from cents to dollars. It is important to track the cost invested in supplements and snacks.

If you are making milkshakes with supplements for calories or protein, look at your labor cost. How much was the ingredient cost? Did the client consume it? The cost is over a

Glossary

Medical Administration Record (MAR)
Medical Administration Record that is a documentation system for patient and resident med pass

Interdisciplinary Team
A team of healthcare professionals working in support of an individual client

Putting It Into Practice

1. You are working with the Interdisciplinary Team in the nutrition care process for a client who needs additional nourishment to reach a desired weight goal. In spite of being served the nourishment three times a day, she has not gained the desired weight. Upon inquiry, you find that she doesn't like the nourishment. What steps would you take to help resolve this concern?

dollar for each milkshake. Was it consumed or thrown away because it was melted, wrong flavor, no longer needed, etc…?

Floor stock intended for client snacks between meals cost thousands of dollars a year. What are you supplying those units with? How much is needed on a daily or weekly basis?

Consider the example above of Mrs. Jones. Has the use of supplements and between meal snacks for her resulted in her being served two different diets a day; a regular diet on the table which she does not eat and a liquid diet of supplements which she finds easier to consume? What is the cost of the double meal service? What is the nutritional impact on her medical outcome?

Sometimes our best intentions have unintended consequences that come at an unexpected price.

Quality Improvement (QI) Monitoring Between Meal Snack and Supplements

Client needs change, their health status changes, taste fatigue sets in, staff availability changes. Lots of events can impact the making, passing and consumption of the between meal snacks and supplements.

Since supplements are prescribed with the intent of impacting the client's medical condition it is important to conduct regular audits to verify their use. Tracking of the supplements should include:

- Order is appropriate to client needs and follows the decision tree process
- The item is prepared according to the recipe (ensure the nutritional composition)
- The item is delivered on time to the client
  > Appropriately refrigerated if needed for a delayed service time, i.e. late night or bedtime snack
- All items served to clients, and/or held in the refrigerator, are dated and current
- The item is within reach of the client and ready for consumption
- The amount consumed by the client
- Client comments when appropriate
- The medical record and recommendations for change are entered when appropriate

Conducting the QI audits on a quarterly basis helps keep the focus on the client's needs.

Legal Implications

CMS (Centers for Medicare & Medicaid Services) is a federal agency that administers the Medicare programs and monitors the Medicaid programs offered by each state. CMS provides Investigative Protocols that define guidelines for the surveyors. CMS guidelines use **F-Tag** numbers to identify specific guidance for long-term care. Healthcare facilities also have differing levels of mandatory state licensing requirements.

A Certified Dietary Manager is responsible for making sure that clients know what their diet is and offer a choice of whether to receive the diet (e.g., a choice about whether to receive nourishments or tube feedings). If the client refuses a tube feeding or additional nourishments, the client, facility, Medical Care Provider and Registered Dietitian collaborate to identify pertinent alternatives.

During a survey, an F-Tag was issued for a tube-fed client who had asked to receive food and drink by mouth. (F 151: The facility failed to address one resident's right to refuse

---

Glossary

F-Tag
Numbers used by CMS to identify specific guidance for long-term care

---

Putting It Into Practice

2. An audit of your nourishment delivery systems shows that nourishments are being delivered to the floors/wings but clients are not receiving them. What are some steps you should take to address this concern?

a physician ordered treatment.) With the CMS guidelines (revised 2014), you have to acknowledge the following:

- Promote care in a manner and in an environment that maintains or enhances each resident's dignity and respect. CMS F-241 Interpretive Guidance: Promoting resident independence and dignity in dining

Figure 6.2 Sample Policy and Procedures for Delivery of Between Meal Snacks

POLICY: Between-meal feedings will be available at established intervals, upon request, or when prescribed to meet the specialized nutritional needs of the resident/patient.

DATE EFFECTIVE: _____

DATE REVISED: _____

DATE REVIEWED: Annually

APPROVED BY: _____

ISSUING DEPARTMENT: Nutritional Services

APPROVE FOR USE IN: _____

PROCEDURE

1. A variety of nourishments/snacks is available at each Nursing Unit daily. Each Nursing Unit will order nourishments/food supplies for residents.

2. Planned nourishments are delivered to the nursing unit front desk at 10:00 a.m., 3:00 p.m. and 8:00 p.m. (HS) for nursing staff distribution.

3. Individual patient nourishments will be available when alterations in the usual feeding pattern are required due to the dietary prescription or patient need. These may be made by patient request, by nursing request, or as recommended by the Nutrition Professional (or approved designee).

4. The Nutrition Professional (or approved designee) and nursing staff will routinely refer to the nourishment intake record and MAR to determine if nourishments and supplements are being consumed and at what level. Changes will be made as needed to ensure acceptability by the resident.

5. Rotation of stock and sanitation of the nursing pantry areas is the responsibility of the respective nursing units and Nutritional Services.

6. Procedures for cleaning and care of the nursing pantry area have been developed by Nutritional Services and are posted in each pantry area.

7. All individual nourishments should be covered for transport to residents. Each is labeled with the resident's name, room number, date and time of delivery.

8. Nourishments or snacks are defined as food and/or drink singly or in combination from the kitchen that are offered between meals to all residents whose diet order allows it. These foods are from the basic food groups.

9. Nutrition services personnel will maintain a log of residents who receive between-meal nourishments and supplements. This list will be used to prepare nourishments. Nursing staff will distribute the nourishments and record intake.

10. The Nutrition Professional will refer to the MAR to determine if supplements are being consumed at what level (i.e., percentage). The Nutrition Professional will refer to the approved facility form to determine if nourishments/snacks are being consumed and what amount.

11. If a nourishment or supplement is not being consumed, the Nutrition Professional should review the meal pattern and overall care plan approaches; visit with the resident and/or family member; and make changes to help ensure intake and acceptability by the resident as much as possible.

Source: Nutrition411.com (used with permission)

- The resident or representative has the right to make informed choices about accepting or declining care and treatment, CMS F-325.

- Decisions about the appropriateness of tube feeding for a resident are developed with the resident, his/her family, surrogate or representative as part of determining the care plan. This requirement is also intended to prevent the use of tube feeding when ordered over the objection of the resident, CMS F-322.

Check with your administrator to review the regulations that cover dining services. Make sure you and your staff are aware of all regulations and their implications for meal service, including the service of nourishments and tube feedings.

Evaluate Food Acceptance and Satisfaction

Overview and Objectives

What role food plays in the facility and even what role your department plays is defined by the clients. Use the information in this chapter to examine how clients' needs influence the foodservice operation. You will identify techniques for gathering meaningful data about your clients and their needs. A successful foodservice department knows who their clients are and routinely surveys each group. Survey results will lead to recommendations and changes to improve the level of service. After completing this chapter, you should be able to:

✓ Identify client food preferences and food problems

✓ Define data needs for judging food preferences

✓ Develop and conduct food acceptance surveys

✓ Analyze data and make recommendations/changes

Who are your clients? They are those who buy your goods or services. In the foodservice environment, goods are generally meals or foods, and services can range from the dining experience to the provision of nutrition counseling. How would you describe your clients?

Everyone you provide meal service to is considered a client. Each of them has different needs and different expectations. Your clients may be called patients, clients, residents, students, inmates, or employees. A successful dining service department knows who their clients are and routinely surveys each group.

If you are in healthcare and started describing the hospital patients or nursing home clients, you would be partially correct. They are a very important part of the client base. Another segment is the staff that work and eat in your facility. Members of the community, such as those receiving meals on wheels, or participating in congregate dining services are also your clients. Special functions and catering events expand the clientele base to family members and conference/meeting attendees. What other groups that you serve aren't mentioned here?

Most operations have a variety of client groups. Along with primary clients, who may comprise the largest group of people you serve, there are others. In a school, for example, services are usually provided for teachers and employees as well as students. In a hospital you may be serving employees, physicians, visitors, and even the community at large. Figure 7.1 lists examples of additional client groups you may serve in various foodservice settings.

Figure 7.1 Additional Client Groups: Examples

PUBLIC SCHOOL
- Teachers
- Other employees
- Visitors
- Consultants
- Professional groups (meetings, seminars)

UNIVERSITY
- Faculty members
- Other employees
- Visitors and guests
- Prospective students and families
- Sports teams
- Consultants and inspectors
- Sales representatives
- Professional groups (meetings, seminars)
- Attendees of conferences

CORRECTIONAL FACILITY
- Guards and other employees
- Consultants and inspectors
- Sales representatives

SKILLED NURSING FACILITY
- Potential residents and families
- Employees
- Physicians
- Community members
- Consultants and inspectors
- Sales representatives
- Professional groups (meetings, seminars)

BUSINESS DINING
- Consultants and inspectors
- Visitors and guests
- Clients and prospective clients
- Professional groups (meetings, seminars)
- Children enrolled in onsite daycare

HOSPITAL
- Visitors
- Employees
- Physicians
- Community members
- Students (in training)
- Consultants and inspectors
- Sales representatives
- Outpatients
- Professional groups (meetings, seminars)

CHILD DAY CARE CENTER
- Teachers
- Other employees

REHABILITATION CENTER
- Potential residents and families
- Employees
- Physicians
- Community members
- Consultants and inspectors
- Sales representatives
- Professional groups (meetings, seminars)

Why Are Clients Important?

In a non-commercial environment (hospitals, senior living and residential facilities), clients are almost always named in the mission statement. Regardless of the specifics, it is clear that the facility exists to take care of its clients. This alone dictates the need for a clear focus on clients in dining services.

To plan a dining service operation some of the key questions to ask are:

- Who are our clients and what are their primary needs?
- What type of service do our clients want?
- What types of foods should we include (or exclude)?
- Where will we serve people?
- What range of meal services will we provide?
- How many meals should we serve?
- What time should we serve meals?
- What will the presentation and environment look like?
- How will we accommodate unique client needs and preferences?

Needless to say, there are many more questions like these. In fact, a multitude of options controlling nearly every aspect of menu and service need to be considered. So much boils down to choices and the decision process. To make these decisions, you need to consider your clients. Ultimately what constitutes a good decision for one group of clients may not be a good decision for another.

The bottom line has to be that the sum total of your decisions creates a dining services operation that gives the clients exactly what they need, the way they need it, and when they need it. In other words, it's really your clients who define the answers to the questions. They do not tell you how to accomplish the job, but they do tell you what the results need to be.

Often the challenge a Certified Dietary Manager faces is how to satisfy clients' needs, while also addressing many additional constraints. Some of these constraints may include budgetary limitations and requirements from external factors such as laws, regulations, and accreditation standards. Non-commercial dining operations perform a continuous balancing act to work within all established limits while using available resources most effectively to meet the needs of clients.

Managers in non-commercial dining services are quickly abandoning the traditional view of their clients as a captive audience. Successful players in the field, including successful foodservice contract companies, have adopted a new outlook. While the presentation and quality of the dining services may not be the deciding factor for most clients, it is a consideration and has become a marketing opportunity for the organization. Recognizing the client as a true customer is changing the provision of services to better meet the client's needs and expectations of their dining experience.

Central to this concept are two dimensions: inward looking and outward looking. Outward looking means looking outside your department, and in some cases, even outside the facility. For example what new service is your competition implementing? Inward looking means self-examination by looking at satisfaction, image, participation rate, and client loyalty.

Inward Looking

Unique Needs of Clients. What do your clients need? What do they like? Answers vary. This is because many factors affect clients' food-related needs, meal expectations, service needs, and even their ability to enjoy food. Clients' unique needs may relate to likes and dislikes, expectations, variety, choice, appetite, sense of taste, drug therapies, allergies and intolerances, cultural and ethnic influences, lifestyle, routines, timing, religious convictions, emotional overtones and personal values about food and nutrition.

Putting It Into Practice

1. During your weekly inservice meeting, some of your staff complains about all the additional work involved with a new room service menu. What would you tell them to help them accept the changes?

In addition further needs may be dictated by presentation, environment, disabilities, language, literacy, culinary trends, and health status. Beyond these factors, some clients have very specific foodservice needs and follow special diets (therapeutic diets). See Figure 7.2 for a closer look at these factors.

Satisfaction and Image. In some situations, the element of choice works a bit differently. In a hospital or a skilled nursing facility, for example, the clients may not have the option of eating somewhere else. However, their satisfaction is still critical to the operation. In these environments competition jumps to the next level. The hospital meal service may not be competing with the doughnut shop next door. However, the hospital itself may very well be competing with the hospital a few miles away.

How will clients choose which hospital to use? Choices may hinge on previous experiences in the hospital, impressions of the hospital, and reputation within the community. Since 2006, The Centers for Medicare & Medicaid Services (CMS) has conducted the Hospital Consumer Assessment of Healthcare Providers and Systems Survey (HCAHPS) of discharged hospital patients to measure their perspectives of hospital care. A portion of the hospital's Medicare Reimbursement is directly tied to the facility's HCAHPS score. Although dining services and food specifically are not included in the survey, two questions relate to the patient's overall rating of the hospital which does reflect on their dining experience. So patient satisfaction relates to reimbursements and competition between hospitals, rather than between foodservice operations.

For a skilled nursing facility a similar model applies. Among other things, when a potential client and their family are selecting a facility they will evaluate the quality of the environment and care they can expect from each option. Dining Services is a major contributor to the image a facility builds, to community perceptions of quality of care, and ultimately—to the decision-making process of potential clients of a facility.

In healthcare, physicians are also clients of the dining services department. A physician brings business to the facility and often has the choice of selecting one facility or another. Although insurance coverage may dictate which hospital the patient is admitted to, the physician's perception of patient satisfaction based on patient comments is certainly a consideration.

In prisons, satisfaction takes on yet a different aspect. An inmate most certainly has no choice of one facility over another. Yet satisfaction looms as a critical issue in ensuring smooth operations. Richard B. Dansdill, a Certified Dietary Manager with Fremont Correctional Facility in Canon City, Colorado notes, "If you study correctional history, you will learn that a large number of the serious riots in correctional facilities started with problems in foodservice." (Dietary Manager, June 2000)

School and university clients have a totally different view of what they expect of dining services. The need to balance food preferences with current fads and nutritionally sound dining options in the meal plans is a challenge. The school and university clientele often want more variety in their choices while maintaining easy access to the popular grilled items.

Essentially, know what your client needs are and then work to satisfy them. It sounds simple; it is anything but simple. Once you have identified your clients and their needs, you can continue to improve satisfaction and image by adopting and implementing standards. For instance, the Disney Institute recommends adopting service standards such as, "safety, courtesy, efficiency, and show."

Figure 7.2 Factors that Influence Client Dietary Needs

Likes and Dislikes	The most powerful influence on food choices are personal preferences. Find out what they are for your clients.
Expectations	Your dining room and foodservice paint a picture that shapes the expectations of your clients. Do you have an elegant dining room? Are your signs scribbled or neatly lettered? Is your staff smiling during service? What picture are you painting?
Variety	You know the old saying, "Variety is the spice of life." Offering variety is especially essential in healthcare, school, and correctional foodservice.
Choice	Room service, selective menus, restaurant style service, self-service bars, coffee kiosks, and food courts all improve client satisfaction through increased choices.
Appetite	Your clients may be impacted by both physiological and emotional factors that may affect their appetite. Offering a variety of portion sizes will help to meet client needs.
Sense of Taste and Smell	Your client's sense of taste and smell greatly factor into their enjoyment of food. Know your client's condition and work with them to add additional herbs and spices.
Drug Therapies	Medications may impact taste and smell. It is important to note and beware of that clients taking several medications may request additional salt or sugar to achieve the same taste sensations. This may not comply with the diet order. Consulting with the Registered Dietitian Nutritionist may be necessary.
Allergies and Intolerances	Lactose intolerance (the inability to digest milk sugar) and allergies (such as nuts or wheat) mean providing accurate identification of products that may contain allergens. Know the allergies and intolerances of your clients.
Cultural and Ethnic Influences	Cultural and ethnic foods, ingredients, and/or seasoning styles relate to familiarity and comfort. These play a part in clients' expectations and perceptions of meal services.
Lifestyle	People are busier today and often eat on the go. You may meet your client needs by offering take-out food, sack lunches, and even room service.
Religious Convictions	For any clients whose religious beliefs influence eating choices, it is essential to acknowledge those choices and offer suitable options. Chapter One of the *Nutrition Fundamentals and Medical Nutrition Therapy* textbook offers a full discussion of cultural, ethnic, and religious influences on menu options.
Personal Values	Both food choices and service concepts relate to clients' personal value systems. An example of this is vegetarianism or people who feel strongly about healthy eating. You will be expected to identify these needs and develop services and alternatives that accommodate them.
Language and Literacy	Language or literacy barriers may require you to evaluate carefully how best to communicate with clients, to relate menus, to offer services, and to gather requests and choices.
Dietary and Clinical	Medical conditions may dictate food restrictions and/or limitations, for example significant protein restriction for renal patients or texture modifications for clients with swallowing disorders.

Participation Rate. Participation rate refers to the proportion of a potential client group that patronizes non-commercial foodservice. In an assisted living community, the question would be: What percentage use the onsite restaurant? If 70 of 100 use the restaurant, the participation rate is 70 percent. If you are in a hospital and are serving employees, you may be concerned with participation rate for lunch in the hospital cafeteria. If half of employees eat in the cafeteria, you have a participation rate of 50 percent. Participation rate is very important in the school foodservice market, where a key impetus is to encourage more students to use school meal services. This also ties into satisfaction and image. Likewise, in universities, the drive is often to encourage students to use the campus dining plan.

Higher rates of participation in non-commercial foodservice can have significant impact on operational revenues. With certain costs being fixed—such as the cost of operating a large food production kitchen and the cost of paying managers—an operation can often achieve greater economy of scale through increased participation. Once the participation rate is high enough to cover the fixed costs, each additional customer adds to the incremental increase in revenue due to increasing participations rates. In turn, this can bring about an improved profitability of the financial bottom line.

In some facilities participation rate is also important for meeting other aspects of the mission. For example, a public school that strives to meet children's nutritional needs would also want to boost participation rates in order to ensure sound nutrition for the students.

Client Loyalty. If a foodservice operation does a successful job of appealing to clients' needs, it can gain a following. Just like a "favorite restaurant," the operation develops a sense of loyalty from clients. They want to keep coming back and choose this operation over an alternative.

Loyalty is very valuable to any business and non-commercial foodservice is no exception. Loyalty means repeat patronage, and a certain level of security in ongoing revenues to the operation.

As you can see, competing in the marketplace, bolstering satisfaction and image, boosting participation rates, and developing loyalty all feed into the mission and objectives of many facilities. Success in each of these areas requires a serious commitment to clients and their needs. Furthermore success requires making the effort to get to know your own client groups, understand their needs, and respond to their preferences. The more effectively you do this, the more readily you can achieve a valid competitive edge in this evolving marketplace.

Looking Outward

Competition. In many cases, non-commercial dining services are competing side-by-side with other forms of commercial and retail operations. For example:

- Employees of a large company can eat in the employee cafeteria or food court.
  - > Take advantage of the growing fast-food industry and walk to the chicken franchise around the corner.
  - > Go to the doughnut shop next door.
  - > Pack their own lunch (brown bag).
- College students may choose to eat in the dining hall
  - > Order a pizza for delivery to his residence hall.
  - > Run to the local convenience store for a take-out submarine sandwich.

- A resident of an assisted living community who wishes to go out to eat may choose the community's onsite restaurant.

  > Drive a mile to a different, privately-owned restaurant.

- A professional group holding a meeting in your facility may have the option of bringing in refreshments from a private catering service, or using yours; likewise with a fund-raising group holding a black-tie dinner.

Professional programs can help identify your client base and improve service through knowing the needs of your potential clients. One such program is the *Disney Institute*. The *Disney Institute* defines "Guestology—knowing your guests (demographics) and understanding your Guests (psychographics)." Information and course descriptions for the various programs is available online at www.disneyinstitute.com.

Another program that helps you focus on your clients and identifying their needs is the Diamond 7Cs, a quality improvement program. To remain competitive today, your facility and ultimately your department, need to define your customers/clients, their needs, and customize innovative methods to meet those needs. See Management in the News at the end of this chapter for the full article about implementing the Diamond 7Cs program at your facility.

Learning About Your Clients

There is much to learn about your clients. Client needs and expectations do not stay the same over time. An effective Certified Dietary Manager continues to monitor clients and obtain feedback and suggestions. Furthermore, it's important to realize that a manager needs to address diversity among clients. One of the strategies used in dining services planning is to look for ways to give everyone what they need.

How can you learn more about your clients? There are multiple methods both formal and informal. Figure 7.3 lists examples.

Client Satisfaction Survey. A client satisfaction survey provides an excellent means of learning more about your clients. The results of a survey, examined carefully, can assist in refining menu offerings, service mechanisms, and more. What is a satisfaction survey? A satisfaction survey is a series of questions designed to elicit feedback from clients in a systematic fashion. Among the considerations for implementing a survey are: the method you choose for offering the survey, the way you select clients to participate, and the actual questions you ask.

There are many methods for offering a survey.

- Print a questionnaire and deliver it with meals
- Allow clients to "grade" the dining services with a menu scorecard for 5 items served in the last week
- Visit clients in person and ask them to answer a series of questions through a brief interview process
- Telephone clients to ask questions
- Send a mailing to past clients asking them to answer questions
- Offer a questionnaire on your dining services website and invite clients to complete it
- Use other technology, such as a computer-based kiosk (free-standing station), or a handheld computer at tables

Glossary

Satisfaction Survey
series of questions designed to elicit feedback from clients in a systematic fashion

Figure 7.3 Ways to Learn About Clients

INFORMAL METHODS	FORMAL METHODS
• Be present during meal times and observe.	• Create a suggestion box for use by both clients and employees. Review suggestions carefully.
• Talk to clients during meal times and ask friendly questions about the meal.	• Provide a comment card on tables where clients dine.
• Talk to dining services staff involved in serving and ask about feedback and requests they receive from clients.	• Tabulate plate waste. This is the food that is left on a plate returned with soiled dishes. Systematically calculate what is left uneaten, and examine percentages of uneaten food for each menu item. Sometimes, uneaten food gives you a good measure of what clients did not enjoy.
• Accept any complaint as valuable feedback and use it to evaluate needs.	
• Talk to related staff, such as wait staff, nurses, or other staff, and ask what they are noticing or hearing.	• Monitor menu mix and product sales. Sales figures often provide a good indicator of what menu items clients are enjoying.
• After a catered function, talk to the person(s) who requested the catering and ask for feedback.	• Use technology to provide an interactive method for clients to provide feedback from tables or bedsides (in a healthcare facility).
• Wear a name tag that identifies your role or title in the facility and make eye contact with people you see. This makes it easy for clients to approach you to give you feedback.	• In a healthcare setting, ask clinical staff to gather information about the needs of clients, to pass along relevant needs, and to help assure that individual needs are addressed.
• Talk to your peers in similar organizations and share observations about trends that are developing.	• Create an advisory committee or focus group comprised of clients and ask them to help provide feedback and suggestions.
• Read foodservice trade journals to learn more about trends and issues.	• Conduct formal satisfaction surveys.
	• Using a mix of clients, evaluate test trays for temperature and quality.
	• Use an outside source (e.g., Press Ganey).
	• Mystery Shoppers—individuals to act as guests/clients and then write a report on their experience.

Each method has advantages and disadvantages, and it's important to consider what method will be most effective for your client group. For example: If you are planning to use printed materials, consider whether all your clients will be able to read them and whether you are communicating in a language they know.

If you are planning to use technology, evaluate clients' comfort level with the devices. In a university environment, for example, technology is frequently used to gather feedback from students. This is a natural fit for a population that uses computers and the internet on a daily basis. However, among clients of an eldercare community, a smaller percentage of clients may feel comfortable interacting with the technology.

A printed piece is easy to ignore. It is inconvenient, and may elicit responses only from those clients who have strong positive or negative feelings. In addition, it can leave out anyone who is unable to read and anyone who is not physically strong to complete a form.

A personal interaction offers its own advantages. Clients are keenly aware of your interest in their satisfaction and may also feel free to tell you more. A disadvantage is that some clients worry about hurting the feelings of the survey taker and will therefore hesitate to express concerns.

Food committees have been utilized in many settings. Regular meetings with a team of representative clients can provide information on what the community wants. It can also become a gripe session if issues are not resolved or effectively addressed before the next meeting.

In some situations, a broad-scale client survey mechanism may already be in place. Sometimes the entire survey process is outsourced or administered by an outside firm (such as using Press Ganey). Dining services satisfaction may be one of several topics addressed on a broad-scale survey of satisfaction.

Who receives a survey can have tremendous bearing on the value of information gathered. For example, in healthcare patients who are unresponsive, highly medicated, tube-fed or those not consuming food by mouth do not provide accurate or actionable data.

Past clients may have different reactions than current clients. Clients who use your services may have different feelings than clients who do not participate. For example, in a business dining environment, you might not want to only survey regular clients, you would also want to hear from employees who pack their own meals, or use other food establishments, in order to learn what it would take to attract them to your cafeteria.

The most effective selection method includes a cross-section of clients and potential clients (if relevant). This means you have a representative sample from all groups. You may select all your clients for a survey, or take a like percentage from each group you identify. Figure 7.4 provides an example of this process.

Figure 7.4 Selection of Survey Participants

In Axl Assisted Living Community there are seven residential buildings. Some residents do not receive any meal service to their living quarters. Others receive home-delivered meals on a daily basis. The community also operates an on-site cafe and a convenience store with take-out foods. In all, there are 500 residents in the community. The survey is going to be administered by telephone, and the Certified Dietary Manager has determined he has the resources (staffing) to complete 100 calls. How does the Certified Dietary Manager select clients to participate in the satisfaction survey?

In this case, there are several different services to evaluate: home-delivered meals, the on-site cafe, and the convenience store. The Certified Dietary Manager knows who uses home-delivered meals, but does not know who uses the other services. In addition, the Certified Dietary Manager has no way of knowing which residents (if any) do not use the cafe and the store. Thus, the most useful selection would simply be a random one from among all the buildings. This is likely to pull a representation of all client categories.

The Certified Dietary Manager goes through a complete roster of residents and highlights every fifth one for a phone call.

Putting It Into Practice

2. What considerations should you include when planning a paper survey for clients in a long-term care facility?

What types of questions should you ask in a survey to learn about your clients? And what kinds of choices should you provide for answers? What you ask can make a big difference in the final results.

For starters, each question should be a neutral question. This means the surveyor is not expecting a particular answer. The opposite of a neutral question is a leading question, in which the surveyor attempts to elicit a particular response or seems to "lead" the participant to an answer. Figure 7.5 shows examples of leading and neutral questions.

In addition, there are several ways to allow a participant to answer a question. An **open-ended question** allows the participant to answer freely, saying whatever comes to mind. It cannot be answered with a "yes" or "no," or with a number. It invites free expression. In Figure 7.5, neutral questions 1, 2, and 4 are all open-ended questions. This type of question is especially valuable for learning more information than just what the question is asking. For example, when you ask, "How do you feel about the food we deliver to you?"—you may learn things that come as a surprise. Often answers include comments like:

- It's fabulous, and I could not live here without this service.
- I can't eat it because I'm on a low-salt diet and you keep giving me salty foods.
- The delivery person is so kind; he always sets up the table for me, too.
- The entrées are usually cold when I get them.
- The beef is too tough to chew.
- I know I signed up for this service but I've never received a meal.

Figure 7.5 Ways to Ask a Question

LEADING	NEUTRAL
1. You like the food we deliver to you, don't you?	1. How do you feel about the food we deliver to you?
2. The food reaches you on time, doesn't it?	2. How is the timing of your deliveries?
3. You use the convenience store, right?	3. How often do you use the convenience store?
4. You haven't had any problems with the service in the cafe, have you?	4. How do you feel about the service at the cafe?

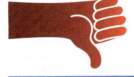
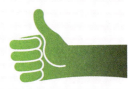

Putting It Into Practice

3. Your facility is interested in getting feedback about the menu selections in foodservice. Which formal method in Figure 7.3 would be the best way to get a good cross section of opinions that would also provide specific information?

There are so many possible responses that without an open-ended question, you could miss some feedback you really need to hear! Realistically there is no way to ask enough questions to cover all the bases and elicit each of these answers without an open-ended question.

On the other hand, a closed-ended question, or closed question, with a limited number of specific answers also has value in a survey. In Figure 7.5, leading question 3 is an example of a closed question. When you ask, "How often do you use the convenience store?"—you can provide choices for the answers, such as:

- Every day
- 2-5 times per week
- Less than once per week
- Never

Answer choices can measure frequency, such as these. Alternately, they can be ratings. A common rating technique uses the **Likert Scale**, which is a system for allowing people to rate how they feel about something by choosing a word or a number. For example, a survey question that says, "Rate your satisfaction on a scale of 1 to 5" is using a Likert Scale. Some surveyors avoid numbers in a survey, because users may make errors in interpreting the numeric scale. Words are more clear. Figure 7.6 shows sample questions from a survey that uses the Likert Scale.

Figure 7.6 Survey Using a Likert Scale

1. How would you rate the offerings in the convenience store? (circle one)

   excellent   good   average   below average   poor

2. How would you rate the quality of food in the cafe? (circle one)

   excellent   good   average   below average   poor

From closed questions with answers that rate frequency or a Likert Scale, you can develop specific figures that identify areas for action and measure trends over time. For example, you can calculate participation rates in the use of the convenience store. Or, you can calculate how many clients feel their hot foods are hot enough when they are served. If you ask the same closed questions again in a few months, you can measure the success of any corrective actions and interventions.

Another advantage to closed questions is that they are easier to ask than open-ended questions. Closed questions can be delivered on a survey form. Too many open-ended questions on a survey require participants to do a lot of writing, and some simply won't do it. Yet another advantage of closed questions is that they elicit answers that are easy to tabulate and summarize.

To learn about your clients, use both types of questions on a survey. If a survey that offers answers on the Likert Scale, for example, you may wish to include one open-ended question at the end, such as, "What other comments would you like to make about the foodservices?"

Glossary

Likert Scale
A common rating technique that uses words or numbers

Let's consider those situations where you are interacting with clients, as opposed to delivering a formal survey. Here, your best tool is the open-ended question. For example, while walking through the cafe during lunch service, the Certified Dietary Manager of Axl Healthcare stops by tables and asks clients, "How is your service today?" or "How is your food?" or "What do you think about today's menu?"

A Certified Dietary Manager who is focused on clients will use a variety of formal and informal techniques, as well as a mix of question types, in order to gather feedback and keep in touch with clients.

Evaluating Survey Results

As you gather information from formal and informal interactions, how can you summarize and evaluate it?

- As you receive answers to open-ended questions the most important thing to do is listen and think about the responses one by one
- Follow through on anything that surprises you, and make your own observations
- Notice similarities among answers.
  - > Group answers and tally them
  - > For example, if 11 people say that the convenience store closes too early in the day, you can tally this information and use it in your planning
- If you are sharing answers with your boss or others in your organization, you may also just make a list of responses so that reviewers can read them one by one

How about closed questions? Here, you can tally answers to each question and calculate rates of responses. Figure 7.7 shows how to calculate percentage rates for responses to a closed survey question.

What do the results of the question in Figure 7.7 tell you? Overall, they indicate that you are doing a great job of offering items the clients want to see in the convenience store. They also tell you that a small proportion of clients are looking for something they are not finding at the store. Hopefully, on this same survey, there are open-ended questions that generate client comments. You may want to look through these to see if anyone has named items they wish you would carry.

What follow-up would be appropriate for these results?

- Work with employees staffing the convenience store and ask them what clients are looking for
- Provide scripting for them to ask each client, "Are you finding everything you need?"
- Have the staff maintain a list of items that clients ask for but do not find
- Meet with vendors to select new items for the store to carry
- Ask clients to participate in an advisory committee to help evaluate product availability

After a period of time, re-survey clients to measure the effectiveness of actions you have taken.

Thoughtful interpretation of a survey can help you improve products and services, identify client needs, and even develop new concepts. As an ongoing process, use surveys to keep a pulse. Surveys are not only useful in solving problems but are helpful in preventing them too. They also ensure successful competition, quality client participation and customer loyalty.

Figure 7.7 Calculating Percentages for a Survey Response

First ask: How many people responded to the survey?

Next, ask: How many people gave each answer to a question?

Then for each possible response, divide the number of responses by the total number of people who responded to the survey. If you do this on a calculator, you can generally round your answer to two decimal places. If you remove the decimal, now you have a percentage.

Example: A sample survey given to clients of Axl Healthcare included the following question.

How would you rate the offerings in the convenience store? (circle one)

excellent   good   average   below average   poor

Your count says 65 people completed the survey.

On this question, 41 answered "excellent;" 12 answered "good;" 6 answered "average;" 4 answered "below average;" and
2 answered "poor."

<u>**Your summary shows:**</u>

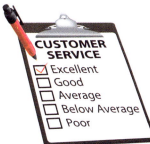

Excellent	41 ÷ 65 = 0.6308 or about 63%
Good	12 ÷ 65 = 0.1846 or about 18%
Average	6 ÷ 65 = 0.0923 or about 9%
Below Average	4 ÷ 65 = 0.0615 or about 6%
Poor	2 ÷ 65 = 0.0308 or about 3%

Note: The percentages add up to 99% due to rounding; i.e. 0.0923 was rounded to 9%. Either round the 0.1846 up to 19% (then the total equals 100%) OR accept (and know) that the total is 99% due to rounding.

In addition, as part of a Business Plan for new or expanding services, surveys help to better understand the market segment being considered. Customer identification and survey of their needs may determine if you go forward with a planned project. This becomes a valuable basis for planning.

The Quality Process

Overview and Objectives

Quality of products and services is the aim of virtually every organization. Quality is adherence to standards, processes, and outcomes. In this chapter you will discover why a Certified Dietary Manager needs to take a proactive approach towards managing quality and identify techniques for verifying quality. After completing this chapter, you should be able to:

✓ Define the Quality Management Process

✓ Identify specific quality indicators for Dining Services

✓ Develop audits to monitor procedures and effectiveness of quality indicators

✓ Evaluate the data collected and recommend changes

✓ Identify the key certification agencies

✓ Describe the role of the Dining Services Manager in the certification process of the facility

Quality initiatives in healthcare have been around for decades. Avedis Donabedian's 1966 article described ways to evaluate the quality of healthcare. He proposed a broad definition of quality and three areas in which to measure it:

- **Structure**—the physical and staffing characteristics of caring for patients
- **Process**—the method of delivery
- **Outcome**—the results of care

This system is still in use today although there is greater emphasis on process and outcomes. In the past, measuring quality meant measuring whether you were meeting certain pre-set standards. For instance, you may have a pre-set standard that all hot food leaving the kitchen be a minimum of 150°F. The measurement would be to take the temperature of a certain percentage of hot foods prior to leaving the kitchen.

Today, while that is still important, the focus is on the outcome- how many clients are satisfied that their hot food is hot? And the attention is on the process—how do you know clients are satisfied that the food is hot, what process is used to measure their satisfaction, and how are you addressing their dissatisfaction.

The pre-set standard of measuring the temperature of hot foods as it leaves the kitchen now becomes part of the process to achieve the outcome. In 2006, Centers for Medicare & Medicaid (CMS), revised F 520 Surveyor Interpretive Guidance and put forth the following definitions:

- **Quality Assessment** is an evaluation of a process and/or outcomes of a process to determine if a defined standard of quality is being achieved.
- **Quality Assurance** is the organizational structure, processes, and procedures designed to ensure that care practices are consistently applied and the facility meets or exceeds an expected standard of quality. Quality assurance includes the implementation of principles of *continuous quality improvement (CQI)*.
- **Quality Improvement (QI)** is an ongoing interdisciplinary process that is designed to improve the delivery of services and resident outcomes.

Quality Assurance Processes

In healthcare, there have been many names for quality assurance processes. (e.g., CQI, QI, QA, PDCA, LEAN, QAPI). Today, healthcare is realizing that quality is an essential element of organizational strategy, not a single initiative. CMS calls it QAPI (Quality Assessment and Performance Improvement). Your facility probably has some type of quality initiative. Whatever your facility calls the quality initiative, it should have these characteristics:

- Focus on clients and what they need, rather than on employees or departments and what they do
- Be a team approach that is cross departmental
- Use and evaluate the data
- Is proactive and continuous
- Do not wait for a problem to occur; continuously look at processes and ways to improve the processes
- Contain a performance improvement segment

Quality initiatives use some key terminology. One term is outcome. An **outcome** is the end result of work such as the results of client interactions. Using the temperature of food example from above, the outcome of serving hot food is a satisfied client. In a healthcare environment, a health outcome describes the consequences of clinical interventions. For instance, if members of the healthcare team work together to improve a client's nutritional status, what happens to that client's nutritional status is the outcome of the clinical care plan.

Quality indicators (QIs) are measures of outcomes. According to Centers for Medicare & Medicaid Services (CMS), an indicator is "a key clinical value or quality characteristic used to measure, over time, the performance, processes, and outcomes of an organization or some component of healthcare delivery." If we look at the temperature of food example again, the quality indicator would be that a certain percentage of clients are very satisfied with their foodservice. As you can see by this definition, indicators are designed to facilitate collection and analysis of data. They are objective and measurable.

A general process for implementing QA (Quality Assurance) in healthcare uses two acronyms: FOCUS and PDCA.

FOCUS means:

F— Find a process to improve

O—Organize to improve a process

C— Clarify what is known

U—Understand variation

S— Select a process improvement

Glossary

Quality Assessment
The evaluation of processes and/or outcomes to determine if a defined standard of quality is being achieved

Quality Assurance
The overall structure, processes, and procedures designed to ensure that the facility meet or exceed an expected standard of quality

Quality Improvement
The ongoing process to improve the delivery of food, services and client outcomes

Outcomes
The end result of work

Quality Indicators
A measurement of outcomes

Once you have selected a process to improve, the next acronym relates to the plan itself. **PDCA** means:

P— Plan: Decide what you will do to improve the process. Decide what information you will collect, and how you will measure outcomes.

D— Do: Make the improvements.

C— Check: Collect and review data, and evaluate how the plan is working.

A— Act: Act on what you have learned. If you have made a successful improvement, make sure it becomes part of your policies and procedures. If not, try an alternate plan.

The Institute for Healthcare Improvement (www.ihi.org) has developed a worksheet that can help you with the Plan, Do, Check/Study, Act process for performance improvement. Their tool is shown in Figure 8.1. The Medicare Quality Improvement Community (MedQIC) website is "a free online resource for quality improvement interventions and associated tools, toolkits, presentations, and links to other resources." The Website is funded by CMS to provide a site to share resources based on the CMS scope of work.

Establishing Standards and Quality Processes

Measuring quality really means ensuring that your operation is meeting certain standards. These standards become the backbone of the quality processes. A **quality standard** is your facility's definition of what constitutes quality for a product (such as food) or a service. A single product or service may have a list of criteria to meet. For example, a quality standard for steak tenderloin might stipulate that the steak will be tender, the temperature will be 145°F or higher, and the food will be neatly presented on a plate, with a garnish.

A quality standard for cafeteria checkout might stipulate that the customer will be able to check out within three minutes, the transaction will be accurate, and the customer will receive a receipt. A quality standard for nutritional assessment might specify that an assessment will be completed within three days of admission to the facility. The same standard might also specify what types of information will be included in the assessment.

For food production, some operations use photographs to show how products should look upon completion. Along with photos, specific standards may be listed. These standards may include both qualitative specifications and food safety or Hazard Analysis Critical Control Point (HACCP) specifications.

It is not always necessary, or even worthwhile, to write a quality standard for everything your operation does. However, through ongoing communications with both clients and superiors, it is practical to target specific products and/or services for which to specify standards. Standards themselves may need to be revisited and revised periodically.

Once quality standards are defined, you can evaluate and monitor quality. Standards also provide support to the process of training employees. In other words, every time you train an employee about what to do, also train the employee about what the results of the work should be. Incorporate the quality standards into the ongoing in-service education for all staff. This sets up a clear expectation and provides essential direction.

Glossary

PDCA
A cycle of process improvement: Plan, Do, Check, Act

Quality Standard
A facility's definition of what constitutes quality for an item or service

Figure 8.1 PDSA Worksheet for Testing Change

AIM: Overall goal you wish to achieve. Every goal will require multiple smaller tests of change.

Describe your first (or next) test of change	Person responsible	When to be done	Where to be done

PLAN:

List the tasks needed to set up this test of change	Person responsible	When to be done	Where to be done

Predict what will happen when the test is carried out	Person responsible	When to be done	Where to be done

DO: Describe what actually happened when you ran the test.

STUDY: Describe the measured results and how they compared to the predictions.

ACT: Describe what modifications to the plan will be made for the next cycle from what you learned.

Source: Institute for Healthcare Improvement

Effective Foodservice Quality Control Processes

Effective control of the quality process requires a proactive approach. Rather than waiting for a complaint or a set of poor survey results to surface, a quality-oriented Certified Dietary Manager monitors and improves quality continuously.

Quality management stems from clearly defined operating objectives and relates to all other aspects of the operation, including things like:

- Service and delivery systems
- Menu development
- Purchasing specifications
- Standardized recipe development
- Food production
- Scheduling of employees and tasks
- Employee performance standards
- Employee training
- And even the budget

Figure 8.2 illustrates the broad picture of how quality management fits into a manager's responsibilities.

In Step 1, the dining services department objectives are established. These should be in harmony with the broad purposes of the organization. In Step 2, strategies to attain objectives are planned. In Step 3, specific operating procedures are developed. Procedures may relate to product specifications, standardized recipes, equipment specifications, schedules, delivery procedures, and much more. Developing good initial procedures requires knowledge of the full scope of the dining operations as well as good judgment.

In Step 4, quality standards are developed. It is helpful to clarify these before beginning a new procedure. Objectively, these standards help define how you will know whether a procedure is effective. They provide a way to begin measuring effectiveness immediately.

Essential to the success of any quality management program is the involvement of employees. In Step 5, employees become aware of specific outcomes that you as a team need to achieve. By knowing what these outcomes are, employees can more readily help with adjusting the process down the line. Training is essential to ensure that everyone is working towards the same objectives.

After specific operating procedures have been developed, they must be implemented Step 6. In Step 7, the Certified Dietary Manager begins to evaluate the effectiveness of the dining services. Types of questions that will help in this evaluation include:

- How do quality results compare with the standards established?
- Did a procedure produce any unintentional or unexpected results?
  > If so, which of these is acceptable/not acceptable?
- Where results do not meet quality standards, what is the cause (or causes)?
- What interventions will address these causes?
- Is the procedure itself sound, or does it need to be revised?

Following evaluation, a Certified Dietary Manager needs to assess any revisions or adjustments that may be in order. Any intervention or procedural revision should be evaluated again. Sometimes several rounds of edits or revision are required to achieve intended results. In addition, involvement of employees and a team-oriented quality effort are typically the most effective in raising the quality of services or products. When employees are engaged in the process they have greater ownership of the outcomes.

With this big picture in mind, let's examine some of the tools a manager can use to gather information related to quality standards. These include taste panels, test meals, temperature, satisfaction surveys, plate waste studies, performance standards and checklists or self audits. Employee Performance Standards will be addressed in Chapter 12.

Figure 8.2 Quality Management Overview

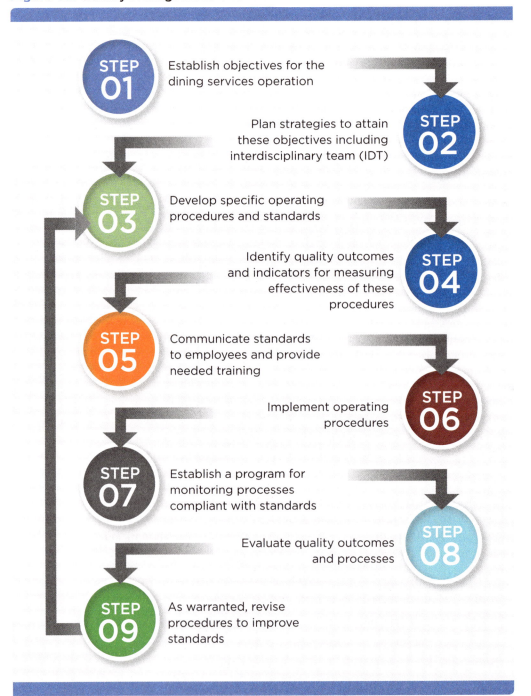

STEP 01 — Establish objectives for the dining services operation

STEP 02 — Plan strategies to attain these objectives including interdisciplinary team (IDT)

STEP 03 — Develop specific operating procedures and standards

STEP 04 — Identify quality outcomes and indicators for measuring effectiveness of these procedures

STEP 05 — Communicate standards to employees and provide needed training

STEP 06 — Implement operating procedures

STEP 07 — Establish a program for monitoring processes compliant with standards

STEP 08 — Evaluate quality outcomes and processes

STEP 09 — As warranted, revise procedures to improve standards

Taste Panels

A taste panel can help determine whether a product meets the given standards. It can also help you achieve an improved outcome of client satisfaction with food. The people on the panel should have knowledge about food standards and the ability to distinguish flavors. When practical, it may also be appropriate to include a few clients in a taste panel. For example, a dining services committee composed of clients in an assisted living community may be an excellent source of panelists.

In a formal taste panel, participants rate each product using a score sheet, such as the one shown in Figure 8.3. The score sheet notes taste, odor, flavor, color, texture, and appearance of the sample product.

The tastes, such as sweet, salty, bitter, and sour, along with the smell of a food, contribute to how people experience flavor. Taste sensitivity decreases with age, increasing the need for seasoning.

Color is also important. Many foods have characteristic colors closely identified with certain highly acceptable qualities. For example, the desired color of an apple is the color present when the fruit is at its peak of maturity. If the color is darkened or faded, the fruit is not perceived as being high in quality. Color sometimes does not reflect quality, as in the example of oranges. They may be mature in flavor but still be green in color. Thus, color is often a subjective—but very important—evaluation.

Texture is judged by the food item's characteristic texture, which may be stringy, smooth, crisp, mushy, tough, tender, or hard.

Glossary

Taste Panel
The evaluation or rating of items by a group of tasters

Figure 8.3 **Product Score Sheet**

Name: _____ Date: _____ Name of Product: _____

(Person on Taste Panel)

		Extremely Poor	Very Poor	Poor	Between Poor & Fair	Fair	Between Fair & Good	Good	Very Good	Extremely Good
TASTE	Sweet								✔	
	Salty									
	Bitter									
	Sour									
	Odor							✔		
	Flavor								✔	
	Color									✔
	Texture							✔		
	Appearance								✔	

Appearance refers to the exterior, interior, and portion size in a bowl or on a plate. Factors to consider include a characteristic and/or regular shape, unbroken pieces, correct portion size, proper moistness level, and good color. Is the interior appealing in terms of texture and color? Does the portion look attractive? Does it fit the container in which it is to be served?

Figure 8.4 outlines suggested quality standards for common food products. Realize that evaluation of a product is somewhat subjective and will reflect individual tastes and preferences. The information or feedback received through a taste panel, however, is very valuable. A manager can use taste panel feedback to adjust recipes and impact the quality of individual food products.

Several tips can help with managing food product quality. Both training programs and use of standardized recipes help an operation to produce food that is consistently high in quality. It's a good idea to interact with employees during food production, and to involve them in the evaluation process. To achieve a consistent food quality, several things must happen:

Figure 8.4 Suggested Quality Standards for Common Food Products

Yeast Bread	Golden brown color, symmetrical, uniform shape, rounded top, good volume, free of tunnels, moist, elastic crumb, nutlike flavor
Muffins	Golden brown color, well shaped with slightly rounded top, moist crumb, light and tender, good flavor, bumpy crust (smooth crust for cake-style muffins), free of tunnels, moist, elastic crumb, nutlike flavor
Cake	Golden brown color (except chocolate cake), smooth surface, slightly rounded top, high volume, fine grain, light but not crumbly, soft/moist texture, tender crumb, delicate sweet and well-blended flavor
Cookies	Uniform shape and color, good flavor, crisp or chewy texture (depending on type of cookie)
Pastry	Golden brown color, blistery surface, uniform and attractive edges, fits pan well, flaky or mealy texture, cuts easily, pleasant/bland flavor
Cream of Vegetable Soup	Thin white sauce base with off-white color; smooth texture that coats a spoon lightly, well blended flavor; vegetables should be finely chopped but have a shape.
Scalloped Potatoes	Potato slices uniform in size, potatoes are tender yet firm, has creamy white sauce, finely chopped onions cling to the potatoes, mild potato flavor with delicate flavor of sauce
Pasta	Cooked al dente, uniformly moist and tender to the bite, not sticky, mild starchy flavor
Oatmeal	Grains are tender, consistency is soft and forms a soft mass in the bowl; not gummy or sticky

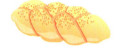

Adapted in part from Molt, M. Food for Fifty, 13th ed. Pearson Education, Inc., 2011.

- An expectation (standard) must be established and communicated to employees
- Employees need to be provided with products or ingredients consistent with the quality standard
- Employees must receive proper operational support to make quality possible.
  > This means you furnish the proper tools and equipment for the job, and schedule employees in such a way that necessary procedures and time frames are feasible
- All recipes need to be tested, scaled and standardized prior to inclusion on the menu
- Before being served, the final product must be checked for quality
  > Work with employees if the product does not meet the standard to coach them through problems and questions

Client reactions to the final product should be shared with employees. When the product receives praise, do not hesitate to pass this recognition on to the staff members who produced the food item. Information about a product that has been overcooked or over-seasoned should also be shared. Discuss whether the equipment is at fault, the recipe is a problem, or human error played a part in the unacceptable product.

Test Meals

Periodically, it is a good practice to prepare a **test meal** as a way of evaluating the service and the quality of foods as handled through a normal meal assembly system. A test meal (tray) is one assembled as part of the usual process, specifically for the purpose of quality evaluation. Some managers create a test meal by inserting a "dummy" tray card or menu ticket into the stack for meal assembly. For a realistic measure, a manager often does not identify this to tray employees as a test.

One strategy in preparing test meals is to make one that will test the outer limits of quality, or the worst case that may be occurring in the process. To evaluate the outer limits of quality, some managers position a test tray as one that will be created late in the tray assembly process, and/or one traveling the greatest distance for delivery.

Give this tray of food the same treatment as other trays receive. Deliver it to the service area and evaluate the tray. You can compare the tray to standards asking questions such as:

- Are hot foods served at or above 140°F?
- Are cold foods served at or below 41°F?
- Are colors bright?
- Are items on the tray in the correct locations?
- Are products served accurately (according to diet order)?
- Is food palatable and enjoyable?
- Is the meal attractively plated?

If "no" was the answer to any one of the questions, you can research the causes and make corrections.

Temperature and Quality

Note that temperature also plays a role in quality, even aside from food safety issues. Temperature often affects the texture of foods and it even affects flavor. Keep in mind that temperature affects the aromatic characteristics of food and smell contributes to taste. A hot food that has cooled may give off less aroma and prove less flavorful. A cold

Glossary

Test Meals
The evaluation of a sample meal as it is served

Putting It Into Practice

2. The test tray came back with the hot foods at 120°F. This is a concern because of client satisfaction and food safety. What are the steps you should take to correct this problem?

food that has warmed can also lose something; think of a warm soda pop with less fizz. This may help explain why seniors rate temperature over flavor in defining food quality.

Temperature and food quality are issues throughout the holding and service process. For example, frozen sweet peas placed in boiling water or steamed to an internal temperature of 200°F for 1-1/2 minutes will be hot and tasty. They will have a bright green color and be slightly crunchy. Frozen sweet peas held on a 212°F steam table for 80 minutes will look pale green and be mushy in texture. This is one reason for batch cooking vegetables and other products that are sensitive to the holding process.

Always check the temperature of the food during preparation and service:

- When panning up the food for the service line
  - > Do not transfer hot food to the trayline if the product is below standard
  - > Plan ahead and preheat the hot wells to avoid temperature loss on the line
- Check the temperature of food just before serving
- Take the temperature again midway through service
- Recheck the temperatures of backup items in a "hot-box"/oven before restocking the service line

Another aspect of temperature management is the balance between food safety guidelines and food preparation guidelines. In efforts to comply with food safety requirements, employees sometimes overcook foods by bringing them to temperatures that are too high, or cooking for excessive periods of time or both.

An example is a burger. To meet 2013 FDA Food Code recommendations, it must reach 155° for 115 seconds. To be safe, a standard practice is to overshoot the mark, and cook to a higher temperature. However, if the temperature goes much beyond 165°F, the burger may begin to become dry and unappealing. This is a delicate balance that requires careful planning and management. Some operations establish both minimum and maximum temperatures for certain products, especially for meats.

Satisfaction Surveys/Process Improvement

Identifying individual clients' food preferences should be a continual process and a component of clinical nutrition care in a healthcare facility. Beyond the individual care plan information or tray cards generated for healthcare clients, a manager needs to monitor trends in preferences and food acceptance. As a manager, one's role is to be continually alert to the changing expectations of the dining experience. For example, if a high number of clients request a substitution for meatloaf at lunch, this may be a clue that the meatloaf suffers a quality issue, or that the menu item itself is not a good choice for this group. Chapter 7 provides a more in-depth discussion of food acceptance surveys.

Plate Waste Studies

A **plate waste study** can also provide valuable information about food acceptance. Figure 8.5 illustrates a format for collecting plate waste information. In this process you review soiled trays before breaking them down and tabulate wasted or uneaten food. To make this information meaningful, it's important to randomly select a good proportion of soiled trays at any single meal. The benefit from conducting a plate waste study is the overall information you receive about specific food products. One example was a plate waste study where shrimp was served. Many plates contained wasted shrimp. Further investigation showed that too many shrimp were being served so the serving size was changed.

Glossary

Plate Waste Study
The evaluation of un-eaten food items returned for disposal

Putting It Into Practice

3. As you observe plate waste, you notice that many plates are returning with the green beans uneaten. What is the first step you should take to correct this problem?

Figure 8.5 Plate Waste Information

In the second column, tally the number of people who refused the product; use the third column to show how many plates came back with half the product, and the fourth column for empty plates.

CYCLE MENU:			
Wk 1, Day 3, Meal 3	**Plate Full of Product**	**Half the Food Consumed**	**Empty Plate**
Soup	III	IIII	IIII IIII II
Juice			
Salad	I	II	IIII IIII IIII II
Entrée	II	IIII I	IIII IIII II
Vegetable	IIII II	IIII IIII	III
Dessert	I	II	IIII IIII IIII II

If a product is repeatedly refused you may reassesses its quality, make adjustments, and re-check its acceptance in another plate waste study. Or maybe take it off the menu. You can also use this method to document the intake of specific clients being monitored through the nutrition care process. This would help you achieve an outcome for a specific client who needs to gain weight.

Plate waste studies are particularly helpful in identifying items to be replaced when planning a new menu and evaluating the approval of new items on the menu. In addition to the formal plate waste study is an ongoing dialog with, and observation of, the dishroom crew. They can tell you on a daily basis what food items are coming back on the trays as poorly eaten or not even touched.

Another source of plate waste information is the diet office. Frequent requests for second trays or substitute items for particular meals is a clear indication of a problem menu.

Checklists and Self-Audits

To ensure ongoing compliance with standards and regulations a Certified Dietary Manager can use checklists and **self-audits**. An audit is a systematic, documented method of evaluating an operation in comparison with established standards. When you perform a self-audit, your own operation (rather than surveyors from the outside) is conducting the audit as an internal quality management activity.

Formalizing the audit process with a tool such as a checklist helps ensure that you are reviewing every practice that contributes to quality processes in the operation. With a well-planned audit form, there is no question whether you've observed everything you should. The audit reminds you point by point.

A self-audit identifies exceptions or problems that can lead to an immediate plan to correct them. The benefit of performing a self-audit is that you can proactively identify problem areas and correct them without waiting for a surveyor to point them out.

Glossary

Self-Audit
A systematic internal "self" review of a process or procedure

By establishing a scheduled routine for self-audits, you can assure ongoing compliance. In fact, the best preparation for a survey—whether by a health department, **The Joint Commission (TJC)**, or a **Centers for Medicare & Medicaid Services (CMS)** survey team—is simply to comply with standards all the time. One example is consistently following the set of quality standards for common food products listed in Figure 8.4.

To create a self-audit tool, you can use the following steps:

1. Review all the standards with which you need to comply, along with your internal quality standards, and list criteria for quality and compliance.

   > When you have multiple standards, such as some from CMS, some from the health department, and some from your own facility, your job as a manager is to consolidate them into one list.

2. Translate each standard into clear, specific, measurable/observable inspection criteria that identify what you need to see to know that the criteria have been met.

   > It is not enough to say: The dining room will be pleasant. Instead list the factors that make the dining room pleasant, such as adequate lighting, cleanliness, minimal noise, attractive table settings, etc. By doing this, you develop a tool that leaves nothing to judgment or imagination. Your criteria can be applied consistently with clear expectations.

3. Group these inspection criteria by logical or functional area to create several different audits.

   > For example, you may develop a meal service audit, a food production audit, a food sanitation audit, a safety audit, a clinical care audit, and perhaps a few others. Ultimately, each tool you create should be clear-cut and easy to use. It should not be so long that no one wants to complete it!

On the next two pages, see Figure 8.6 for an example of a self-audit tool.

A Certified Dietary Manager typically delegates some auditing responsibilities to work teams. For example, an audit of the dining room service can include a supervisor and/or a few employees in this service area. Any time you place the audit into the hands of employees, you empower them to manage quality within their own realms of responsibility. You also give them the message that they are expected to work together to make quality a reality. An audit tool can also be a very effective training tool for new employees, and an aid for reviewing required procedures with experienced staff members.

In conducting a self-audit the assigned person should review the criteria, use a checkmark or other system to indicate whether the criteria are met, and add a plan for corrective action if warranted. Often, a problem can be corrected on the spot, and this is ideal. The employee who completes an audit should also date and sign the document, acknowledge responsibility and accountability, and return the form to the supervisor or manager.

Even when audits are conducted by others in your department it is important to review every completed audit document. Sometimes an audit will reveal chronic problems with procedures, training, equipment, or other issues that a manager needs to address. Ultimately, the manager is responsible for compliance with all established standards. Also, the manager should maintain completed audit documents for future reference and for surveyors who may request to see them.

In all, an ongoing self-audit procedure is an essential tool for managing quality. To ensure that audits occur, it is a good idea to create a schedule for audits and assign responsibility

Glossary

The Joint Commission (TJC)
A voluntary for-profit "accreditation organization (AO)" approved to provide the routine surveys to determine compliance for Medicare certification

Centers for Medicare & Medicaid Services (CMS)
The governmental agency responsible for the administration and management of Medicare and Medicaid

Figure 8.6 Meal Service Self-Audit Tool

Dining and Foodservice Audit	Yes	Sometimes	No	Correction Plan
1. Food complaints from residents, family, and others are routinely investigated.				
2. Results of food complaint investigations are appropriately documented.				
3. Dining room(s) has/have comfortable sound levels.				
4. Dining room(s) has/have adequate illumination.				
5. Dining room(s) has/have appropriate furnishings to meet resident needs and quality of life.				
6. Dining room(s) has/have adequate ventilation.				
7. Dining room(s) is/are absent of inappropriate odors.				
8. Dining room(s) has/have sufficient space.				
9. Resident rooms (where residents eat meals) have comfortable sound levels.				
10. Resident rooms (where residents eat meals) have adequate illumination.				
11. Resident rooms (where residents eat meals) have appropriate furnishings to meet meal service needs and quality of life.				
12. Resident rooms (where residents eat meals) have adequate ventilation.				
13. Resident rooms (where residents eat meals) are absent of inappropriate odors.				
14. Resident rooms (where residents eat meals) have sufficient space.				
15. Tables are adjusted to accommodate wheelchairs where meals are served.				
16. Appropriate hygiene is provided prior to meals.				
17. Resident eyeglasses, dentures, and/or hearing aids are in place prior to meals.				
18. Resident chairs, wheelchairs, gerichairs, etc., are at an appropriate distance from tables or tray tables.				
19. Assistive devices/utensils are identified in care plans.				
20. Assistive devices/utensils are provided and used as planned.				
21. Dishware and flatware is appropriate for each resident.				
22. Single-use disposable diningware is not used except in an emergency.				
23. Each resident has an appropriate place setting including water (except those with fluid restrictions).				
24. Meals are attractive (color, shape, presentation).				
25. Meals are palatable.				

Figure 8.6 Meal Service Self-Audit Tool *(Continued)*

Dining and Foodservice Audit	Yes	Sometimes	No	Correction Plan
26. Meals are at appropriate temperatures.				
27. Meals are served within 30 minutes of scheduled meal time.				
28. Substitutes are offered to residents as needed.				
29. Substitutes arrive within 15 minutes of request from resident.				
30. Diet cards list food preferences.				
31. Food preferences are honored.				
32. Correct portion sizes are served according to the menu.				
33. Condiment requests are honored.				
34. Residents are promptly assisted with eating.				
35. Appropriate verbal cuing is provided at meal times.				
36. Residents at the same table are served concurrently.				
37. Resident concerns regarding taste, temperature, quality, quantity, and appearance are addressed promptly and appropriately.				
38. Mechanically altered diets are prepared appropriately (ground, National Dysphagia Diet).				
39. Resident refusals of food items are addressed to determine reason(s) for refusal.				
40. Food placement, color, and textures address resident needs or deficits.				
41. Test tray sent to furthest unit is palatable and at correct temperatures.				
42. Medication pass does not interfere with quality of meal service.				
43. Pain medications are given prior to meals so that meals can be eaten in comfort.				
44. Foods served are not routinely or unnecessarily used as vehicle to administer medications.				
45. Meal intakes for food items are monitored accurately and in a timely manner.				
46. Intakes for fluids are monitored accurately and in a timely manner.				
47. Plates are returned to dining services with 75 percent or more of meals consumed.				
48. Dining Services staff are prepared to discuss dietary services with surveyor (staff assignments, meal monitoring procedures).				
49. Resident care plans regarding meals, feeding, dietary needs are followed at meal service.				

Note: This tool provides some audit criteria based on CMS standards, but is not comprehensive. Please consult your current standards to ensure all applicable criteria are met.

on a calendar. Then monitor to ensure that audits are completed on a timely and thorough basis and problems are addressed.

The Role of Expectations/Outcomes

Outcomes and expectations are related. When determining outcomes as a facility look at what your clients are expecting. Outcomes should address both their needs and their expectations.

To understand how clients perceive and rank quality it's critical to understand the role of expectations. Part of the evaluation of taste and quality boils down to whether a food matches what a client expects. Individually, we each have an idea of what a food should be like, and these ideas vary among all of us. Being different or putting a new twist on a traditional product is sometimes effective, but only if it is communicated in advance, so that the client will not be unhappily surprised.

Often quality becomes a gauge of whether the food a client receives is the food he expected. In any facility, this factor merits special attention. A recent poll of restaurant customers found the #1 reason for dissatisfaction was not receiving food as ordered or expected.

In serving clients who have given up some control of their own meals, it's especially important to evaluate expectations and plate accuracy. Tray assembly service systems require attention to how meal choices are gathered and honored. The move to restaurant service and room service models have improved client satisfaction results simply by offering more choices and allowing the client to select the meal as they want it.

In surveys, sometimes clients will comment that meals are not "accurate." This affects your client satisfaction outcomes. When this occurs, carefully evaluate what this means. Possible sources of a comment such as this include:

- The client did not complete a selective menu
- The client completed a selective menu, but did not understand which meal it indicated
- The client selected foods from a menu or by placing a phone call, and clinical staff had to adjust selections to meet a diet order
- The client has experienced a change in diet order that affected food choices on the tray
- The client asked the nurse for a specific food, and the request was not passed on to the dining services department
- The client asked for foods that are not available ("write-ins")
- A clinical staff person has not taken food preferences for the client or has not communicated them to tray assembly employee
- An error was made in processing orders, tray tickets, or plates
- An error was made in tray assembly
- A food shortage occurred, and the manager had to make a substitution
- A tray was properly assembled according to client's order and food was removed during transit or delivery

Clearly, many factors contribute to a perception of accuracy. When concerns about tray/plate accuracy arise, a manager should track the meal service process and identify the breakdown. Feedback in this area can also help to pinpoint areas that require stronger communications.

Consider this example: You learn that clients rated meal accuracy poorly for a certain meal. In tracking the service, you note that a macaroni and cheese was substituted for scalloped potato casserole. Two questions should come to mind:

- How did this occur, and what steps can be taken to prevent this in the future?

  > A solution may be as simple as revising the forecast figures for this product.

- Was the substitution explained to clients?

  > If it wasn't, then from a client's perspective, the switch was a mistake.

Although substitutions are not desirable in meal service, they are occasionally unavoidable. Some operations keep small substitution cards on hand and place these on trays when a substitution has to occur. This at least tells clients that the dining services department recognizes the change and that it was not an error. A substitution card may say something like:

> "Sorry! The item you requested was not available today, and we had to make a substitution. For further assistance with your meal service, please call extension 404."

Outcome measurements help bring the focus of all you do back to the client's needs and expectations.

External Standards for Quality

Some standards begin with sources external to your operation. In fact, both governmental and private associations may be involved in the evaluation of dining services—and thus, with the establishment of standards. For example, to support a healthcare facility with maintaining accreditation, you will need to assure that the dining services operation meets standards established by The Joint Commission (TJC). If your facility receives Medicare reimbursement for services, you may also be subject to certain standards enforced by the Centers for Medicare & Medicaid Services (CMS). In addition, you may be responsible for complying with specific standards for state and local agencies, as well as with sanitation standards as enforced by a state and/or local health department.

External standards form a backdrop for quality management in many healthcare organizations.

In a correctional facility, there may be other sets of standards affecting the dining services operation. For example, federal law stipulates religious freedom for inmates, and this carries through to honoring food choices related to religious convictions. State departments of corrections may also apply certain standards.

In a public school setting, standards for menu planning and program management come from the USDA for schools participating in the National School Lunch Program and seeking reimbursements and commodity foods.

The Joint Commission

There are several for-profit agencies that offer voluntary accreditation according to their established standards of care. They are not to be confused with the requirements of a state license or for the requirement to certify for federal funds. The most well known is The Joint Commissions (TJC).

Originally, The Joint Commission only accredited hospitals but it has moved into other healthcare facilities such as long-term care. CMS recognizes The Joint Commission as an "accreditation organization (AO)" approved to provide the routine surveys to determine compliance for Medicare certification. According to the Joint Commission, their mission is: *To continuously improve healthcare for the public, in collaboration with other stakeholders, by evaluating healthcare organizations and inspiring them to excel in providing safe and effective care of the highest quality and value.* The Joint Commission has established standards that each facility is measured against.

To comply with TJC standards, it is essential to review the current standards with others in your own organization. Check those labeled as pertaining to nutritional services, and then review those labeled under other categories too, as many standards are somewhat universal throughout the organization. For example, one standard will explain how to verify staff credentials and assure that they are up-to-date. Another will address disaster planning which is a facility-wide function.

Next clarify any standards that are unclear. Your own standards, in-house experts, a consulting dietitian, and colleagues may be sources of information.

Governmental Agencies and CMS

The National Social Security Act mandates that facilities participating in Medicare and Medicaid programs meet minimum health and safety standards. Medicare is a federal entitlement program where those 65 or older or people in other categories receive health insurance. Medicaid is a state administered, federally aided entitlement health and medical care program for certain people with low income or limited resources. The requirements pertain to hospitals, skilled nursing facilities, and a wide range of other providers and suppliers of health services.

The Medicare program is administered by CMS, which is an agency of the U.S. Department of Health and Human Services. States may also establish additional requirements under the Medicaid program. Typically the federal government sets minimum standards; states may develop more specific standards, and those that provide the greatest degree of control will apply.

An agency is designated in each state to carry out the requirements of the Social Security Act. Among other requirements is the need to visit facilities to assure that minimum standards are met and to complete various records.

While state-level officials are generally responsible for conducting on-site surveys for Medicare and Medicaid requirements, the federal government has several responsibilities:

- Review survey and certification reports submitted by state agencies
- Evaluate fiscal, administrative, and procedural aspects of its agreements with the states
- Conduct some on-site surveys of Medicare and Medicaid facilities
- Review and approve state budgets and expense reports dealing with survey/certification activities.

The Survey Process

Both TJC and CMS use surveys as part of their accreditation or enforcement effort. CMS contracts with state agencies for surveys of healthcare facilities. As part of its enforcement effort, CMS and its contracted state agencies conduct on-site surveys of healthcare facilities. Each time a team of surveyors arrives to evaluate compliance of a healthcare facility with CMS regulations all managers become involved. A survey is typically unannounced and may occur on any day of the week. A standard long-term care (LTC) survey is designed to review compliance with CMS regulations, including all the detail of the various F-Tags. A new survey process for long-term care was beta-tested in six states. It is called the CMS **Quality Indicator Survey** or QIS. National implementation of the QIS is progressing state-by-state as resources are available to conduct training of state and federal surveyors. The QIS process provides for the review of larger samples of clients based on the **Minimum Data Set (MDS)**, observations, interviews, and clinical record reviews.

A Certified Dietary Manager is involved in many quality management issues. Interdisciplinary effort is a strong focus of quality management and CMS regulations. Thus, neither surveyors nor administrators, divide up CMS regulations and hand a section to a single manager for response. Nonetheless, the manager is often the most accessible person during a survey. You need to understand the regulations, your facility's quality assessment process, and how your data supports your performance improvement.

Each state agency designated to administer the Medicare and Medicaid programs has several duties, which taken together, are referred to as the certification process. Since the standards used will change, they are not included in this text.

These basic standards may be combined into an overall facility requirement. The state agency is responsible for the following:

- Identify as many qualified providers and suppliers of health services as possible. There must be eligible facilities on a state-wide basis.

- Conduct investigations and fact-finding surveys to determine how well participating facilities comply with requirements. Often this investigation is done in conjunction with the state's own licensure and other regulatory programs.

- Complete certification, re-certification, and periodic follow-up reports dealing with whether facilities are qualified to participate in programs.

- Provide consultative services to providers and suppliers and to those seeking eligibility for the program in order to help them maintain required standards and qualify for participation.

As a Certified Dietary Manager, it is your responsibility to be very familiar with the rules and regulations established in the state for the type of facility where you work. It is also your responsibility to work collaboratively and cooperatively with the Interdisciplinary Team (IDT).

In the most general terms, the manager must provide a nutritionally adequate diet. The diet should supply the nutrients for the age group being served. The modified diets ordered by the doctor, or medical care provider, should be followed using the guidelines set forth in the diet manual approved at the facility. The authorized clinical nutrition representative (certified dietary manager, registered dietitian nutritionist or dietetic technician, registered) may make suggestions for diet changes in the medical record, but the individual who has ultimate responsibility to issue an order should be carefully

Glossary

Quality Indicator Survey (QIs)
Automated review of client data to help systemize the survey process

Minimum Data Set (MDS)
A standardized record of client screening and assessment required for Medicare clients

Putting It Into Practice

4. What are some steps you can take to help prepare your staff for a state survey?

considered; in some states and/or facilities, this choice may be dictated by licensure laws and/or policies of the facility.

There are food and nutrition related guidelines incorporated throughout the Medicare and state requirements for certification. F-Tags related to residents dignity and the use of tube feedings were examples in Chapter 7. In addition, the minimum time allowed between the last meal in the evening to the first meal in the morning may be specified in requirements (e.g., 14 hours between the evening meal or major evening snack and breakfast).

A facility that participates in Medicare must also meet the conditions established by the federal government. Discuss these conditions with the administrator in order to understand the role that dining services plays in meeting the requirements.

Surveys and Certification

There is a close relationship among the certification process, state license requirements, programs for professional accreditation (such as TJC), and medical assistance standards. Typically, the relationships among these standards require close coordination and information exchange. For example, healthcare facilities cannot qualify for Medicare assistance unless they have first been licensed by the state. Standards used by TJC generally meet many of the standards issued by the federal government. Thus, the facility is not faced with sets of conflicting standards which make compliance with any defined standards impossible. The guidelines, recommendations, standards, and interpretations of each regulatory agency and professional association interface to provide guidelines for managing healthcare facilities.

It is important to be up-to-date with a set of current requirements. CMS regulations change continuously. Unlike TJC, there may be variations in standards administered from one state to another, so your state must be used as a source of information. To verify the standards for which you are responsible, work with your own administrator or IDT, and ask for copies of the standards. Also be aware that the CMS website (www.cms.gov) provides information and clarification. One of its features allows users to request clarification about specific standards and to review questions and answers from others. An entire section specifically addresses the "kitchen/food service observations".

CMS standards address many basic requirements, such as the need to establish menus, to assure that required nutrients are provided, and that food is palatable and safe. They also emphasize honoring the needs of individual clients and providing substitutions or alternates when requested. In addition, they stipulate a maximum time that may elapse from dinner to breakfast. They address staffing, dining room environment, and more. Like TJC standards, the CMS survey protocol includes a section about foodservice, as well as information in other sections that is pertinent to foodservice. Consider the following examples:

- Clients' rights and the right to refuse case apply to dietary choices and the right to refuse nutritional support
- Confidentiality procedures relate toe everyone handling client information, which of course includes foodservice staff
  > **HIPAA** is the federal Health Insurance Portability and Accountability Act of 1996 with the goal to protect the confidentiality and security of healthcare information
- Standards relating to infection control have cross-over implications for sanitation and food safety in a foodservice operation

Glossary

HIPAA
1996 law on Health Insurance Portability and Accountability Act

Putting It Into Practice

5. When the surveyors arrive at your facility, what should you do?

- A number of standards relating to nutritional status, hydration, and feeding assistance (if required) are truly interdepartmental issues

  > For example, in honoring a diet order for thick liquids, both nursing and dining services staff need to work together to assure this is carried through

  > In tracking weight changes or malnutrition, staff must also work together closely to monitor progress and implement therapeutic plans

In a long-term care environment, it is easy to understand that clients' clinical needs may change over time. So, CMS documentation requirements stipulate a schedule for assessing clients. For example, an admission assessment must be completed within a resident's first five days in the facility. Another assessment is required at approximately a two-week point, and then approximately monthly afterwards. Any major clinical change also signals the need for an assessment.

Certification, Surveys and Quality Management

While all of this activity serves to ensure critical reimbursements to an institution, it also has an interesting bearing on quality management. A protocol for assessment serves as a type of quality management tool, and a way of ensuring that services are (dynamically) geared towards what each client needs. Clinical assessments are a very client-specific, proactive quality management tool.

CMS also uses quality indicators for tracking and benchmarking care. Quality indicators highlight issues relating to clinical care. Several quality indicators are very specific to nutritional care, as implemented by the healthcare team. For more information about quality indicators and CMS standards for clinical nutritional care and documentation, please consult *Nutrition Fundamentals and Medical Nutrition Therapy* (ANFP, 2015) or the CMS website. As a Certified Dietary Manager, you can weave this into your routine quality management procedures and evaluate this information as you would any other quality data.

The Centers for Medicare & Medicaid Services (CMS) initiated a five-star quality rating system for nursing homes in December 2008 that resembles the "star" rating system that measures quality in hotel chains. Clarity and public awareness is what CMS is hoping to provide from this initiative. Giving consumers a recognizable scale to search for quality elder care is what prompted the creation of the five-star quality ratings. The ratings are based on three separate categories:

1) Health Inspections

2) Quality Measures

8) Staffing Levels

Each category is assigned from one to five stars, with one star being the lowest rating and five stars the highest. CMS includes this statement when describing the rating's merits.

> *"Nursing homes with five stars are considered to have above average quality compared to other nursing homes in that state. Nursing homes with one star have quality much below the average in that state (but the nursing home still meets Medicare's minimum Requirements)."*

Legal Implications

Surveyors look at what you do for quality assurance and at how you are using the data for performance improvement. CMS has language in both the hospital and long-term care regulations that facilities must:

- Develop, implement, and maintain an effective, ongoing, facility-wide, data-driven quality assessment and performance improvement program
- Involve all departments and services
- Focus on indicators related to improved health outcomes.

At the time of a survey, a Certified Dietary Manager may be asked to provide documentation and pertinent information. Surveyors will focus on quality indicators. They will review medical records and interview clients. Part of the survey may include a detailed tour of foodservice areas. A manager should accompany a surveyor and cooperate fully. When the survey concludes, the survey team will state any deficiencies noted and reference F-Tag numbers.

A deficiency is a finding that the facility is not in compliance with CMS Guidelines. The facility is cited and instructed to correct the deficiency. Deficiencies are categorized by the level of risk/harm that may occur. If a problem is identified, the manager and other members of the interdisciplinary team need to follow up promptly and effectively to correct them. If deficiencies are not corrected within a reasonable amount of time, the facility may be shut down.

In all, a Certified Dietary Manager plays a critical role in assuring that quality of dining services meets the needs of the clients and that the end results of care are excellent.

Position Analysis and Staffing Needs

Overview and Objectives

Planning for staffing needs involves anticipating the future, and what it will require in personnel. Tools such as job descriptions and job analyses help define the staffing needs in the facility. Calculating the number of FTEs, planning for appropriate staff in response to changes in census and the impact on the budget are all functions of Personnel Needs. After completing this chapter, you should be able to:

✓ Differentiate between Job Descriptions, Workflows and Job Routines

✓ Assess the Staffing Needs

✓ Conduct a task analysis through a Workflow Process

✓ Write job descriptions

✓ Prepare an organization chart for the department

Staffing is one of the major functions of a Certified Dietary Manager and is defined as the selection, training, management and development of employees to fulfill the Dining Services department needs. Determining current and future personnel demands is done through a needs analysis by reviewing staffing history data and trends. In many dining services departments with long-term staff it will be especially important to consider future hiring needs. When conducting a personnel needs analysis there are several factors to consider.

Strategic Plan

Most facilities today have some type of strategic plan in place that outlines the goals and objectives for the future. Your personnel needs analysis has to fit within that strategic plan. For instance, let's say one objective of the facility's strategic plan is to *expand community outreach*. One way to implement that would be to expand your cafeteria to serve community residents. That would impact the dining services personnel needs analysis as your need for human resources/staffing would likely increase.

Full-Time Equivalents (FTEs)

As part of the job of organizing work, a manager must coordinate job descriptions, staffing plans, and **full-time equivalents (FTEs)**. FTEs, discussed in greater detail in Chapter 12, are a way of measuring how many hours of work go into an overall labor budget. One person working full-time translates into one FTE. The definition of how many hours constitutes a full-time employee can vary from organization to organization.

Glossary

Full-Time Equivalents (FTEs)
One person working full-time translates into one FTE. The number of hours that constitutes full-time can vary. The most common definition is 40 hours per week or 2080 per year

Typically the benchmark is 40 hours per week, times 52 weeks is a total of 2080 paid time (scheduled work time, vacation, holidays and sick time) in a year. Some companies define full-time as 32 or 35 hours a week. This makes labor comparisons based on FTEs between organizations difficult when their definitions vary.

The number of FTEs in a department is a simple math calculation based on:

$$\frac{\text{Total number of hours paid in a year or week}}{\text{The number of hours in your FTE definition}} \quad \textbf{OR} \quad \frac{495 \text{ hrs.}}{40} = 12.4 \text{ FTEs}$$

The number of FTEs is not equal to the number of employees in a department. Often employees are part-time staff members and do not work a full-time schedule.

For budgeting purposes, the Certified Dietary Manager may be held to both the hours paid for department staff **and** separately the total dollars paid. The Certified Dietary Manager must ensure that the master staffing pattern matches the budget for FTEs and labor costs.

Budget

As you analyze your personnel needs keep in mind that whatever staffing needs you determine will have to be consistent with the budget. One way to minimize adding staff is by analyzing the tasks that each position performs. Many of the tasks may work well for utilizing cross-trained staff from other departments, such as the environmental department who may also be able to assist with dining room service. Cross-training your staff can allow you to more efficiently use your labor budget.

Trends and Forecasting

As part of the budget planning process related to labor and staffing, the Certified Dietary Managers should be flexible as staffing needs develop. Today's fast-changing dining services may foster personnel concerns you are not even aware. Participating on a work team, comprised of human resource department representatives, top dining services department staff, and other management staff within the department, is useful. As you look at trends and forecasting future staffing needs, use the data that either your department or human resources department should have:

- Turnover rate
- Staffing levels
- Retirement eligibility.

If your human resource department does not calculate turnover rate you can easily calculate that for your own department. Decide what length of time you want to consider. Six months or a year is typically used. Determine the average number of employees over that time. Total the number of employees who left your employment during that time. Divide the number of employees who left by the average number of employees to determine your turnover rate.

January 1 – December 31 Average number of employees = 16

January 1 – December 31 Number who left employment = 2

2 ÷ 16 = .125 x 100 = 12.5% turnover rate

A 12.5% turnover rate is considered very low in comparison to the restaurant industry where turnover rate can be as high as 80%.

Forecasting the staffing needs allow you to plan for recruiting, hiring and training before the issue becomes a crisis.

- Anticipate the number of staff retirements in the coming year
- Recognize long-term illness or surgical concerns
- Identify the number of employees returning to school in September
- Calculate the turnover rate
- Define the labor impact of planned new services or reductions in services (i.e. 3rd floor is scheduled for four months of renovation starting in May)

External Environment

Employment laws also affect your staffing levels. The Certified Dietary Manager mustmake sure that all policies dealing with staffing and human resources are developed within the framework of the employment laws. If you have an HR (human resources) department, work with them to develop goals and developmental programs for staff members who are new, in training, or in career advancement modes. If you don't have an HR department work with your administrator to make sure you are following the employment laws.

Another external influence on your staffing will be the CMS (Centers for Medicare & Medicaid Services) regulations. For instance, both state and federal regulations may address staffing in your department. An example of the regulations in the State of Texas reads as follows:

> "The facility must employ a qualified dietitian either full-time, part-time, or on a consultant basis…"

> **§19.1103 Sufficient Staffing**

> "The facility must employ sufficient dietary support personnel who are competent to carry out the functions of the dietary service."

It will be very important to pay attention to these considerations as you analyze your personnel needs. The basic steps are shown in Figure 9.1.

In staffing the bottom line is that planning for the future is the only effective way to ensure that the number of surprises will be minimal. While no one can predict what will happen in the future, a great deal of your human resources requirement can, in fact, be predicted. By planning and taking appropriate action, you help to ensure that your operation will continue to function smoothly now and in the future. A Certified Dietary Manager is perpetually thinking about these steps on a daily basis in order to meet ongoing staffing needs.

In contrast to the broad issue of staffing, a manager must also consider the finer detail involved in scheduling, or planning employees' specific activities and assignments from day-to-day.

Tools that help a manager with scheduling include a staffing pattern, a job analysis and a job description.

Putting It Into Practice

1. Your department has a staff of 55. If your turnover rate has been about 15%, your staffing level is 95%, and you know of four employees who will retire next year, forecast your hiring needs for next year.

Figure 9.1 Steps in Personnel Needs Analysis

1 Forecast future personnel needs—The forecasting of future needs should be in harmony with growth

2 Determine base staffing pattern needs—What are the minimum positions and hours needed on a daily basis

3 Conduct inventory of current staff—What are the skills, abilities, interests, and needs of currently employed staff members?

4 Assess staff planning needs—Consider planned vacancies or changes

5 Develop internal training/education activities—Depending upon your needs, retrain staff *OR*

6 Plan for new recruitments, selection and training procedures—Recruit, select and train new staff

7 Design program monitoring systems—Develop a way to monitor your progress (how many staff were hired, trained, etc.?)

8 Control and evaluate planning systems—Evaluate how your analysis is working and make adjustments if necessary

Staffing Pattern

The **staffing pattern** defines what positions are needed each day of the week. Employee names and tasks are not included. The staffing pattern is based on the optimal number of positions to meet production and meal service needs. Typically Saturdays and Sundays are staffed lighter than during the the typical five day work week, so some positions may be covered only five days a week instead of every day.

The staffing pattern may also adjust for increased labor needs on the scheduled foodservice vendor delivery days. Evaluation of the menu may indicate that a staff person is needed on Mondays only. Likewise, coverage of a position needs does not always require an 8 hour shift.

The sample staffing pattern shown in Figure 9.2 is for an organization with a small cafeteria that is open for breakfast and lunch only on the weekends. See how the staffing needs change from day to day which in turns affects how many employees are scheduled each day.

Comparing the desired staffing pattern to your current schedule can help identify where the plan does not match the reality.

- How well does the Staffing Pattern compare to the actual number of positions you schedule and the total hours paid each week?

Glossary

Staffing Pattern
The base schedule of positions needed each day

Figure 9.2 Sample Staffing Pattern

Position Title	Short Title	Start-Stop Times	HOURS NEEDED EACH DAY							Total Hrs/ Wk	40 Hr. FTEs
			Mon	Tues	Wed	Thu	Fri	Sat	Sun		
AM Cook	CK1	5:30-1:00	8	8	8	8	8	8	8	56	1.4
Patient Cook	PtCk	7:30-4:00	8	8	8	8	8	8	8	56	1.4
Late Cook	CK2	10:30-7:00	8	8	8	8	8	8	8	56	1.4
Grill Cook	CrCK	10:00-2:00	4	4	4	4	4			20	1.4
Salads & Desserts	S&D	9:00-5:30	8	8	8	8	8			40	1
Salads Weekends	S&D2	9:00-2:00						4.5	4.5	9	0.2
Storeroom Aide	StRm	7:00-3:00		8			8			16	0.4
Trayline Supervisor AM	TLSup1	5:30-1:00	8	8	8	8	8	8	8	56	1.4
Trayline Supervisor PM	TLSup2	11:00-7:30	8	8	8	8	8	8	8	56	1.4
Foodservice Worker 1	FSW1	6:00-2:30	8	8	8	8	8	8	8	56	1.4
Foodservice Worker 2	FSW2	6:00-2:30	8	8	8	8	8	8	8	56	1.4
Foodservice Worker 3	FSW3	6:00-2:30	8	8	8	8	8	8	8	56	1.4
Foodservice Worker 4	FSW4	6:00-2:30	8	8	8	8	8	8	8	56	1.4
Foodservice Worker 5	FSW5	6:00-2:30	8	8	8	8	8	8	8	56	1.4
Foodservice Worker 6	FSW6	4:00-7:30	3.5	3.5	3.5	3.5	3.5	3.5	3.5	24.5	0.5
Foodservice Worker 7	FSW7	4:00-7:30	3.5	3.5	3.5	3.5	3.5	3.5	3.5	24.5	0.5
Foodservice Worker 8	FSW8	4:00-7:30	3.5	3.5	3.5	3.5	3.5	3.5	3.5	24.5	0.5
Foodservice Worker 9	FSW9	4:00-7:30	3.5	3.5	3.5	3.5	3.5	3.5	3.5	24.5	0.5
Foodservice Worker 10	FSW10	4:00-7:30	3.5	3.5	3.5	3.5	3.5	3.5	3.5	24.5	0.5
Cafeteria Cashier	FSW1	6:00-2:30	8	8	8	8	8	8	8	56	1.4
Cafeteria Server	FSW2	10:00-2:00	4	4	4	4	4			20	0.5
Cafeteria Cashier	FSW1	11:00-7:30	8	8	8	8	8			40	1
Catering	CTR	6:30-3:00	8	8	8					24	0.6
		Total Hours	138	146	138	130	138	110	110	907.5	
		Total FTEs	17.2	18.2	17.2	16.2	17.2	13.8	13.8		22.7
		Total Positions	21	22	21	20	21	17	17		

- Are you right on or do you find that there are some days that you have coverage and others that you are really short?

- Do you have the right staff to cover the positions as needed or are you short in some areas?

- If you need to make some changes and rearrange the employee schedule to better meet the Staffing Pattern, where and how will you do that?

- Often labor and staffing is the target of expense reduction. Can you reduce your staffing schedule?

All of these questions are wrapped up in the Job Analysis or Position Workflow. What position is assigned to complete specific tasks and are all needed tasks assigned to some position?

Workflow and Job Analysis

A detailed Job Analysis starts with looking at everything that needs to be done and assigning the appropriate amount of time to completing the tasks. The easiest way to see the whole day is to lay it out in what is called a **Gantt Chart** or a timeline.

Figure 9.3 is an example of a **Job Analysis Workflow** being developed.

- Each position is listed with start & stop times
- Time sensitive deadlines (meal service times) are highlighted
- Major tasks to be completed by the different positions are entered
- The planned time needed to complete the task is blocked out

This is an exercise without employee names or "Sally always does xyz…." Tasks are assigned to the position not the person. The tasks are individual events to be sorted into a logical workflow for the day. By reducing a lot of back-tracking and creating a workflow of related tasks the job analysis can improve the daily task assignments to flow more logically throughout the workday.

A well done job analysis workflow identifies what each position is assigned to do and confirms how many positions are needed to complete the assigned tasks. If large blocks of unassigned times are identified the workflow can be used to develop a position consolidation and reduce hours on the schedule. Likewise, if there are a number of unassigned tasks with no open labor time available, the workflow can help justify the need for an added position in the department.

Figure 9.4 shows a summary of an individual job analysis for a Hot Foods Cook. Notice that it divides the job of preparing food into individual tasks. A job analysis summary lists tasks specifically and concretely but does not spell out procedures for doing the work. For example, if you are writing a job analysis for a receiving clerk, it is appropriate to list tasks such as: "Checks food deliveries against invoice" or "Rejects food deliveries that do not meet established standards for quality and sanitation." However, it is not useful to write tasks such as: "Uses good judgment," because this does not tell what the employee actually does.

Glossary

Gantt Chart
A spreadsheet with a timeline to design task assignments by staff position

Job Analysis Workflow
The completed Gantt Chart for all positions and all tasks within the department

Figure 9.3 Sample Job Analysis Workflow

Job Workflow Spreadsheet for:

Date Revised:

Position	06:00	06:15	06:30	06:45	07:00	07:15	07:30	07:45	08:00	08:15	08:30	08:45	09:00	09:15
Supervisor 6-2:30	Opening set up & staffing assign				Breakfast									
Supervisor 11-7:30														
Diet Office 5:30-2	Review Diet Order		Prep Menus		Phone, Computer, Late Trays									
Diet Office 10:30-7														
Trayline 6-2:30	Prep Cold Food		Set Line		Breakfast				Clean	Break	Dishroom			
Trayline 6-2:30	Wrap Silver/ Trays		Set Line		Breakfast				Clean	Break	Dishroom			
Trayline 6-2:30	Prep Cold Food				Breakfast				Clean	Break	Dishroom			
Café 6-2:30	Set-Up		Café Breakfast Service											
Café 6-2:30	Set-Up		Café Breakfast Service											

Figure 9.4 Job Analysis Summary

- Withdraw ingredients from food stores and document on requisition form
- Use food production sheet and standardized recipes to measure ingredients per standard procedures
- Complete food preparation of all assigned hot food items per standardized recipe instructions
- Create pureed versions of assigned products per procedures
- Complete HACCP records for food prepared
- Arrange presentation and garnish food per recipe
- Cover and label food products; take foods to hot holding area
- Clean up work area
- Complete pre-prep for next day
- Complete leftover records after meal service
- Discard or label and store leftovers per procedures

Job Routines

Based on the Job Analysis Workflow for each position, you can develop the individual Job Routines. While the Gantt Chart of the workflow helps the team see that all of the tasks are assigned and the flow through the day is smooth and balanced, it is not easy to read and follow. **Job Routines** are the daily workflow for an individual position.

The level of detail can be fairly general, such as "7:30 to 8:15 serve meals" or highly specific, such as "2:00 to 2:15 deliver snacks" on 4 West. Anticipated times for Breaks and Lunch are usually included as well as "Side-Work" like: clean and restock Starter's Station for next meal. Each position should have a thought-out workflow and assigned tasks for the day defining the primary duties and assigned side-work.

Competencies or Skills Needed By Staff

Once the staffing pattern is defined and the job analysis workflow has been completed you need to determine the skill sets required of each position. A potential employee's skills and knowledge must match the requirements of the job. For example, an upscale catering service will require the expertise of someone trained in culinary arts. The job of serving clients in the dining room will require excellent customer service and people skills, along with an ability to work in an organized and efficient manner. It is important to identify what skills would be considered essential for each type of staff position based on the type and style of facility you manage.

Job Descriptions

What exactly is a job? The word "job" or "position" describes the tasks an employee is responsible and accountable for performing. Positions have titles to help you refer to them. Titles are shown on organization charts, on schedules, and in descriptions of the job themselves. Jobs are not the same thing as individual people.

For example, you may have a job titled Morning Cashier. This is a position with a set of assigned responsibilities. One day, an employee named Mary may fill this position. The next day, a different employee, named Carlos, may fill it. The job title simply refers to the set of assigned work.

Tasks are the individual activities that, together, comprise a job. For example, the morning cashier job may involve tasks such as:

- Setting up the cash register or point of sale system.
- Counting the bank and verifying that it is accurate.
- Checking out clients; and many others.

The job of a trayline employee may involve tasks such as:

- Transporting food and supplies to the trayline.
- Portioning food.
- Cleaning the tray assembly line and work area after other tasks have been completed.

Tasks such as these are outlined in a **Job Description**. A job description is the official, written account of an employment position. It tells what the employee is responsible for doing. It defines to whom the employee reports. It specifies the typical working hours of the job and generally where the person works (such as dining room, receiving dock, trayline, dishroom, etc.).

Putting It Into Practice

2. Your facility is going to renovate the east wing reducing your meals by 15% for the next 6 months. What tools can you use to plan for this reduction in service?

A job description also documents the qualifications a person must meet to be placed in this job and the salary range for the position. It forms the basis for evaluating employees' performance. Duties and expectations defined in the job description help managers structure coaching activities and will aide in the discipline or termination of an employee.

What to Include in the Job Descriptions

The job description is a written documentation of the general responsibilities and duties of a job category. A well written job description defines for the employee, and the employer, what is expected of them. You need enough detail to provide a clear picture of the job but not so detailed that a separate job description is needed for each position or title within the department.

A job description should be written for each type of position in the dining services operation. For example, there should be a job description for Cook with a list of the tasks and responsibilities which could include the morning cook, main line cook, late cook, patient cook and possibly even the grill cook. The different positions represent all of the locations that the Cook may be assigned to but they are not different job descriptions. Likewise a Dining Services Worker may be assigned to the trayline, passing trays, the dishroom or cut & plate in cold food. While these are very different tasks they typically are not different job descriptions.

A sample job description appears in Figure 9.5. The exact format of a job description is usually set by your organization, and may include most or all of the following sections:

- Job title
- Section or department
- Supervisor's title
- Brief summary of basic responsibilities
- Description of duties
- Working conditions (e.g., heavy lifting involved)
- Employment qualifications or minimum job requirements
- Education and experience requirements
- Conditions of employment (e.g., health and drug screening)
- Wage scale
- Date developed or last revised

Job descriptions answer several questions, such as: What are the tasks an employee in this position must perform? Who supervises an employee in this position? What knowledge and skills must a candidate possess to qualify for this position? What is the pay scale for anyone who holds this position?

Managers can use job descriptions as tools because they clarify who is responsible for what, e.g., who receives food deliveries—the dining services supervisor or the cook. Occasionally, a manager may need to reference job descriptions with employees to clarify disagreements. Most managers use job descriptions as a communication tool to help define expectations of employees during job interviews, new employee orientation, and later in performance evaluation.

Job descriptions also indicate how each position relates to other positions in the dining services department. As such, they lay the foundation for the flow of communication,

Figure 9.5 Job Description: Certified Dietary Manager (Sample)

General Summary of Work: Responsible for the daily operations of foodservice department according to facility policy and procedures and federal/state regulations. Provides leadership and guidance to ensure that food quality, safety standards, and client expectations are satisfactorily met. Maintains records of department personnel, income and expenditures, food, supplies, inventory levels, and equipment.

PRINCIPLE TASKS

Operations Management

- Recruit, interview, hire, train, coach, evaluate, reward, discipline, and when necessary, terminate employees
- Develop job descriptions and job duties for each level of foodservice personnel
- Develop work schedules to ensure adequate staff to cover each shift
- Create and monitor budgets for a cost-effective program
- Manage revenue generating services
- Use forecasts, food waste records, inventory and equipment records to plan the purchase of food, supplies and equipment
- Justify improvements in the department design and layout
- Work cooperatively with clients, facility staff, physicians, consultants, vendors, and other service providers

Foodservice Management

- Specify standards and procedures for preparing food
- Participate in menu planning including responding to client preferences, substitution lists, therapeutic diets, and industry trends
- Inspect meals and assure that standards for appearance, palatability, temperature, and servings times are met
- Manage the preparation and service of special nourishments and supplemental feedings
- Assure that foods are prepared according to production schedules, menus, and standardized recipes

Food Safety

- Assure safe receiving, storage, preparation, and service of food
- Protect food in all phases of preparation, holding, service, cooking, and transportation, using HACCP Guidelines
- Prepare cleaning schedules and maintain equipment to ensure food safety
- Ensure proper sanitation and safety practices of staff

Nutrition and Medical Nutrition Therapy

- Process new diet orders and diet changes; keeps diet cards updated
- Complete the assigned MDS section according to required timeline
- Determine client diet needs and develop appropriate dietary plans in cooperation with RD and in compliance with physicians' orders
- Review plan of care related to nutritional status; document concerns that can be resolved, improved or addressed to improve client's nutritional status and eating function
- Review, revise, and implement, in cooperation with the IDT, the client's nutrition assessment and plan of care
- Supports Registered Dietitian Nutritionist duties as needed

GENERAL KNOWLEDGE, SKILLS AND ABILITIES

- Skill in motivating, coaching, and supervising foodservice personnel
- Intermediate computer skills
- Mathematical and numerical skills; mechanical aptitude helpful
- Has effective written and oral communication skills
- Demonstrated organizational skills
- Has current awareness of legislation and regulations influencing the practice of standards of care

EDUCATION REQUIREMENTS

- Graduate of Dietary Manager's Program, 2-yr, or 4-yr foodservice program
- Successful completion of Certified Dietary Manager exam
- Two years' experience in foodservice management
- Prior experience in healthcare foodservice preferred

PHYSICAL DEMANDS/WORKING CONDITIONS

- Able to lift and carry in excess of 50 lbs.
- Able to withstand extreme temperatures, hot and cold
- Able to work long hours, including some evenings, weekends, holidays, as needed
- Able to interact positively with a variety of personalities and populations

authority, and responsibility throughout the organization. They help a manager organize positions into work sections to form a basis for developing effective labor control systems.

Note that many organizations end a list of duties in a job description with this point: "Other duties as assigned." This addresses the fact that some flexibility is required. There may be one day when your department has an unexpected need to serve coffee and breakfast rolls to an ad hoc Board of Directors meeting in your building. To whom will you assign the work of providing this food? It may not fall under anyone's job description. There may be another day when two employees call you early in the morning and say they are unable to report to work. You may have to divide their responsibilities among other employees who are working today.

These are just examples of why flexibility is important. From a management perspective, it is best to communicate your expectation of flexibility from the beginning with every employee. This minimizes surprises and possible resistance down the line.

From the general to the specific, job descriptions and job routines guide management and staff in completing the tasks at hand and reaching the department goals: Service to our clientele. Figure 9.6 shows how these concepts relate.

Another benefit of the job analysis and a well written job description, is that it helps identify what standard operating procedures you should develop. The performance expectations also help determine what the audit monitors should track for the Quality Improvement Process.

Figure 9.6 Job Description to Job Routines

JOB DESCRIPTIONS	• General description of what a job can encompass • Foodservie worker: generic title • Cook: includes grill, patient, cafe
POSITION/ TITLES	• More detailed "sub-categories" of what the job actually does • A foodservice worker can be a trayline server, cafeteria server, dining room assistant, dishroom attendant, tray passer
JOB ROUTINES	• Specific daily assignment of tasks to individual positions • A trayline server can be on the hot-line, starter, loader, cart delivery, etc. • Based on a Gantt Chart of the daily workflow

You should maintain a reference of all job descriptions in your department. This may be on your computer network, as well as in a notebook. As jobs change, it is important to review, and if needed, update job descriptions. The survey process and Quality Assurance Plans often specify annual dated and signed reviews to ensure that Job Descriptions are current.

An Organization Chart

As you write job routines for new positions you add them to your organization chart. An **organization chart** is a fundamental management tool that represents task groupings and responsibilities in a graphical form. An organization chart (often referred to as the "org chart") shows the names of task groupings as departments or something similar. In a few words, it defines responsibilities.

Boxes representing groupings and/or positions (managers) are connected with solid lines signifying responsibility, authority, and accountability. In a traditional organization chart authority flows from the top of the chart to the bottom. This tool does not tell everything, however, it provides a useful framework for organizing the structure of an facility. An organization chart may show an entire facility or a close-up view of a given area, such as a dining services department. Figure 9.7 shows a sample organization chart for a hospital.

In this example the departments are named in boxes. These include Admitting, Information Services, Human Resources, Medical Records, Quality Assurance, Public Relations, Audiology, Clinical Labs, and more. You can see that the hospital is organized into two main sections: administrative and medical. You can also see that there are three assistant administrators, who have responsibility for the department of groups of departments. The Dining Services department falls under one of these assistant administrators.

Now, who reports to whom? Six people report to the hospital administrator: an administrative assistant, a secretary, three assistant administrators, and a director of finances. These relationships are illustrated by solid lines connecting the boxes. Does the secretary supervise anyone? No. There are no lines connecting the secretary to more boxes below.

Does the Department Manager for Dining Services supervise anyone? Yes, but this chart shows only the major areas. Another, more detailed chart would show the divisions and relationships within the Dining Services department.

The flow of formal power may go through several hierarchies or levels. An organization chart graphically illustrates a concept called **chain of command**, which means the flow of formal power through organizational lines. In any organization chain of command has to be clearly defined. As you look through an organization chart, you should be able to trace the chain of command for any area from top to bottom or from bottom to top. If you are in charge of the Dining Services department in this hospital, you know that your supervisor is the Assistant Administrator of Support Services. That person's supervisor is the Administrator. Furthermore, the Administrator reports to the Board of Trustees.

Another key management term is **delegation**. Delegation means passing authority downward through the organization. The ability to delegate is one of the essential features of a manager. The act of delegating recognizes that you do not do everything yourself and that you cannot do everything yourself. For example, if you manage the Dining Services department, you know that you cannot cook all the food for all the meals. You delegate the authority downward through the chain of command to a group of cooks. Along with the job, you delegate responsibility and accountability to the cooks.

So, the lines on the organization chart designate responsibility, authority, and accountability throughout the organization. You are responsible for the department and have the authority and formal power to make things happen. You are also accountable to the Assistant Administrator of Support Services for the work performed in Dining

Glossary

Organization Chart
A graphical management tool that shows job relationships in a facility

Chain of Command
The flow of formal power through organizational lines

Delegation
Passing authority for tasks or assigning duties downward through the organization chart

Figure 9.7 **Organization Chart for a Hospital**

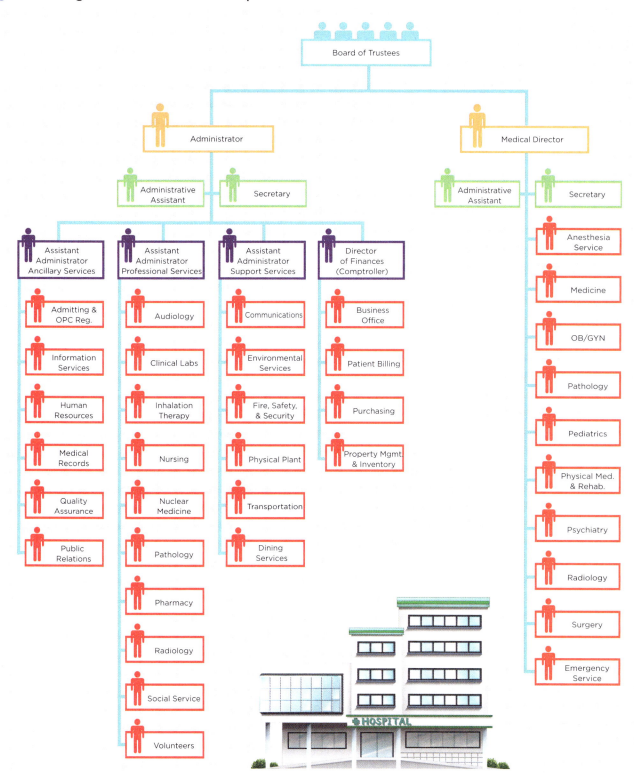

Services. Meanwhile, this Assistant Administrator is accountable to the Administrator for Dining Services, and so forth.

In any organization, people are expected to respect and follow the chain of command. In this hospital, it would be poor business etiquette (professionally inappropriate) for you to call the Administrator directly to discuss your new idea for the employee cafeteria or to complain about a problem you are having with the Purchasing department. Instead, you should be discussing these matters with your own boss, the Assistant Administrator of Support Services. It is up to your boss to work through the next level up in the organization as needed.

You also notice in an organization chart that each person has only one boss. This is called unity of command, which means each person reports to only one superior. Management experts suggest that this is a sound idea. Multiple bosses can lead to conflicting command and a breakdown of functioning.

From the portion of the hospital's organization that is apparent on this chart, you may also notice that there is a limit to the number of lines flowing down from any one person. Realistically, one person can directly supervise only so many staff. What if the hospital administrator did not have the help of assistant administrators and a director of finances? Could one person effectively supervise these 26 departments? Of course, the answer is no. A consideration in organizing work is the ratio of managers to other employees.

Figure 9.8 Organization Chart for a Hospital

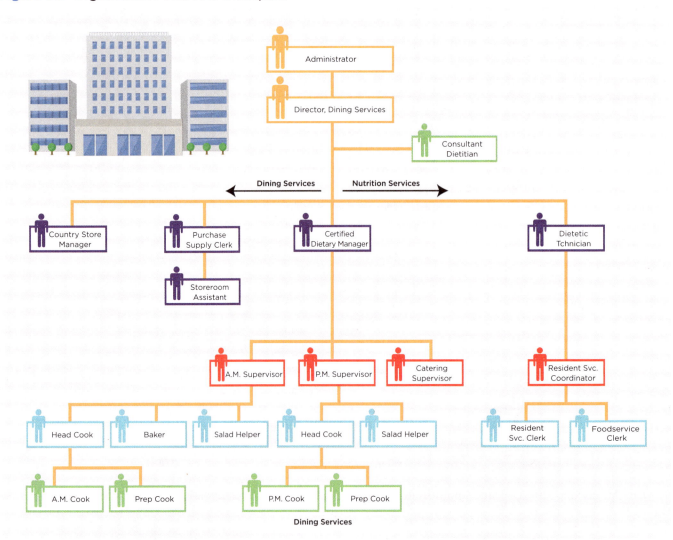

Now, let's take a closer look at the finer picture, the organization of a Dining Services department. Figure 9.8 shows a sample of a dining services department for a retirement community serving about 165 people.

In this example, you can see that the person in charge of dining services reports directly to the administrator of the organization. Furthermore, the Dining Services Department are split into two areas, which represent two main purposes. First, there is a Dining Services section. This group clearly purchases and produces food for the residents of the retirement community. There are several levels of supervision, and there is an established chain of command.

Secondly, there is a Nutrition Services section. This section addresses the nutritional needs of residents (beyond food itself). Notice that within this area, there is also a Consultant Dietitian who reports to the Director of Dining Services, but does not directly supervise anyone at all. This type of relationship is sometimes called a staff relationship.

A **staff position** provides advisory or consulting support to a manager who is in the chain of command. This person is not a supervisor and is not in the chain of command, but provides valuable expertise that the manager needs. In this example, the Consultant Dietitian provides expertise in nutrition on a periodic basis to assist with the tasks of evaluating the individual needs of residents. Typically, a consultant dietitian in this setting may assist with planning menus to assure needs are met and with planning, monitoring, and reviewing the nutritional care of individual residents. A staff position may be filled by an outside consultant or even by an employee of the organization. The important point is that someone in a staff position supports a manager.

Figures 9.9 and 9.10 show additional examples of organization charts for a small hospital and a large university dining service.

For the hospital Dining Services department in Figure 9.9, there is a nutrition services section, although it does not use this name. Much like the retirement community, this healthcare organization delivers clinical nutritional services in addition to dining services.

Glossary

Staff Position
Provides advisory or consulting support but is not in the chain of command

Putting It Into Practice

3. Using Figure 9.8 Sample Organization Chart for Retirement Community, if the PM Cook is having a problem with the Prep Cook and the Head Cook is on vacation, who should he go to for assistance?

Figure 9.9 Organization Chart for Small Hospital Dietary Services (200 Beds)

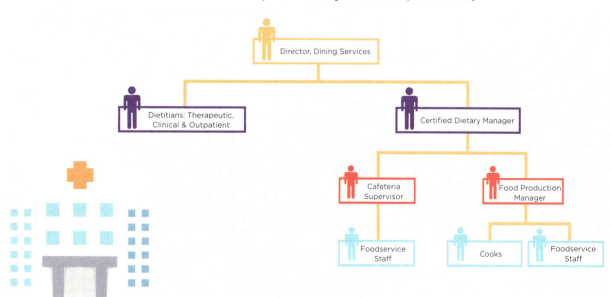

The dietitians delivering this service report to the Director of Dining Services and do not have a supervisory role over other employees. In this organization chart, the dietitians are employees of the facility, not outside consultants.

This difference probably reflects the scope of service. Often, an acute care environment requires a high level of nutrition expertise applied intensively with shorter turnaround requirements. Clients in an acute care setting typically stay for a short time, and have healthcare needs that may change significantly from day-to-day.

The structure of the university dining services in Figure 9.10 is significantly different from that of the previous example. Clearly, the organization chart has been developed differently to reflect the purposes and tasks of this university dining services operation. Notice that Dining Services fall in with a cluster of activities that relate to residence halls. Why is dining services bundled with sanitation employees and a building supervisor? In this environment, all of these functions relate closely to a single purpose of providing housing for students.

You might also imagine that employees throughout this chart will need to coordinate their efforts, interact with each other, and work as a team to fulfill the purposes of the residence halls department. A manager shown at the top of this chart bears responsibility for assuring that the sum total of tasks related to housing are accomplished.

Figure 9.10 Organization Chart for Large University Foodservice*

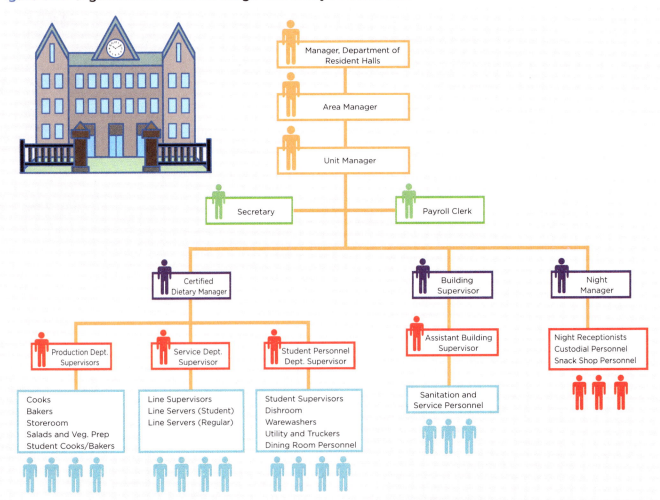

Some facilities and corporations are utilizing a circular organization chart. While it is more difficult to represent distinct reporting relationships, it encourages the integration of all employees on the chart and can be useful for representing team-based organizations. In this format, the Director of Dining Services is within the center circle representing the position of the Corporate Dining Services Director with direct (solid lines) responsibility to two Certified Dietary Managers on the next circle out from the center.

These managers could be on different campuses, in different regions of the country or responsible for unrelated dining venues within a single campus. The Certified Dietary Managers are in turn directly responsible for two Head Cooks on the next (4th) circle out from the center. The Head Cooks are in turn responsible for the Wait Staff and Dining Services Assistant within their dining venues.

See Figure 9.11 for an example of the circular organization chart.

Figure 9.11 **Circular Organizational Chart**

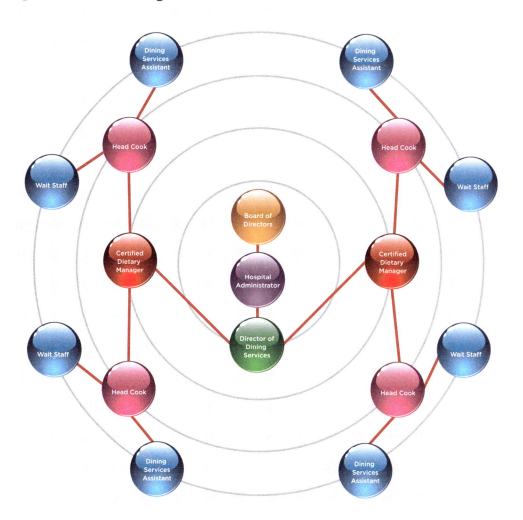

Notice that organization charts for dining services operations bear many similarities with each other. This is because many basic tasks of a dining services operation are universal. Someone needs to plan a menu, order food, manage inventory, prepare food, and manage delivery of services. In a small organization, one person may have responsibility for many functions. In a larger operation, individual managers may have a more specialized role.

However, in each of these examples, you can see that organization follows a logical task list that varies from one facility to another. It bundles related tasks. It pulls together similar resources and skills. It defines the responsibility, accountability, authority, legal power, and chain of command.

Consult with your facility administration for assistance in editing, or if need be developing the organization chart for the Dining Services department. All department staff members should know how their position relates to the activities of the department and how the department relates to the other departments in the organization. The organization chart clarifies the chain of command and reporting structure, which is also part of the written job description.

Recruit, Select, and Hire Employees

Overview and Objectives

Because of high employee turnover rates, effective recruitment and interviewing becomes an important staffing tool. After initial recruitment efforts, you may be able to predict how well candidates will perform through a structured interview process. This chapter will review employment laws, interview, and hiring techniques. After completing this chapter, you should be able to:

✓ Identify fair employment laws and practices that affect the Dining Services department

✓ Document department-based selection procedures and policies

✓ Develop and document relevant interview procedures for the department

✓ Identify and explain department procedures and policies to applicants

✓ Develop written decision criteria for applicant selection

✓ Design an orientation program for new employees

Before establishing policies and practices related to human resources management, it is important to be aware of certain constraints imposed by sources external to the organization. These take the form of federal and state employment laws that affect what a manager can and cannot do. In this chapter, we will explore several federal regulations. State regulations vary by location, so it is important to investigate these in your own state. In addition, the human resources department and/or legal counsel of a facility can serve as an excellent resource for understanding the obligations with regard to personnel management.

Federal Equal Employment Opportunity (EEO) Laws

The U.S. **Equal Employment Opportunity Commission (EEOC)** provides the oversight and coordination of all federal equal employment opportunity regulations, practices, and policies. Figure 10.1 shows some of the important employment legislation that has been passed making it illegal to discriminate in hiring based on a person's race, color, religion, sex (including pregnancy), national origin, age (40 or older), disability or genetic information. The EEOC does not enforce the protections that prohibit discrimination and harassment based on sexual orientation, status as a parent, marital status and political affiliation. However, other federal agencies and many states and municipalities do. An organization may be held liable for the discriminatory acts of its employees, even if administrators were unaware of those acts. Not only does a Certified

Dietary Manager need to be aware of the legislation contained in Figure 10.1, but the employees also must realize that they are under a legal obligation not to discriminate. If there is a human resources department, work with it whenever there are employment concerns or questions.

Figure 10.1 Federal Laws Affecting Employment Management

1963 Equal Pay Act	Protects men and women who perform substantially equal work in the same establishment from sex-based wage discrimination.
1964 Civil Rights Act	Protects against employment discrimination based on race, color, religion, sex or national origin.
1967 Age Discrimination in Employment Act	Protects individuals who are 40 years of age or older.
1973 Rehabilitation Act	Prohibits discrimination against qualified individuals with disabilities who work in the federal government.
1990 Americans with Disabilities Act	Prohibits employment discrimination against qualified individuals with disabilities in the private sector, and in state and local governments.
1991 Civil Rights Act, amended	Provides monetary damages in cases of intentional employment discrimination; established glass ceiling.
1993 Family and Medical Leave Act (FMLA)	Provides up to 12 weeks leave, unpaid and job-protected, per year to an employee for birth or adoption; or to care for a spouse, parent, or child with a serious health condition.
1994 Uniformed Services Employment and Reemployment Act	Protects individuals who leave work to fulfill their military service obligation.
1996 Health Insurance Portability and Accountability Act (HIPAA)	Protects confidentiality of medical records and provides for transfer of medical coverage of existing illnesses to another employer's insurance plan.
1996 Illegal Immigration Reform and Immigrant Responsibility Act	Provides for severe restrictions on persons who remain in the United States longer than permitted by their visa and/or who violate their nonimmigrant status.
2008 Genetic Information Nondiscrimination Act (GINA)	Prohibits employment discrimination based on genetic information about an applicant, employee, or former employee.

Source: www.eeoc.gov accessed 3-17-15

These laws apply to all facilities that employee 15 or more people. The laws prohibit discrimination practices that are associated with any aspect of employment, including:

- Hiring and firing
- Compensation, assignment, or classification of employees
- Transfer, promotion, layoff, or recall
- Job advertisements
- Recruitment
- Testing
- Use of company facilities
- Training and apprenticeship programs
- Fringe benefits
- Pay, retirement plans, and disability leave
- Other terms and conditions of employment

Discrimination

Discrimination is treatment or consideration based on class or category, rather than individual merit. In essence, discrimination puts people in categories based on personal factors, and treats everyone within a category the same. Since this treatment is based on ignorance of the individuality of employees, it can generate unjust managerial policies, decisions, and actions based on stereotypes and prejudices.

Discrimination includes practices where the effects may not have been intended, such as using human resource tests that have not been validated as a selection device. In addition, there are certain questions that may not be asked on an employment application or during an interview. Care in structuring questions included in application forms is important. Figure 10.2 summarizes what a potential employer may and may not ask of a job applicant.

Dress codes and standards for personal appearance also have discriminatory implications. For example, if a facility requires employees to be clean-shaven in the Admissions department, this requirement should probably be standard for all service employees, including those in foodservice and gift shop areas. There should be consistency throughout the organization in the interpretation of what is appropriate for employees.

Individual departments or managers should not set conflicting dress codes. Exceptions may be needed for specific department requirements, such as hair restraints in foodservice, jewelry restrictions in surgery and others. The same general dress code standards apply to men and women; the standards must be reasonable, appropriate, and consistent.

Religious discrimination must be avoided. Employees must be scheduled so their work requirements will not conflict with religious commitments/beliefs, and it is necessary to make whatever schedule and other adjustments are necessary to meet these special requests. An employee's personal appearance may reflect religious heritage (length of hair, for example), and human resource policies must accommodate these special circumstances.

Certified Dietary Managers must not discriminate on the basis of sex. For example, personnel specifications such as weight or height, that may be perceived as based on gender, are unlawful unless they reflect essential attributes required for performing the job. These essential attributes are called **bona fide occupational qualifications**

Glossary

Discrimination
Treatment or consideration based on class or category, rather than individual merit

Bona Fide Occupational Qualifications (BFOQ)
Allowed personal or physical characteristic normally considered discriminating

Putting It Into Practice

1. You are interviewing a prospective employee who is visibly limping. During the interview, your head cook asks, "Can you tell me what happened to your leg?" Is this a legal question? Why or why not?

Figure 10.2 Pre-Employment Inquiry Guide

SUBJECT	LAWFUL PRE-EMPLOYMENT INQUIRIES	UNLAWFUL PRE-EMPLOYMENT INQUIRIES
Name	• Applicant's full name. • Have you ever worked for this company under a different name? • Is any additional information relative to a different name necessary to check work record? If yes, explain.	• Original name of an applicant whose name has been changed by court order or otherwise. • Applicant's maiden name.
Address or Duration of Residence	• How long a resident of this state or city?	
Birthplace		• Birthplace of applicant. • Birthplace of applicant's parents, spouse, or other close relatives. • Requirement that applicant submit birth certificate, naturalization or baptismal record.
Age	• Are you 18 years old or older?*	• How old are you? What is your date of birth?
Religion or Creed		• Inquiry into an applicant's religious denomination, religious affiliations, church, parish, pastor, or religious holidays observed. • An applicant may not be told "This is a Catholic (Protestant or Jewish) organization."
Race or Color		• Complexion or color of skin.
Photograph		• Requirement that an applicant for employment affix a photograph to an employment application form. • Request an applicant, at his or her option, to submit a photograph. • Requirement for photograph after interview but before hiring.
Height		• Inquiry regarding applicant's height.
Weight		• Inquiry regarding applicant's weight.
Marital Status		• Requirement that an applicant provide any information regarding marital status or children. • Are you single or married? Do you have any children? Is your spouse employed? What is your spouse's name?
Sex		• Mr., Miss or Mrs., or inquiry regarding sex. • Inquiry as to the ability to reproduce or advocacy of any form of birth control.

* *This question may be asked only for the purpose of determining whether applicants are of legal age for employment.*
Source: State of Michigan, Michigan Department of Civil Rights, Lansing, MI.

(Continued)

Figure 10.2 **Pre-Employment Inquiry Guide** (Continued)

SUBJECT	LAWFUL PRE-EMPLOYMENT INQUIRIES	UNLAWFUL PRE-EMPLOYMENT INQUIRIES
Health	• Do you have any impairments (physical, mental, or medical) which would interfere with your ability to do the job for which you have applied? • Inquiry into contagious or communicable diseases which may endanger others. • If there are any positions for which you should not be considered or job duties you cannot perform because of a physical or mental handicap? Please explain.	• Inquiries regarding an applicant's physical or mental condition (which are not directly related to the requirements of a specific job, and which are used as a factor in making employment decisions in a way which is contrary to the provisions or purposes of the Civil Rights Act). • Requirements that women be given pelvic examinations.
Citizenship	• Are you a citizen of the United States? • If not a citizen of the United States, do you intend to become a citizen of the United States? • If you are not a United States citizen, do you have legal right to remain permanently in the United States? Do you intend to remain permanently in the United States?	• Of what country are you a citizen? • Whether an applicant is naturalized or a native-born citizen; the date when the applicant acquired citizenship. • Requirement that an applicant produce naturalization papers or first papers. • Whether applicant's parents or spouse are naturalized or native born citizens of the United States; the date when parent or spouse acquired citizenship.
Natural Origin	• Inquiry into languages applicant speaks and writes fluently.	• Inquiry into applicant's (a) lineage; (b) ancestry; (c) national origin; (d) descent; (e) parentage, or nationality. • Nationality of applicant's parents or spouse. • What is your mother tongue? • Inquiry into how applicant acquired ability to read, write, or speak a foreign language.
Education	• Inquiry into the academic, vocational, or professional education of an applicant, and the public and private schools attended.	
Experience	• Inquiry into work experience. • Inquiry into countries applicant has visited.	
Arrests	• Have you ever been convicted of a crime? If so, when, where, and nature of offense? • Are there any felony charges pending against you?	• Inquiry regarding arrests. Have you ever been arrested?
Relatives	• Names of applicant's relatives, other than a spouse, already employed by this company.	• Address of any relative of applicant, other than address (within the United States) of applicant's father and mother, husband or wife and minor dependent children.

Source: State of Michigan, Michigan Department of Civil Rights, Lansing, MI.

(Continued)

Figure 10.2 Pre-Employment Inquiry Guide (*Continued*)

SUBJECT	LAWFUL PRE-EMPLOYMENT INQUIRIES	UNLAWFUL PRE-EMPLOYMENT INQUIRIES
Notify In Case of Emergency	• Name and address of person to be notified in case of accident or emergency.	• Name and address of nearest relative to be notified in case of accident or emergency.
Military Experience	• Inquiry into an applicant's military experience in the Armed Forces of the United States or in a state militia. • Inquiry into applicant's service in a particular branch of United States Army, Navy, etc.	• Inquiry into an applicant's general military experience.
Organizations	• Inquiry into the organizations of which an applicant is a member, excluding organizations, which by name or character, indicate the race, color, religion, national origin, or ancestry of members.	• List all clubs, societies and lodges to which you belong.
Transportation	• Do you have reliable transportation to get to work by 7:00 a.m.?	• Do you own a car?
References	• Who suggested that you apply for a position here?	

Source: State of Michigan, Michigan Department of Civil Rights, Lansing, MI.

(BFOQ). An example of a legitimate BFOQ might be that storeroom employees must be able to lift or move heavy boxes of canned goods. Since this task can be done by a female employee, you might have difficulty defending a discrimination charge filed by a woman if all of these positions were filled by men. Discriminating against pregnant women or refusing to hire women (or men) because of uniform, locker space, or other problems are examples of unlawful practices.

The Discrimination in Employment Act of 1967 was enacted to prohibit arbitrary discrimination based upon age. It applies to persons over the age of 40. Offering different fringe benefit packages to older employees, refusing to train or promote them, and mandating their retirement are all examples of illegal acts.

Federal Privacy Act

Federal and state laws also protect employees against invasion of their privacy. The **Federal Privacy Act** covers employee records, locker and personal inspections, background investigations, and other matters. Normally, employees are entitled to a reasonable expectation of privacy and, if this is denied, legal liability can result.

Americans with Disabilities Act (ADA)

The **Americans With Disabilities Act (ADA)**, passed in 1990, requires covered organizations to take steps to accommodate disabled persons, including employees, and to employ qualified disabled job applicants.

The law's definition of **disability** is important: "A physical or mental impairment that substantially limits one or more major life activities of such individuals; a record of such an impairment; or being regarded as having such an impairment." This definition includes

Glossary

Federal Privacy Act
Protects employees against invasion of their privacy in the workplace

Americans With Disabilities Act (ADA)
Requires reasonable accommodation for disabled persons

Disability
A physical or mental impairment that substantially limits one or more major life activities of such individuals; a record of such an impairment; or being regarded as having such an impairment

persons with a wide range of disabling conditions, such as blindness, hearing impairments, arthritis, heart conditions, emphysema, shortness of stature, amputation, and others.

Regulations state that organizations must make "reasonable accommodations" as long as doing so does not create an "undue burden." Issues such as costs, financial resources of the facility, and its relationship, if any, with a parent corporation are all taken into account as these and related issues are assessed.

Generally, public accommodations must remove architectural barriers in existing facilities if such removal is readily achievable (easily carried out without too much difficulty or expense). Each public accommodation must evaluate its facilities and determine what can be done. If a problem exists, the organization typically must provide goods, services, facilities, and accommodations through alternative methods.

In regard to the facility itself, there are several priorities:

- The first priority is actual access to the public accommodation (doorways, entrance ramps, etc.).
- The second priority is access to goods and services. (For example, do all disabled visitors have access to the cafeteria?)
- The third priority is access to restroom facilities.
- The fourth priority is access to any other services, goods, or facilities offered by the organization.

A wide range of regulations apply when there is new construction or alteration to existing facilities. Likewise, enforcement provisions include opportunities for victims of discrimination to go to court.

Most healthcare facilities have been designed to accommodate persons with disabilities and, in fact, exist to provide health services for them. However, healthcare facilities may be confronted with the same types of issues as other organizations relative to the employment of persons with disabilities.

Figure 10.3 reviews major concerns that must be addressed in the personnel policies and procedures of most employers.

Figure 10.3 Americans with Disabilities Act Requirements Fact Sheet: Employment

- Employers may not discrimininate against an individual with a disability in hiring or promotion if the person is otherwise qualified for the job.
- Employers can ask about one's ability to perform a job, but cannot inquire if someone has a disability or subject a person to tests that tend to screen out people with disabilities.
- Employers will need to provide "reasonable accommodation" to individuals with disabilities. This includes steps such as job restructuring and modification of equipment.
- Employers do not need to provide accommodations that impose an "undue hardship" on business operations.
- All employers with 15 or more employees must comply.

Sexual Harassment

Today, **sexual harassment** in the workplace receives significant attention and is one of the most frequent reasons for employee litigation (lawsuits). In March 1980, the EEOC issued specific guidelines dealing with sexual harassment. Sexual harassment is a violation of Title VII. Simply stated, in order for conduct to be considered sexual harassment:

1. The conduct must be sexual in nature.
2. The conduct must be unwelcome.

Sexual harassment may be physical, verbal (including suggestive comments), or visual (for example, displaying pornographic photographs).

While the laws and their interpretations may vary, some principles are well established. The Certified Dietary Manager and/or employer will probably be held liable for sexual harassment if an employee is deprived of a tangible job benefit (e.g., promotion) because of a refusal to provide sexual favors. If an employee's work environment is negatively affected (in the employee's opinion) by the sexual harassment of a supervisor or co-worker, and if the employer knows or should have known of this conduct and does not take immediate action, the employer will probably be held liable. The manager and the facility can also be found liable for the harassment of employees by clients or their guests if unwanted activities occurred, facility personnel were aware of them, and immediate corrective actions were not taken.

A facility must exercise reasonable care to prevent sexual harassment. In the event a manager is informed that an employee is being sexually harassed, the EEOC Guidelines on Discrimination Because of Sex indicate that the following steps should be taken:

1. Notify your own superior.
2. Investigate the situation according to your organization's policy.
3. Seek legal advice before further action is taken.
4. Confront the accused party and get the accused party's side of the story.
5. Take any necessary disciplinary action(s).

To deal effectively with the issue of sexual harassment:

- The facility or organization should have a formal written policy specifically addressing the step-by-step procedures to be followed regarding sexual harassment. As a corporate or system-based policy, the approving signature is typically that of the senior administrator and a lawyer or the facility Risk Manager.

- All managers should be familiar with the policy. This policy should include disciplinary guidelines for both the individual who is guilty and guidelines for harassers who retaliate against those who report them. The policy should include a formal complaint procedure for employees to use if they think they have been victims of sexual harassment, with provisions for immediate investigation and prompt disciplinary action when appropriate.

- Employees should be educated on how to recognize sexual harassment, how to report it when it occurs, and the steps that will be taken if an employee is guilty of sexual harassment. All cases of possible sexual harassment must be investigated according to this policy set by management.

- Follow-up needs to be provided after all instances of sexual harassment. Victims must be contacted and witnesses need to be asked if the sexual harassment has indeed stopped and that no retaliation is taking place.

Glossary

Sexual Harassment
Workplace conduct that is:
1. Sexual in nature and
2. Unwelcomed

Putting It Into Practice

2. Your male cook has a habit of calling the females with whom he works "honey." Is this a violation of the sexual harassment law?

Fair Labor Standards Act (FLSA)

The **Fair Labor Standards Act (FLSA)** addresses the idea that an employee deserves to be paid fairly. It defines:

- Minimum wage
- A 40-hour work week
- Requirements for overtime
- Restrictions on child labor

Individual states also have provisions relating to these standards. What is legally acceptable varies from state to state. The FLSA specifically includes state and local hospitals, as well as educational institutions. Among other things, the law requires that employees exceeding a 40-hour work week receive overtime pay.

The overtime pay requirement does not apply to an exempt employee. An **exempt employee** is on salary (as opposed to receiving an hourly wage). An exempt employee does not receive overtime compensation. In a facility where employees belong to a union, an exempt employee may have a broader definition. Employees who meet the following criteria can be exempt from the overtime provisions of the Wage and Hour Law as executives:

- They supervise two or more other employees.
- Their salary is the minimum amount determined by the Wage and Hour Division (which changes periodically).
- They have the power to hire and fire, or their recommendations must carry significant weight.
- Their primary duty is management. They cannot do non-exempt work more than 40 percent of the time in any given work week. Generally, they cannot do the work of the people they supervise.
- They are able to exercise discretionary powers and set policies on the job.

Often only the department manager can set policies within that department, and all others follow those policies. If so, only one person in a department is usually considered exempt as an executive. However, the Wage and Hour Division has been interpreting this rule to allow an assistant manager who is working on an entirely different shift from the manager to be exempt if the other requirements are met.

Definitions regarding what determines full-time versus part-time status, eligibility for benefits and "paid time off" are not specifically defined by FLSA or other federal regulation.

Workers Compensation

The concept of workers compensation is to limit liability of the employer if an employee becomes injured on the job. It also provides income to an employee who is unable to work due to injury on the job. The federal government has laid the groundwork for workers compensation through the **Federal Employment Compensation Act (FECA)**, which is administered by state governments. Each state has its own policies and legislation and administers the program.

Family and Medical Leave Act (FMLA)

The **Family and Medical Leave Act (FMLA)**, enacted in 1993, requires employers to provide at least 12 weeks of leave to a qualified employee who has specific family or medical reasons to request time off. This time may be paid or unpaid, according to the employer's policy. The law requires that this leave be available once during a rolling, 365- day, one-year period.

During the leave, the employee should still be eligible for health insurance benefits (even though the employee may be required to pay for these benefits). Upon returning to work, the employee should be reinstated into his or her previous position.

The types of situations that qualify for family and medical leave include:

- Birth of a child
- Adoption of a child
- Serious health condition of employee's spouse, parent, or child
- Serious illness experienced by the employee

The law applies to businesses with 15 or more employees, and to all public agencies and schools. The law can also protect an individual employee who is unable to work because of a personal health condition. This has created a bit of legal confusion, because the legislation overlaps with the ADA (Americans with Disabilities Act). For example, cancer is considered both cause for medical leave and a disability. So, an employer might need to grant a 12-week leave to an employee with cancer according to the FMLA, and then grant additional leave or other accommodations afterwards to comply with the ADA. Rulings and statutes are evolving to address issues such as these.

Federal Unemployment Tax Act (FUTA)

Another form of protection provided by law is the financial protection awarded to employees in case they become unemployed through no fault of their own. The law providing this protection is the **Federal Unemployment Tax Act (FUTA)**. FUTA provides a right to unemployment compensation to protect the income of former employees while they seek new employment. It does not apply to an employee who was terminated through a disciplinary process.

For example, if a facility determines that it needs to eliminate a set of jobs, the employees who lose their jobs may be eligible to receive unemployment compensation. How much and for how long depends on a number of factors. State entities are involved in administering the legislation, and employers pay a tax to help provide funding for this program.

These are some examples of employment regulations, but this section does not present an exhaustive list. For information about federal employment regulations, visit the U.S. Department of Labor website Compliance Assistance section (www.dol.gov) to review regulations by name or topic. Furthermore, the human resources department is the best authority on all the employment laws (federal and state) that may affect your actions as a manager.

Reviewing the human resource policies and procedures of the organization assists a Certified Dietary Manager in understanding the standards for the department. These policies affect how to recruit new employees and manage existing team members.

Selecting Employees

The best employees start with the hiring process!

Selecting employees involves several steps: recruitment, screening, checking references, interviewing and making a hiring decision. Some facilities may use their human resources department to coordinate the selection process. It is important to have standardized

Glossary

Federal Unemployment Tax Act (FUTA)
Provides a right to unemployment compensation to employees who become unemployed through no fault of their own

Putting It Into Practice

3. Your head cook, who supervises the p.m. cook and the assistant cook, receives an hourly wage. She recently put in extra hours to help prepare for a special meal. Is she entitled to overtime pay?

procedures for each of these steps, as they are covered by the EEOC. The government provides free guidelines for the selection process titled, *Uniform Guidelines on Employee Selection Procedures* located at this URL: http://www.uniformguidelines.com/. If there is no HR department, be sure and consult these guidelines, including the questions and answers found on the website.

The Recruitment Process

The recruitment process helps to build a pool of applicants for open positions. The Certified Dietary Manager will need to decide if they are going to recruit from within the facility or search outside the facility. The Human Resource Department can assist in the recruitment process, based on the open positions and the availability of qualified candidates in the facility. If outside recruitment is needed, the Human Resource Department can assist in obtaining candidates via newspapers or online job sites.

After initial recruitment efforts, the manager is faced with the task of predicting how well candidates will perform on the job. Much of the information for a final decision is gathered during a structured screening and interview process. This determines who is selected as the new employee.

The Screening Process

Many businesses now use a screening process to select the applicants to be interviewed. Screening means comparing each applicant's qualifications to the job description. To be protected by the EEOC and follow the Uniform Guidelines for Employee Selection, use a screening committee that compares each applicant in the same way to the job description. Some facilities have a written form for the screening process that is used for each applicant, such as shown in Figure 10.4. Using the same template with each applicant helps to reduce discrimination.

Figure 10.4 **Screening Template for Foodservice Employees**

QUALIFICATIONS	EDUCATION	EXPERIENCE					OTHER
		Sanitation	Record Keeping	Food Protection	Notification	Customer/ Client Service	
Applicant #1							
Applicant #2							

Some organizations have implemented a **pre-employment testing** process consisting of some or all of the following:

- Aptitude testing evaluates a candidates' critical thinking and problem solving skills.
- A personality questionnaire tests for behavioral characteristics related to customer service and other workplace performance.
- Skills testing for basic competencies needed in the workplace or specific skills required for the position.

The testing may be a general evaluation of candidates required for all positions within the organization or highly specific to individual job descriptions. When there are too many applicants for consideration, use of both the paper screening process (match to the job description and results of pre-employment testing) and a formal interview should be considered.

The Interview Process

Much information about job applicants can be gained from application forms, reference checks, selection tests, and medical exams.

- Reference Checks—Without a human resources department, use a standard form for all candidates that asks for: dates of employment, reporting relationship, reason for leaving.
- Pre-employment Selection Tests—If used for any applicants, it should be used for each applicant.
- Medical Exams—The American with Disabilities Act requires that this be directly related to employment and cannot be required until employment is offered.

This may not be enough information for determining whether an applicant will be suitable for the available position. One or more pre-employment job interviews may also be essential to match a candidate with a job vacancy.

A second manager that has not been part of the preliminary interview may want to conduct a second meeting with the candidate prior to the selection process. The purpose of an interview is to assess the abilities, attitudes, and compatibility of the applicant for the position. It is very important that the immediate supervisor be involved in the applicant selection process. Figure 10.5 identifies some basic questions that may be useful during an interview.

An interview is really a planned conversation and provides a structured discussion of relevant topics for both parties. Generally, an interviewer works from a pre-determined list of questions in order to assure fairness in assessing candidates. However, the best interview process puts a candidate, at ease and allows them to open up and tell more. Figure 10.6 provides additional interviewing tips.

When interviewing a prospective employee, you are indirectly setting the tone for the relationship that may follow if that individual is hired by the organization. The interview can ultimately be construed as a legally binding description of both the job opportunity and your company's value system (or lack of it).

Types of Interview Questions. There are three basic types of interview questions: directive, non-directive and situational. Directive interview questions are specific questions formulated in advance and asked in a checklist fashion. Questions asked should solicit important information.

Glossary

Pre-Employment Testing
Aptitude, personality or skills testing conducted prior to employment as part of the screening process

Figure 10.5 Frequently Asked Interview Questions

- Why did you choose to interview with our organization?
- Describe your ideal job.
- What can you offer us?
- What skills have you developed?
- What did you enjoy most about your last employment?
- What did you enjoy least about your last employment?
- Have you ever quit a job? Why?
- Why should we hire you rather than another candidate?
- What do you consider to be your greatest strengths?
- Would you be successful working on a team?
- What do you know about our organization?
- Have you worked under deadline pressure? When?
- How do you feel about working in a structured environment?
- How do you feel about working overtime?

- How did you get along with your former co-workers?
- What are your expectations for rate of pay?
- Tell me about yourself.
- Do you have any computer experience?
- Would you be willing to take a drug test?
- How does your past experience apply to this position?
- How does this job match your interests?
- What skills do you have which will help in this job?
- What are your main strengths for this job?
- What major weaknesses will need to be overcome for you to do this job adequately?
- Will you have any problems getting to work?
- What other information can you provide which will help me to understand your capabilities for this work?
- What questions do you have about the job?
- When would you be able to begin work?

Examples of directive interview questions include:

- What did you do in your last job?
- Why did you leave your last position?

Directive interview questions solicit facts and do not seek opinions. All topics of directive questions should directly impact on how well the applicant can perform the job. Any other questions may be in violation of EEOC or other laws. When directive interview questions are used, it is important that the job applicant be given time to ask questions and that the interviewer provides basic information about the job. Generally, the interviewer should record responses to questions as they are given.

The second type of interview question is **non-directive**. While these questions are also planned and perhaps written down in advance, they are less structured and more non-directive so that the interviewee can provide creative responses. Examples of non-directive questions include:

- Why do you think you'll like this job?
- What elements do you consider important when you consider a new position?

Many interviewers like to use responses to non-directive questions as springboards for additional questions formulated on-the-fly. With this approach, the interviewer can go on in depth and learn more about the applicant. Applicants who are encouraged to speak on their own will usually provide much more information than they will in response to closed-ended, yes-or-no questions.

Glossary

Directive Interview Questions
Pre-planned interview questions seeking specific information

Non-Directive Interview Questions
Pre-planned open-ended interview questions seeking more expansive responses

Figure 10.6 Interviewing Tips

- Respect a candidate's feelings and self-esteem at all times. Strive to put the candidate at ease.
- Begin with a pleasant, professional introduction and appropriate light conversation.
- Remember that to the candidate, you are the organization.
- Don't give excessive encouragement, verbally or nonverbally, at any point.
- Examine candidate evidence in areas of past performance and achievement, as well as work philosophies and beliefs.
- Use verbal rejoinders to trigger additional response in crucial areas, such as "Tell me more...," "Give me another example," etc.
- Use nonverbal reminders, such as nodding, facial gestures, etc. to maintain a steady flow of information.
- Take notes as needed and in a natural sequence. Don't make a final appraisal of notes until the interview is concluded.
- If you don't see a desired characteristic, ask for it specifically. If it is still not apparent, score the applicant accordingly.
- Make yourself thoroughly knowledgeable about the candidate prior to the interview and use that knowledge throughout the meeting.
- Portray the available position adequately and accurately; question candidate to determine specific qualifications.
- Have a set questioning process prepared prior to the interview; seek specific data to match against the job description.
- Don't wander into EEOC-sensitive information unless you are seeking BFOQ—Bona Fide Occupational Qualifications. Avoid areas such as age, race, marital status, and any other sensitive areas unless information is volunteered by candidate.
- Let the candidate do the majority of the talking.
- Listen attentively, accurately, and actively.
- Postpone all final judgments until after the interview.
- Interrupt the candidate only when necessary, and then with tact and brevity.
- Ask candidate for permission to take notes, or merely inform candidate you will do so.
- Control excessive applicant rambling by introducing the next question or a rejoinder.
- Ensure the candidate answers a question at hand completely before moving on to another area.

Use of **situational interview questions** is an excellent way to further evaluate how well a candidate will fit in with the department. These questions ask a candidate to describe a type of situation and related decisions and/or actions. Here are some examples of situational questions:

- Tell me about a time when you knew a co-worker was not following work procedures. What happened, and what did you do?
- Describe a personal conflict that you had with a co-worker. What happened, and how did you respond?
- If you knew someone was stealing, what would you do?
- Can you think of a time when you disagreed with a company policy? Tell me what you decided to do.
- If you saw an unsafe situation, what would you do?

Glossary

Situational Interview Questions
Questions designed to describe an event or situation

During an interview, a Certified Dietary Manager can combine directive, non-directive, and situational questions to help build an understanding of the candidate's suitability for a job. To encourage the applicant to tell you as much as possible, avoid leading questions.

Leading questions can also influence a candidate's response and interfere with receiving valid information. Here are some examples of leading questions to avoid:

- "You would like to work here, wouldn't you?"
- "You wouldn't argue with a client, would you?"

Preparing For and Conducting An Interview

Needless to say, there is much more to an interview than just asking questions. The interviewer must properly prepare for it.

- A private environment free from interruptions is best.
- Set a beginning time and stick to it.
- Read over the application form and any other information available about the applicant.
- Provide enough time so that information can be solicited without the need to rush.
- Review the checklist of questions and be sure that all questions are relevant to the selection decision.

Some basic principles help develop good interview techniques. It is essential to put the applicant at ease. Candidates are likely to be nervous, so some friendly, opening conversation can be helpful in developing the rapport necessary for a good interview. A friendly handshake, a hospitable greeting and perhaps a cup of coffee are always good ways to start.

Once the interview begins,

- Ask simple questions first.
- Be aware of the time and don't allow yourself to feel rushed.
- Listen to what is being said.
- When the interviewee is speaking, concentrate rather than thinking ahead.
- Strive to maintain excellent eye contact and observe the candidate's nonverbal behavior.
- Listen open-mindedly.

Recognize that the candidate is probably very eager to learn about the position and the facility. A rule of thumb is to listen for about 75 percent of the interview, and talk for about 25 percent. Most of the facility information can wait until the late stage of the interview. Again, relating the details of your philosophy and standards may influence an applicant to simply say what he thinks you want to hear.

Follow-up after the interview is necessary. If there is no human resource staff assisting, it is a considerate gesture to notify the applicant that they are not being considered for the position. Perhaps there is another vacant position for which the interviewee will be eligible. Put yourself in the interviewee's place. Wouldn't you like to know about the interview results as soon as possible?

If you believe the applicant is qualified but want to interview others, it is fair to inform the interviewee. Name a time by which you will relate the selection decision. Adhere to the schedule or apprise the interviewee of any changes in the timetable. If the interviewee is qualified and there are no other applicants to consider, you may inform the interviewee that a job offer will be extended.

If working with a human resources department, each interview team member may be asked to rank the candidates based on the selection criteria. The human resources department will follow up with the candidate after the interview.

Putting It Into Practice

4. Why is it a good idea to have an advance checklist prepared for interviewing multiple candidates?

Now let's look at some additional pointers:

- Watch for the halo effect, which means hiring people who are just like you. An effective manager recognizes the value of building a team with complementary skills.

- Take your time. If you are not prepared for an interview or feel pressure to make a decision immediately, you are likely to obtain incorrect or incomplete information about the applicant.

- Follow legal guidelines, such as EEOC and other applicable laws throughout the process.

- Be upbeat about your organization, but refrain from making false promises or unrealistic commitments. Always tell the truth and let the applicant make decisions based upon a fair and reasonable expectation.

- Tell the applicant everything he or she should know to make a decision.

- Leave the applicant with a positive impression of your organization. Even if you will not be offering a job, the applicant is likely to be a member of the community, and your actions may have a public relations impact.

- Thank the candidate for meeting with you.

- Use reasonable standards for comparison. For example, if you compare an applicant with another employee with many years of experience, perhaps no applicant will seem acceptable. Instead, compare the job applicant's skills with the job specification.

The Hiring Decision

To make a selection decision, review the notes from interviews and weigh them carefully. In certain cases, you may have picked up some red flags indicating a candidate may not be able to take direction, or work with others, or perform in a reliable manner. You will probably want to remove these candidates from the list.

At the same time, there may be a list of multiple candidates who seem to be well qualified and may fit in well with the job requirements. Who should be offered the position? Typically, this decision is made by reviewing applicant information, considering the relevance of training, experience, education, assessing how well the candidate is likely to work with others on the team, and making a prediction of how likely the candidate is to become a successful long-term employee. Checking references at this point may provide additional decision information.

Sometimes, you may feel that there are no qualified candidates for an open job. While there may be pressure to fill a job, it is usually worth waiting to make a solid match. Bringing in the wrong person may seem easy and expedient for the moment, but it is likely to create more work down the line. In fact, if the candidate does not work out, you will find yourself again at the point of recruiting. A better approach is to be able to say no and immediately increase your recruitment efforts to find more candidates.

All information developed from the recruitment and selection process should be maintained on file in the new employee's personnel records. Sometimes reasons applicants were not selected may also be important. Documentation of applicant information is very important and must be emphasized as permanent files are developed.

The Onboarding and Orientation Process

All employees need to complete an initial orientation process as new hires. This may include required tuberculosis screening, fitting for respirator masks, and completion of a formal training period regarding facility and department policies. Often, the orientation program conducted by the human resources department addresses the system-wide policies required by the regulatory agencies but does not refer to the policies specific to food handling and service.

Development of your own **onboarding** process helps ensure that the departmental expectations and standards are communicated to all staff members. Consistent, clear expectations minimize the confusion of "I'm not sure how I am supposed to do this task" or "I don't know if I am doing a good job", which is a common reason for losing new employees. The onboarding process may last throughout the probationary period, and may include multiple learning tasks and/or on-the-job training sessions.

The onboarding and orientation process should be clearly defined in both the Human Resources and the Dining Services policies. Documented success, or failure, to complete the tasks may determine whether employment will be continued. Documentation in the employee's personnel file verifies the training provided and proficiency achieved by the staff member. These documents can also support you in the event of future performance issues.

A comprehensive orientation and step-by-step onboarding process will improve your employee retention and increase their job performance from the first day.

Glossary

Onboarding
The process designed to educate new employees to the department's, expectations and standards

Ongoing Employee Education

Overview and Objectives

A key part of developing personnel is education and training. Training builds the value of people in the facility through motivation, positive morale and superior performance. Planned and focused education is designed to achieve results and behaviors that align with the facility's needs and objectives. After completing this chapter, you should be able to:

✓ Orient new employees to facility procedures

✓ Develop and implement training programs

✓ Identify training resources and needs

✓ Conduct/arrange in-service and on-the-job training with a focus on food and dining services activities, such as
- Safe food preparation practices
- Sanitation
- HIPAA guidelines
- Hospitality and customer service
- Physical and workplace safety

✓ Document completion of training and orientation

Teaching employees involves training content, techniques, evaluation, and the trainers themselves. Training improves all aspects of the foodservice department. It is important to remember as you review this material that training is not a one-time event, it is an ongoing process.

The Onboarding Process

The retention of skilled staff and new hires starts with the orientation process. As discussed in Chapter 10, onboarding of new employees often starts with human resources-developed education and orientation requirements. This may not include information specific to the Dining Services department.

Federal, state and local guidelines often stipulate specific training programs on food safety and sanitation, medical confidentiality, equipment usage, disaster preparedness plus food service fire and safety training. Remember that new employees do not know where the fire pull box is located, or the safest route for evacuation of residents from the dining room. Developing a dining services orientation program, with a comprehensive checklist, will help ensure that all staff members are fully aware of policies and expectations that affect them.

Start thinking about all of the information a new employee needs to get through Day 1 and then what they need to know generally to do their job.

- Introduction to supervisors and co-workers
- Tour of the department and all relevant areas of the facility
- Map of the department with fire pulls, extinguishers, exits, break room and locker room
- First day policies
  > Fire and Weather Safety
  > All needed phone numbers
  > Attendance/call-in policy/tardies/etc.
  > Schedule locations and shift swap process
  > Relevant job routines
  > Dress code
  > Reference HR department policies
  > Food service sanitation and health code policies
- Review of their specific job description
  > Temporary or probationary limitations
- Employee health sign-off for TB testing, mask fitting, and any physical restrictions

Orientation also includes the training and skills testing essential for the specific tasks they will be performing. A Diet Clerk does not need to be approved for use and cleaning of the meat slicer, but a new cook needs that skill validation plus demonstrated proficiency with the fryer, char-broiler, and knife safety, etc.

- Equipment competency checklist
- Skills testing

The Onboarding Process is the sum of all the orientation activities, and is often planned to cover the first 30-90 days of employment (the typical probationary period). Completion of the different activities frequently includes a signed checklist and often a test of some kind. Documentation validates that each employee has been given the information they need to appropriately perform their assigned tasks.

It is helpful to use an orientation checklist to organize the content, to ensure that everything is covered, and to develop documentation of the orientation. An example appears in Figure 11.1. Some facilities require two sets of initials next to each item on a checklist: the supervisor's initials to verify that this content has been covered, and the employee's initials as a way of accepting responsibility for having learned this content.

Many managers have developed a New Hire Training Manual or three-ringed binder system that employees can build during their onboarding process. This may include copies of all relevant policies, department and facility maps, schedules, contact information, job descriptions, etc. Retaining the employee-signed receipt for the materials and training post-tests verifies the completion of each step in the process.

An additional scheduling consideration relates to the length of time for orientation. Realize that a new employee is virtually bombarded with information. It is not realistic to expect a new employee to learn everything in one sitting. If possible, a useful approach to this problem is to schedule orientation in short blocks of time.

Figure 11.1 **Orientation Checklist**

Employee's Name: _____ Starting Date: _____

Job Title: _____ Supervisor: _____

TOPIC	DATE DISCUSSED	SUPERVISOR'S INITIALS	EMPLOYEE'S INITIALS
Introduction to supervisor and co-workers			
Orientation to work areas			
Locker room location and use			
Dress code and uniforms			
Employee schedule			
Request for time off			
Attendance policy			
Timeclock procedures			
Meal and break policies			
Payroll procedures			
Overtime policy			
Handwashing requirements—when to wash hands			
Handwashing procedure			
Employee health policy and illness reporting			
Employee health & wellness (health risk assessment)			
Safety rules			
Safety data sheet (SDS) and chemical safety			
Fire safety procedures			
Confidentiality policies			
Personnel policies			
Critical rules			
Performance standards			
Performance review process			
Probationary period			
Progressive discipline policy			
Grievance procedures			
Job route for: (position)*			
Job route for: (position)*			
Job route for: (position)*			
Equipment operation for:*			
Equipment operation for:*			
Equipment operation for:*			
Policies and procedures for:*			
Policies and procedures for:*			
Policies and procedures for:*			
Policies and procedures for:*			
Temperature recording and logs			
Food requisition withdrawal form			
How to report concerns			
Departmental goals and objectives			
Sanitation program			
Quality management process			
Customer service initiative			
Disaster and emergency procedures			

- On the first day, cover some basic elements related to timeclock procedures, uniforms, and department layout.
- As follow-up on the next day, cover work procedures and routines.
- At yet another time, review safety policies.

Working with content in smaller segments gives the employee time to process new information and improves retention. An additional advantage of this approach is that as an employee begins working, familiarity grows. The employee develops a context in which to understand and store this new information. The employee may also encounter questions and curiosities that enhance learning.

The Dining Services-specific Onboarding Process Record should be kept in the employee's department file for easy reference.

> Some managers have used a color coded system to make recordkeeping easier. The Onboarding Process record is on blue paper, Fire and Safety are on pink paper, Sanitation is on yellow paper, Diet information is on green paper, etc. By looking in a file, they can quickly see if an employee has a signed checklist or post-test for the different training programs.

Training Beyond the Orientation Period

Mastering new skills and realizing potential are tremendous motivators. Training can meet employees' basic needs and foster good morale. Training serves other purposes, too. For a facility, effective training can:

- Reduce the occurrence of injuries, accidents, and mistakes.
- Improve quality of services and/or products.
- Improve productivity.
- Reduce turnover rate and recruitment expenses.
- Bring about better management of resources often with associated cost reductions.
- Improve compliance with regulations and standards.
- Support implementation of new procedures or techniques, new systems, or new equipment.

All foodservice employees, those new on the job and those with years of experience, can benefit from effective training programs. The TJC (The Joint Commission), OSHA (Occupational Safety and Health Administration), most state licensing laws, and many health department regulations require specific ongoing employee training programs for foodservice related employees, which may specify training on topics, such as:

- Sanitation practices
- Employee illness reporting
- Safety and disaster preparedness
- Role in medical nutrition therapy
- Confidentiality
- Safe operation of equipment
- Injury/accident prevention and reporting
- Safe use of chemicals
- Risk management
- Sexual harassment
- Labor laws and employees' rights

A number of regulations and standards stipulate that orientation and training must be provided to all employees from all shifts, and must be planned and conducted for all foodservice personnel. Check with members of the facility to determine specific guidelines that apply to the situation. As new procedures are implemented and new equipment is purchased, there is a need for ongoing in-service (on-the-job) training. Furthermore, tenured employees need periodic (some are annual) updates and refreshers, even for information they have learned in the past, to increase motivation and reinforce work practices.

All training should be documented. Documentation may be required by inspectors or surveyors, and it also helps keep track of what has been done. One way to do this is to ask each attendee to sign an attendance sheet and file this along with the outline of the training session.

Developing and implementing effective training programs is not difficult, but it does require time to develop a plan and procedures to ensure that training is effective.

Steps in Training

Step 1: The first step in training is to determine the need—who and what should be offered.

Step 2: Training content is the second step in training.
How do you determine what content to cover in training? To identify content, you can:

- Check standards that specify content.
- Identify changes in the operation that require training
- Review quality studies and identify areas that require training for improvement.
- Review operating objectives and select items that require training.
- Talk with employees during performance reviews and ask them what they need and want to learn.
- Observe operations and make notes of skills that need to be developed.
- Check with colleagues for new ideas about training content.

As training content is defined, try to focus on specifics. For example, a session about all aspects of safety may be too much. A session about appropriate knife handling and another session about lifting objects safely are likely to generate better outcomes.

Step 3: The third step is to decide on an objective/outcome of the training. To write an objective, start with thinking about what he employees need to do at the end of the training. If a task has been documented as a performance standard, then these tasks become the training objectives. A well-written objective begins with an action verb and should fit the S.M.A.R.T. principle:

- **S**pecific
- **M**easurable
- **A**chievable
- **R**elevant
- **T**imely

Examples of S.M.A.R.T. training objectives for foodservice employees are listed below:

- Describe the importance of and access to Safety Data Sheets (SDS).
- Use proper protective equipment when using chemicals in the kitchen.
- Document food waste using appropriate forms.
- Compute cost of menu items.
- Demonstrate proper handwashing procedures.
- Use proper portion control utensils.
- Define proper cooling procedures for soup.

As you can see, these all begin with a verb and are outcomes of the training session.

Step 4: Once there is an objective, it's time to gather the materials needed for teaching the objective. The materials will depend upon the objectives.

- For example, when training on how to use SDS forms, having actual forms available will improve the training.
- Use proper portion control utensils will require having various portioning utensils and perhaps some food items to practice portioning.
- You can use posters and reminder signs in your department to reinforce training content.

Many training resources are available through trade and industry websites.

Step 5: Decide where to hold the training.

- Does the facility have a conference room where you can be undisturbed and comfortable?
- Consider using the kitchen if there will be equipment demonstrations.
- Make sure to reserve any rooms needed ahead of time.
- Plan to use a stand-up meeting to quickly cover one or two points, or as a reminder of specific activities.
- Consider a roving in-service to briefly meet with staff in small groups throughout the department or facility.

Step 6: Promote the training. Post the date, place and time far enough ahead for every shift to see the information. If it is a facility-wide training, confirm that the staff has received the information.

Step 7: Conduct the training. (See the section later in this chapter on training techniques.)

Step 8: Evaluate the training. (See the section later in this chapter on evaluating the training.)

Who Should Train?

Can anyone train? The answer to this question is no—at least without training to become a good trainer. A trainer must have an ability to teach and be willing to commit the time necessary for training activities.

Since the person selected to train is critical to the ultimate success of the program, the characteristics of effective trainers must be applied to the selection of a trainer. Among the attributes of a good trainer are:

- An interest in training
- Extensive knowledge of the subject matter
- An ability to communicate effectively
- Strong interpersonal skills
- Patience
- A sense of humor
- Respect for trainees
- Confidence in the ability of others to learn
- An enthusiasm for the training assignment.

As with every other task on the job, a motivated individual can develop and refine training skills. As a Certified Dietary Manager, expect to deliver a great deal of training. At the same time, plan to enlist the help of staff members who are showing excellent performance, a positive attitude, and motivation to lead others. This provides recognition to qualified staff members and creates new opportunities for them. In addition, you may find that a staff member who is particularly skillful at a certain task is the best teacher.

Beyond the Dining Services staff, there may be others in the facility and community who can provide training about specific topics. For example, a social worker in your facility may be an excellent resource for providing a training session about dealing with angry clients, or a financial expert may be able to deliver a session about cost control. A local college or university may be able to provide training about almost any topic. A consulting dietitian may provide training about special diets or tube feedings, or many other topics. Vendors and others may also offer training.

When delegating training to others, be sure he or she is aware of the objectives or outcomes set. Discuss the content, and review the outline together before finalizing the program. If applicable, review handouts in advance and assure that they complement internal policies and procedures.

Training Techniques

Several principles of learning should be incorporated into training programs. Educational material, particularly the required annual safety and sanitations programs, can become very repetitive year-after-year. Mixing up the material and trying different techniques can help make the content more interesting.

It is always best when the trainees have a desire to learn. An internal motivating force can lead employees to seek additional job knowledge and/or new job-related skills. Employees cannot be forced to learn, but sometimes, you can create the desire to learn by presenting a thought-provoking question, piece of information, or problem at the beginning of a training session. If you can, relate the training to personal experiences and personal needs. When employees see the benefits in training and recognize how it can improve their performance, their participation levels improve.

Putting It Into Practice

1. Write a S.M.A.R.T. objective for New Employee Orientation, day one.

Typically, employees want to take an active role in the training activities. Everyone learns best by doing, not by passively reading or listening. The more staff members can be involved and active in training, the more effective training will be.

Training should focus on real-world problems which employees face and solve on the job. Trainees can then see how the training activities will apply directly to their own work. Perhaps the most important aspect of adult education is the idea of knowledge transfer. This means relating the training content to the job where participants apply it in actual practice.

People learn differently. For instance, some people are auditory learners (they learn by hearing the information). Some people are visual learners (they learn by reading or seeing a diagram). Many people learn by doing (this is known as kinesthetic learning). When training techniques combine listening, reading and doing, trainees will learn more. It may be important to determine the literacy level of the employees. If employees have low reading skills, use more pictures in the training. With a diverse group of employees, language may also be a barrier that pictures can help overcome.

Furthermore, a trainee's prior experiences influence learning. This concept is especially important in group training, where each employee brings a different background to the training. Trainees learn at different rates and will react differently to specific training experiences. Each person has a unique and individual learning style. For this reason, most trainers use a variety of communication techniques in order to provide something for everyone.

What techniques can be used? Lectures, videotapes and DVDs are examples of one-way flow of information from the trainer to the trainees. Although these methods are inexpensive and require little preparation time, they require the learner to be passive. To use these aids effectively, follow up with activities that help participants transfer the information, such as problem solving, hands-on practice, or role playing.

Computer-assisted instruction adopts the principles of programmed instruction and adds the power and flexibility associated with rapidly expanding computer technology. Today, many food and dining services training programs are available online or on CD. Well designed computer-based training uses two important learning principles—motivation and feedback. If access to computers is not possible, perhaps video/DVD training sessions can be made available during down time or breaks.

Another option is use of case studies that present a problem or situation. Trainees analyze and discuss the problem and devise a set of solutions. Have them work in small groups.

A variation of this is a group activity in which participants have to carry out a task. As an example, Figure 11.2 presents a training aid for a fire safety in-service that sends employees through their own work areas to identify locations of various fire-protection devices.

For any procedure requiring a series of steps, demonstration is a very useful technique. An effective demonstration breaks a task into clear step, and walks trainees through the steps at a comfortable pace. Following a demonstration, each trainee needs to practice the procedure with feedback from the trainer. Then, the trainee should do it again. On the job, the trainee should repeat the process with intermittent feedback and support from the Certified Dietary Manager.

Figure 11.2 Fire Safety Activity: Fighting Fire—Where Is It?

Write down the location of these items closest to your work area.

Smoke detector:

Heat detector:

Fire alarm box:

Silver (water) fire extinguisher for paper, cloth:

Red (carbon dioxide) fire extinguisher for grease, oil, flammable liquids, or electrical equipment:

Evacuation route:

Source: F&N Training Paks. ©The Grossbauer Group. Used with permission.

Types of Training

One type of training is called **on-the-job training (OJT)**. This technique is common in many dining services departments because it is practical and easy to transfer. It involves simply teaching an employee how to do a job while the employee is on location and actually on the job.

To conduct OJT, break down the job into parts, just as you would for a demonstration. In the training, address each part and provide the procedures, performance standards, safety information and all relevant components. Then, demonstrate and allow the employee to practice.

Repetition is important both to make sure that the trainee knows how to do the work and to allow them to build confidence and speed. Coaching, an integral part of training, is also important while the trainee practices. The trainer can observe and make friendly suggestions about the work. The trainer should frequently compliment the trainee for performance that meets quality standards.

The final step in OJT training is follow-up. After the training has been completed, the trainee should be able to do work without constant supervision. However, the trainer should continue to observe the trainee to ensure that no problems arise. At this time, reinforcement and feedback become important. Figure 11.3 lists the steps for on-the-job training.

Glossary

On-the-job Training (OJT)
Involves teaching an employee how to do a job while the employee is on location and actually on the job.

Figure 11.3 Four Steps for On-The-Job Training

01 PREPARE

Arrange work area: Arrange the work area to allow the trainer to stand next to the trainee; collect any needed tools; remove distractions if possible.

Put trainee at ease: Reduce the trainee's anxiety, assure him/her that you are there to help. Encourage the trainee to ask questions if he/she doesn't understand any directions.

02 PRESENT

Demonstrate the job function: Show the trainee how to do the job function by actually doing it and allowing him/her to observe. If the trainee desires, he/she may take notes during this phase.

Explain key points: While demonstrating, explain key points to the trainee. Attempt to answer the questions: Who, What, When, Where, Why, and How.

Repeat the demonstration: The trainer again performs the task as the trainee observes. This reinforcement increases the likelihood that the trainee will retain the new information.

03 PRACTICE

Let the trainee attempt parts of the job: Allow the trainee to practice part of the job. After he/she attempts to do part of the job provide constructive feedback, coaching, and suggestions.

Let the trainee perform the entire job under observation: The trainer now provides feedback periodically rather than frequently, and encourages the trainee to begin acting independently.

04 FOLLOW UP

Conduct periodic progress checks: The trainer steps back and only spot checks the trainee's progress.

Allow the learner to work independently: At this point, the trainee has formally completed the training topic, but is encouraged to seek out the trainer if assistance is needed. Complete the training checklist.

In-Service Training

In-service training is professional development for the employees to improve or update specific skills. It takes place after the employee has started working. In-service training should follow the training steps outlined earlier in this chapter. (See Figure 11.4 for an in-service outline for a HIPAA presentation.)

There are many topics that can be included in the in-service training plans. Some examples are:

- Coping with emergencies
- Dealing with difficult clients
- Professional and ethical expectations for foodservice employees
- Security and confidentiality (HIPAA guidelines)
- Client/Customer Service

As reinforcement for in-service training activities, provide employees with a handout or brochure that summarizes key points. A sample handout for a fire safety in-service appears in Figure 11.5 on page 188.

Putting It Into Practice

2. What types of training materials or resources would be useful when training employees on personal hygiene?

Figure 11.4 HIPAA In-Service Training

Intended Audience: All Foodservice Employees

Content to Cover:

HIPAA (Health Insurance Portability & Accountability Act) was made into law in 1996. The Privacy Rule took effect in 2003 with updates in 2006 and 2013. The primary goal is for people to keep health information confidential and to help the healthcare industry control administrative costs. This in-service identifies how HIPAA applies in the foodservice department.

Resources:

Additional information on the law is found at the Health & Human Services website (www.hhs.gov). General information on HIPAA is available at the following links: (http://www.cms.gov/Regulations-and-Guidance/HIPAA-Administrative-Simplification/HIPAAGenInfo/). Health information privacy. U.S. Department of Health and Human Services website (http://www.hhs.gov/ocr/privacy/) (http://optimalhealthcareinc.com/wp-content/uploads/2012/12/HIPAA-online-in-service.pdf).

Objectives:

- Staff will be able to describe which parts of HIPAA affect their work
- Staff will know how to protect private client information

Outline:

1. What is HIPAA (Health Insurance Portability & Accountability Act)?
   - Protects the privacy of all personal and health information about clients, including written, spoken and electronic.
   - Identifies clients' rights to their medical information.
   - Limits access to client-protected information.
   - Clients can request that no information be shared without specific permission.
2. What does the medical facility have to do?
   - Develop privacy policies and procedures.
   - Train staff on the procedures.
   - Define disciplinary action if information is inappropriately released.
3. How does HIPAA affect the Foodservice Department? What is confidential information?
   - Computerized Diet Information includes name, DOB, diet, medical record number, and often diagnosis.
   - Meal identification menus or cards include name, DOB, diet, and medical record number.
   - Meal delivery sheets include identifiers on all clients on the unit.
   - Clinical and diet office staff can access more detailed information via the medical record.
4. How to manage the privacy of clients:
   - Do not discuss client information with anyone other than those needing the specifics.
   - Do not discuss client information with family members or friends without the client's permission.
   - Keep client information closed, covered or out of sight.
   - Do not access the electronic medical record for information other than what you need to do your job.
   - Discard client related materials in the shredding boxes.
5. Review the HIPAA facility and department policy.

Activity:

As a group create a poster that can be put up in the department, of areas where client information is located and procedures for what they should do with the information.

Evaluation:

Administer the post-test to determine the level of understanding.

Source: dk Foodservice Solutions, LLC. Used with permission.

Figure 11.5 Sample Handout for Fire Safety In-Service

FIRE RESPONSE PROCEDURE	
RACE	**PASS**
R: **REMOVE** everyone from danger	**P:** **PULL** the pin
A: Turn on the **ALARM**	**A:** **AIM** at the base of the fire
C: **CONFINE** the fire	**S:** **SQUEEZE** the trigger and keep the extinguisher in an upright position
E: **EXTINGUISH** the fire if you can do it safely	**S:** **SWEEP** from side to side

Sanitation and Safety Training

This is listed as a type of training because safety and sanitation training is a mandatory program. The 2013 FDA Food Code opening statement is as follows:

Foodborne illness in the United States is a major cause of personal distress, preventable illness and death, and avoidable economic burden. Scallan et al. (2011a,b) estimated that foodborne diseases cause approximately 48 million illnesses, 128,000 hospitalizations, and 3,000 deaths in the United States each year. The occurrence of approximately 1,000 reported disease outbreaks (local, regional, and national) each year highlights the challenges of preventing these infections.

These numbers give us reason to pause. Most foodborne illnesses are preventable. Certified Dietary Managers have an obligation to train every member of the foodservice team in food protection. In fact, the FDA Food Code stipulates that managers must train employees in such topics as:

- The risks of bare-hand contact with food.
- When and where to wash hands.
- How to wash hands.
- How to maintain fingernails.
- Prohibition of jewelry.
- Basic hygiene.

The FDA Food Code also notes that managers must document sanitation training. Many managers document training with attendance sign-in sheets, along with a summary of each training meeting. (This would be a good use of the color coded post-test placed in the employee file, verifying successful completion of the training session.)

Training improves the likelihood of compliance with food handling policies and practices, reduces the need for constant supervision, and improves employee self-esteem and job satisfaction. Training for food safety should include topics such as:

- Personal hygiene
- Restrictions and precautions for illness
- Why, when, and how to take temperatures
- Safe thawing and preparation practices; sanitation techniques
- Other food protection practices that relate to the employees' job responsibilities

Putting It Into Practice

3. You want to cover food safety and sanitation in a training session. With the topic of hand washing, how would you incorporate the three major learning styles (auditory, verbal, and kinesthetic)?

Particularly because of the health and safety consequences, trainers should be carefully selected based on job knowledge and ability to facilitate learning. Training strategies appropriate for sanitation training include new employee orientation, on-the-job training, and group training (in-services). Each of these approaches is important for improving and maintaining the sanitation skills and knowledge of foodservice employees.

For instance, the OJT program for a new dishmachine focuses on the proper steps in manual and automatic dishwashing. The new employee learns how to perform these job tasks by working with an experienced employee. The instruction is accomplished through observation and return demonstration by the new employee, while the experienced employee provides coaching and feedback.

Instructional Materials

The Certified Dietary Manager may need instructional materials to assist in providing food safety training to staff. A variety of resources are available from groups and organizations such as:

- Professional associations in the foodservice and hospitality industry.
- State departments of public health.
- Federal agencies such as the Food and Drug Administration, United States Department of Agriculture, and Centers for Disease Control and Prevention.
- Cooperative extension programs.
- Local colleges, universities, and technical schools.
- Vendors and suppliers to the foodservice industry.
- State and local health departments.

Many free posters, handouts and interactive resources about food safety are available on reliable websites, such as those of the U.S. government and county extension agencies. Many are available in various languages, and some rely on graphics to support the message. These can be useful in training employees who speak English as a second language or have language barriers.

Evaluating Training

Remember that training is a process and that involves evaluation. Two ways of evaluating training are measuring knowledge gains or satisfaction with a written evaluation and by giving feedback.

Witten Evaluation

Some standards applying to non-commercial foodservice operations specify that employees' knowledge should be measured both before and after training. So, the Certified Dietary Managers may use a pre-test and a post-test to measure knowledge. A sample pre-test that doubles as a post-test appears in Figure 11.6. A test such as this does not measure transfer of learning, but it does tell whether employees have grasped the prerequisite information.

Employees should also evaluate the training session. Find out whether participants felt the training was useful, what questions were left unanswered, and how participants rate their own confidence in being able to do something differently on the job. Ask them what they will do differently as a result of training. Ask them what else they would like to learn. A sample in-service training session evaluation appears in Figure 11.7.

Figure 11.6 HIPAA In-Service Training Post-Test

Name: _____ Date: _____

1. **True or False:** When approached by a visiting family member, the dietitian should explain the reason for a cardiac diet to the client's son.

2. What could happen if an employee leaves the unit's Diet Sheet on the counter?
   a. The employee could lose their job
   b. The patient could sue the facility
   c. Both of the above
   d. Neither of the above

3. How should confidential paperwork be managed?
   a. Dispose of expired or unneeded paperwork in the shredder boxes
   b. Keep active information nearby on the desk
   c. Maintain current client information filed in drawers
   d. Throw yesterday's diet sheet in the wastebasket for trash disposal
   e. A and C above

4. **True or False:** Diet Office staff need to know a client's diagnosis and should look up test results.

5. **True or False:** HIPAA really only affects medical and nursing staff in a medical facility.

ANSWER KEY: 1. False   2. c. Both of the above   3. d. A and C above   4. False   5. False

Source: dk Foodservice Solutions, LLC. Used with permission.

The best way to assess the training efforts is to work with the list of objectives and observe what employees are actually doing. If objectives have been met, the training has been successful. If not, it is time to analyze further.

Giving Feedback

Feedback is information about what an employee is doing. It provides perspective, direction, and recognition. During orientation, and in later training activities, it is important to provide staff with relevant and prompt feedback on how well they have mastered a task. An encouraging word or early correction of a misstep may be all that is needed.

Everyone enjoys receiving positive feedback, such as praise for a task well done. At the same time, though, constructive feedback about something that did not go perfectly conveys a critical message. The critical message is: *Your work matters. What you do is important.* All forms of feedback, when handled well, can improve an employee's performance and boost their self-esteem.

Often, Certified Dietary Managers expect training to solve all problems. It does not. When an employee performs poorly, most think the employee needs training. This may or may not be true. An employee may know how to do something, but fail to do it because of factors such as:

- Poor motivation
- Peer pressure
- Obstacles in the workplace

Glossary

Feedback
Information about what an employee is doing. It provides perspective, direction, and recognition.

Figure 11.7 Sample In-Service Evaluation Form (Measuring Satisfaction)

In-Service Session Title: _____ Date: _____

Please answer the following questions to help us improve our training programs.

1. Please rate how well this session relates to your own job:
    ○ excellent match   ○ fair match   ○ poor match

2. Was this material:
    ○ too complex   ○ too simple   ○ just right

3. Please rate the audio-visuals used:
    ○ excellent   ○ fair   ○ poor

4. Please rate the learning activities used:
    ○ excellent   ○ fair   ○ poor

5. Please rate the handouts used:
    ○ excellent   ○ fair   ○ poor

6. What did you like most about this training session?

7. What did you like least about this training session?

8. What topics would you like to see covered in future training?

- Lack of resources (such as time or supplies)
- Malfunctioning equipment
- Poorly designed systems.

Whenever an employee's performance does not reflect the training provided, talk with the employee. Listen, and size up the need. Decide what interventions can be provided and try them out.

The effective use of feedback, Performance Improvement Plans, and disciplinary actions are discussed in Chapter 13.

In-Service Planning

To have an effective in-service planning session with the department supervisors and managers, sketch out the list of topics that need to be covered in the coming year. Often, Human Resources or the Education Department provides the state and federally required in-services, which may **not** provide the foodservice level of detail. A case in point is the Fire Safety training for the kitchen and knowledge of the different types of fire extinguishers. Sanitation in the Dining Services department includes food preparation, holding and storage that are specific to foodborne illnesses, which others may not need.

The following is a sample in-service training schedule of topics frequently addressed in a food preparation and service delivery department:

1. Fire Safety
2. Handwashing
3. Personal Hygiene
4. Time and Temperature Control (HACCP)
5. Portion Control
6. HIPAA, Confidentiality and Ethics
7. Infection Control
8. Therapeutic Diets
9. Customer Service
10. Body Mechanics & Ergonomics
11. Disaster Preparedness
12. Sexual and Personal Harassment

When scheduling in-service sessions, the manager should also assign the task of who will be presenting the information. Often, department supervisors and other department managers can be recruited to provide educational programs.

It is extremely important to maintain a record of each in-service training session to include:

- The objective and lesson plan
- Sign-in attendance record with date
- Results of a post-test to verify understanding
- If appropriate, a color coded Post-Test to be placed in each employee's file

Training and education should be a life long expectation in the workplace. Technologies change, staffing patterns change, basic systems change, and we need to continuously update and train all staff members to the current trends. New views and knowledge reflect on the skills and qualifications of the Dining Services staff.

Putting It Into Practice

4. How can you ensure an employee's competency in using a new piece of equipment?

Employee Scheduling and Assignments

Overview and Objectives

From pay period to pay period, employees need to be scheduled to ensure that the needed personnel are always available to do required work. Scheduling involves assessing the production and service needs, the volume of work or output, and how long it takes to fulfill assigned duties. In Chapter 9, we explored staffing patterns, workflows and job analysis. In this chapter, we will look at how those tools affect the schedule, different types of schedules, time and attendance, and the documentation process. After completing this chapter, you should be able to:

✓ Prepare a time schedule

✓ Maintain time schedule chart/records

✓ Prepare absence/tardy reports for personnel files

A Quick Review

In Chapter 9, we started by setting up the **staffing pattern** for each position in the department and the hours to be scheduled each day of the week. Using the full-time equivalent calculation of 40 hours per week, we were able to calculate how many FTEs were needed to cover the schedule as planned.

The developed Staffing Pattern led into an evaluation of the Job Analysis Workflow of each position's work assignments. This allowed for a potential redesign of the flow of activities and tasks for each position. Once all of the tasks were assigned, defined **job routines** were easy to update. The **job routines** in turn, determined what was included in the **job description** as a summary of duties and responsibilities, which led back to a revised **staffing pattern** and the scheduling of staff. Because the needs of the department are always evolving, the demands on staffing and the scheduling of staff is also changing.

Effective Scheduling

Well-planned schedules are important for:

• Controlling labor costs.

• Ensuring that adequate labor resources are available at the right times and places to accomplish the work.

Keep in mind that the most effective staffing plan and set of job routines may not be the same every day. In many operations, the volume of work and level of services declines on

Saturdays and Sundays. The volume of employee dining services provided would likely also be reduced. As a result, assigned tasks may be combined into a single job routine requiring fewer employees (on the schedule). Holidays typically change the staffing requirements.

The work performed in many positions of the operation should be adjustable to reflect the changes in volume. Seasonal events or changes in the economy may lead to shifts in the client count or census, affecting the daily staffing needs. As numbers reduce, being pro-active by adjusting downward based on staffing needs creates sound management and financial control. Conversely, as the client numbers increase, it may be necessary to step up staffing levels.

Goals for Scheduling

Once it is determined how many people are needed in each position for day-to-day operations, a schedule can be written. This is a task that most managers complete and post about a week before each new pay period begins. A schedule identifies when each employee will work during that pay period, and to what position(s) that employee will be assigned.

When developing a schedule consider the following goals:

- Schedule staff to fit work needs.
- Use creative scheduling plans.
- Use the skill of your staff.
- Address employee schedule requests.
- Use scheduling policies.
- Plan ahead for special events.

Schedule Staff to Fit Work Needs

It is generally not useful for all staff to begin and end shifts at the same time. Referencing the Staffing Pattern developed in Chapter 9, staff should be scheduled at the times needed to meet the work required. This is called **staggered scheduling**.

For example, one dishmachine might be scheduled to begin work one hour before the evening meal period begins. This time may be used to clean up any remaining dishes from lunch and take care of production pots and pans for the dinner period. A second service employee might be brought in 30 minutes before the time of service to perform other duties. Both employees will be ready for the evening rush period.

Likewise, other personnel can be scheduled to meet the need for the various positions at different times of the day. Typically, the first employee in will be the first employee to leave. Staggered ending times also help maximize employee efficiency.

Flex scheduling is a concept used in some organizations to increase staffing as activity increases and reduce labor hours during slower periods. Hospitals may have a planned schedule based on their typical census resulting in defined reductions in shifts for weekends or declining client activity. Identifying the appropriate activity levels that trigger a change in staffing is the first step. Dovetailing responsibilities to reduce the labor hours and still maintain the needed quality of service is the second step. Finally, implementing the reduction, when appropriate, is the last step. Flexing the labor hours to reflect the census or level of activity can have a significant impact on the department budget.

Glossary

Staggered Scheduling
Scheduling staff so they come in at different times instead of coming in at the same time

Flex Scheduling
Designed to increase staffing as activity increases and reduce labor hours during slower periods

Use Creative Scheduling Plans

Part-time staff can be hired to work short shifts, such as three-, four-, or five-hour shifts. Sometimes, a job is designed as a **split shift**, or two short shifts in one day separated by a period of time off.

Temporary or "as-needed" employees can also be used. Many facilities maintain a list of people who don't want steady work but who like to work occasionally. If there is a special event, an employee illness or other need for temporary assistance, these personnel can be very helpful.

In the continuous challenge to do more with less, Certified Dietary Managers are becoming quite creative in devising ways of providing essential human resources to the operation. One idea is to use **cross-training,** which means training one employee to perform more than one job. To a certain degree, cross-training is a given in foodservice operations. Most employees are trained for several positions. This gives the manager the flexibility to adjust staffing on a daily basis.

Branching out, some organizations even cross-train employees between departments. An employee of an environmental services or laundry department, for example, may also learn certain jobs in the foodservice department—and vice versa. Cross-trained employees then become part of a job pool, and can be assigned or re-assigned as needed into various work areas. This flexibility helps managers in all affected departments use human resources very efficiently, and can result in full-time employment for the staff member.

Job sharing might be an idea that works in the community. With job sharing, you divide a full-time job into two or more shifts that are then shared by two or more part-time staff. This often works better in positions that have a fair amount of flexibility in the scheduling, such as the clinical dietitian. Job sharing can be split on the day, by different days of the week or alternating weeks. A drawback of job-sharing is the potential for increased cost of benefits, such as medical insurance.

Another idea used frequently, particularly in healthcare facilities, is to establish a volunteer program. This is done on a facility-wide basis, and an individual is assigned to manage volunteer services. Volunteers are available from all walks of life. The help of volunteers in a dining services department typically is limited to assisting clients with menu selection, transport of items from one area to another, help with some clerical tasks, and other non food contact activities.

Creative scheduling, job sharing, volunteer hours and cross training does not mean scheduling abuse. These are alternative scheduling options that may help the department, and the employee, but need to be managed carefully. Bouncing staff from one position to another, day after day, gets old quickly.

Use the Skills of Your Staff

Consider the skill sets of each staff member. If there is an employee with a pleasing smile and personality, he or she might enjoy helping in the dining room or serving in the cafeteria with high client contact. If an employee does not handle the demanding speed of the trayline, assign them to a less time-sensitive position.

Every department has strong employees and some who are not as skilled or experienced. Plan to schedule the staff to create a balanced team on every day. The goal is to get the job done with the best people available. Cross-training staff for multiple positions allows the flexibility to maximize their value to the organization and raises the performance of the whole department.

Glossary

Split Shift
Two short shifts separated by a period of time off in one day

Cross-Training
Training an employee to do more than one job

Job Sharing
Dividing a full-time position into two or more positions

Recognize Employee Schedule Requests

Consider personnel preferences whenever possible. Have a mechanism for employees to use to communicate special scheduling needs in advance of the time you prepare the schedule.

- If Mary needs to be off on the first Tuesday of the pay period, she should let you know by completing a form.
- If Mark needs to leave by 2:00 p.m. to attend a wedding, he can request to work an early shift.
- If Juanita wishes to take a one-week vacation next month, she needs to request it in advance.

Request forms may be used by personnel for indicating in advance those days/shifts when they wish to be off duty. It is good management practice to honor employee requests when possible.

Establish and Use Scheduling Policies

Operation of a foodservice department typically requires staffing at times that many employees might not consider optimal work hours. The breakfast cook may start at 4:30 or 5:00 in the morning and the night cashier may be working until 2:00 a.m. Holidays and weekends are a normal part of the dining services schedule. When employees work weekends, they often do not enjoy having two days off in a row. A day off might occur on a Tuesday one week, and on a Friday another week.

In addition, the number of employees who can take days off or schedule vacation at any given time is limited. During peak vacation seasons, many employees may wish to take the same time off work. However, rarely can all requests can be approved.

If there is no consistent method for requesting time off and making scheduling decisions, employees may feel that scheduling practices are not fair and equitable. (Scheduling preferences and task assignments are often the source of employee complaints about "favoritism".) Poorly planned schedules become a source of discontent among employees.

To manage these kinds of situations, establish policies relating to working hours, rotation of shifts, scheduling for weekends, holiday assignments, and decision-making regarding requests for time off, make these policies known to all employees, and follow them consistently. Without clear and consistent policies, each scheduling decision becomes a random or arbitrary action, subject to the scrutiny of all employees. (Policies and Procedures are discussed in greater detail in Chapter 14.)

Several factors may affect how you set policies.

1. The first is employment law.
   a. There are limits to how many hours each employee is scheduled.
2. Next, if the department employees belong to a union, there may be stipulations in the union contract with which the policies must comply.
3. If the facility has human resources policies that relate to scheduling, you must comply with these also.

Beyond these constraints, you must develop your own workable guidelines. There may be a history of scheduling preferences or assumed "promises" extended by a prior manager that need to be clarified, in written policy format, with human resources and the employees.

Here are examples of practices Certified Dietary Managers sometimes include in scheduling policies:

- Employees in _____ area are required to work weekends. The schedule is developed such that each employee works every other weekend.

- An employee who works the night shift on one day is not scheduled for the early morning shift the next day.

- For holiday scheduling, each employee completes a holiday request form, indicating a first, second, and third choice for holidays to be scheduled off duty.

  > The manager takes these requests in sequence, honoring as many requests as possible, and with an eye to who worked the holiday the year before.

  > Regularly scheduled days off may need to be changed to accommodate holiday schedules. Consider the following real life example:

  Hazel had worked at the hospital for 10 years, making salads and desserts for both the patients and the cafeteria. Although she worked every other weekend, she had been consistently scheduled off on Thursdays.

  When the holiday request schedule went up for Thanksgiving, Christmas and New Year's, Hazel considered herself lucky because this year Christmas and New Year's fell on Thursday. She knew she would be off all 3 days and not have to take a single vacation or paid holiday because "Thursday was her day off".

  Hazel was stunned when the manager reminded her to enter her preferred holiday off request. As a long-term employee with her schedule of Thursday's off, she took her concerns to the Human Resources Director. To her surprise, Human Resources reminded Hazel that "per the hospital policy" there are no guaranteed days off and that in departments where appropriate, all staff members would be scheduled to work holidays.

  Hazel requested Christmas off, and as luck would have it, also got Thanksgiving off. She was scheduled to work New Year's Day and she volunteered to work the supper line on New Year's Eve as a swap for Thanksgiving Day with another employee.

- Requests for time off are granted on a first-come, first-served basis.

  > If two requests are received on the same day and only one can be granted, the request is granted to the employee with the longest tenure.

  > Establish a reasonable request period to eliminate 20 requests submitted on December 26th for the following Christmas off.

  > Accepting requests a couple of months out allows employees to make travel plans.

Plan Ahead for Special Events

Often, a two-week schedule can be copied and adapted to fit the next two-week pay period. Sometimes, special events and holidays require a totally different schedule. You can use past schedules as a reference.

Planning the staffing needed for the employee holiday dinner, the Foundation Annual Extravaganza, Mother's Day brunch, or even the monthly board of directors meeting can be a lot easier when you reference prior schedules. Keep a history of these events to help plan both the food needed and the staff to make it happen.

Schedules and the Union Contract

Typically, a significant portion of the union contract is focused on the scheduling of union staff members. The contract may specify times, days and frequency with which employees may be scheduled. Often, the contract will specify how replacement staff needs to be scheduled to cover for vacation, holiday and sick time.

Remember that the union contract is another version of the Policy and Procedure Manual. Read it, know it and understand it. Work with the Human Resources Department and the Union Stewart to make sure that management and the employees understand the guidelines and requirements of the contract as it relates to scheduling and task assignments.

Do not let the contract come between you, the staff and the needs of the facility. Use the contract, and the Union Stewart, to help set the scheduling policies and explain them to department staff members.

Schedules and Employee Relations

Work schedules directly affect employees' lives. Whether it is the day of the week, the start/stop times or total hours scheduled, they are expected to adjust their personal lives to meet staffing needs. Few things cause disruption in the department faster than an inconsistent or frequently changed schedule.

Here are a couple of "rule of thumb" scheduling courtesies that are not difficult to follow but are frequently overlooked.

- Post a written schedule at least one week prior to the start of the schedule.
  - > Typically, schedules are based on the two week pay period; some start Sunday and others start Monday.
  - > Post the schedule no later than the Monday prior.
- Covering the schedules is more than filling in the blanks:
  - > Schedule qualified people into the positions.
  - > A dining room server may be willing to make breakfast, but may not be qualified to do so.
- Try to establish regular days off for each staff member.
  - > As a 365-day operation, weekends and holidays coverage is essential
  - > If employees consistently work every other weekend or one-in-three, although not always possible, try to give them the same day off in the week before and after working a weekend (It is important to remind the staff that this is a courtesy and not mandatory. The schedule is developed for the needs of the department and clients and, as such, could change. Also important is to communicate these changes with the staff involved.).
- If there is a change to their regular day off to cover the schedule, make the employee aware before posting the schedule.
  - > They may have a doctor's appointment or family event planned for that regular day off and may not be available for the schedule.
- Try to accommodate employee requests for days off—both paid and unpaid.
  - > Although not always an option, when staff members know that you tried they often become a little more flexible in their requests.

- Avoid scheduling "double back" assignments or too many days in a row:
  - > Many jobs have early and late positions, but it is physically difficult to work a late shift one day followed by an early shift the next morning.
  - > Frequently scheduling more than five days in a row is very taxing for most staff members.
- Do not change a posted schedule without talking to the affected staff members.
  - > Once the schedule is posted, they are responsible for what was posted—not what has been changed without their input.
- Be fair. Rotate weekend and holidays around to all qualified staff members.
  - > Unless there is an organizational policy, or it is written into a contract or job description, all employees within a given job description should experience an equal number of working weekends, holidays and ease of access to vacation time.
  - > Post tentative schedules for Thanksgiving through the New Year's holidays in early November so all staff can plan for travel and family time.
  - > Often, when given the opportunity to work it out:
    - Older staff want Thanksgiving and Christmas Eve off for cooking and family time.
    - Younger staff often prefer New Year's Eve off ,with New Year's Day to relax.
    - Staff with young children want Christmas Day morning off.
- Schedule employees consistent with their employment status.
  - > Full-time employees expect to be scheduled 32-40 hours a weekend depending on your facility's definition of full-time.
  - > 30-, 24-, or 20-hour positions should be scheduled according to their hours and should not be consistently scheduled above those hours.

Employment Status Terminology

Full-time status is typically referenced as 40 hours of work a week and overtime eligible. Some employers define a 32 or 35 hours a week as full-time.

Part-time status is less than the 40 (or 35 or 32) hours per week and with a consistent number of hours, i.e., 16 or 24 hours.

PRN or pool status refers to employees of the facility with no set schedule— they are scheduled "as needed".

Temporary, casual, agency or per diem status refers to staff assigned from an outside agency on a day basis or as independent contractors.

Nonexempt status positions are paid on an hourly basis, covered by minimum wage and overtime guidelines. (The majority of the employees in a facility)

Exempt status positions are paid a defined salary, and excluded from minimum wage protection and overtime regulations (Primarily the management and professional level employees).

Employees need to be able to anticipate how much they will earn in wages to pay their life expenses and, if need be, take on another job. A predictable schedule shows respect for the employee and allows them to better manage their time away from work.

Glossary

Nonexempt Status
Employees paid on an hourly basis and eligible for overtime

Exempt Status
Employees paid a defined salary with no overtime

Creating the Schedule

Scheduling can be a time-consuming task. Managers often develop a scheduling form that has standard details, such as the shift times, names of employees, and the hours of operation already completed.

Some facilities have computer programs for timecard/payroll management and scheduling employees. A typical **electronic scheduling** program allows for entry of facility-defined scheduling guidelines and current employee requests. It generates a schedule based on all available information, and allows for review and edits if necessary.

As with most software programs, the number and types of reports available can be overwhelming.

- Employee scheduling software usually allows you to establish desired staffing ratios that define the number of employees needed based on meal or client counts.
- Advanced reports help verify that the proposed schedule will meet the budget.
- Once the schedule information is set, there are several format options: a master schedule, a daily schedule, an employee's personal schedule, and so forth.
- Most systems track attendance and tardiness within the program. Some systems may notify you when unscheduled absences and/or late work arrival meet the criteria for disciplinary action.
- Employee records within a scheduling program may include contact information to make calling of replacement staff when there are unscheduled absences.
- Typically scheduling packages are available as part of a timeclock system, which then integrates with time-clocks and payroll reporting.

Electronic Scheduling

An alternative to developing the staffing pattern from the Job Analysis Workflows built in Chapter 9 is to work through the process within the electronic scheduling program. The set-up process will take an investment in time, but allowing the computer to help generate schedules and track attendance can be time well spent.

The various scheduling programs offer different features and the manager needs to check with the organization's particular software for specific tasks available. However, electronic scheduling program offers:

- Ability to create a daily, weekly, or pay period schedule that assigns authorized positions to employees.
- An employee work schedule is generated for each individual staff member, including requested days off.
- Provides reports, such as:
  > "Positions requested" which present the same information as the staffing pattern that discussed in Chapter 9.
  > Schedules for posting in the department.
  > Schedules sent to staff via company staff emails.
  > Overtime reports.
  > Position control reports.
  > Vacation and sick time reports that can be used when working with individual staff requests.
  > Tracks absenteeism – including sick calls and arriving tardy.
  > FTE reports based on budget and actual numbers.

Glossary

Electronic Scheduling
Computer based program for scheduling, time and attendance tracking

Putting It Into Practice

1. Two employees have submitted requests to have the same day off. Having both of them gone at the same time would pose a hardship for the department. What should you do?

Calculating Total Labor Hours and FTEs

The computer can easily calculate the number of FTEs (Full Time Equivalent) in the entire schedule or by individual job description. How to calculate FTEs and total hours based on the staffing pattern is covered in Chapter 9. The electronic scheduler makes the process easier and readily available for review by the year, the month, the pay period or by the day.

If the organization functions under a **position control** structure, knowing how many FTEs are in each job description can be a major benefit. Position Control is a finance and human resources concept where each job description in the department is authorized a specific number of positions. This defines the number of hours approved in the budget for cooks or meal servers or supervisors. Each position is assigned a unique number in the human resources system that ties to the financial budget for the number of hours approved for the position.

Position control relates to the hours and number of positions approved in the budget, irrespective of how many staff members are actually on the payroll. When facilities do not implement the control side of position control, approved positions are not being filled while other positions are over-staffed. Following the position control for labor hours approved will keep you on budget.

Using a Productivity Standard

Much of today's foodservice industry estimates staffing needs using a productivity standard, such as meals per labor hour or minutes per meal. If you know your **meals per labor hour** or **minutes per meal**, compare this figure to industry benchmarks. Many of the electronic schedulers will accept a productivity standard for tracking purposes.

For instance, imagine you are a school foodservice manager and have calculated the meals per labor hour to be 9.7. The industry standard is 13-15 meals per labor hour. This example means that the staff is not producing as many meals per labor hour as the benchmark. While that could mean that the number of meals served was not calculated correctly, in reality it probably means you are overstaffed. This information can help identify the opportunity to increase the number of meals served or areas for reduction in labor hours.

The Dietary Manager Professional Practice Standard for Estimating Staffing Needs can be found at the end of Chapter 9 in the Management in the News section. Review this standard to determine the facility's productivity standards. Once there is an accurate standard for the facility, you can compare the staffing to the benchmarks provided.

Types of Schedules

There are generally three types of employee schedules you can use to communicate with staff: Master Schedule, Work Area Schedule and a Shift Schedule.

Master Schedule. The master schedule is for the entire department and includes days on and off, plus vacations days for all employees. The master schedule may be developed for a week, two weeks, or even a month.

Work Area Schedule. In larger departments, or departments with multiple managers/supervisors, a separate schedule may be posted specifically for those employees. For example, a schedule may be posted for the Production Staff while a different schedule is posted for the Dining Room or Cafeteria staff.

Glossary

Position Control
A management system to control the number of positions for each job description

Meals Per Labor Hour
A productivity standard that is a calculation of the total meals served divided by the total number of department labor hours

Minutes Per Meal
A productivity standard that is a calculation of the total department labor minutes divided by the total number of meals served

Shift Schedule. The shift schedule shows the different shifts, and when they begin and end for different positions. For instance, using a small hospital as an example, a shift schedule for the a.m. and p.m. cooks would look like the graph below, Figure 12.1. The shift schedule is useful when interviewing new employees to show them the position coverage.

Figure 12.1 Staff Schedule for Cooks

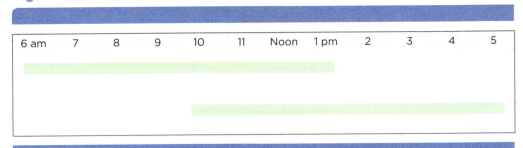

| 6 am | 7 | 8 | 9 | 10 | 11 | Noon | 1 pm | 2 | 3 | 4 | 5 |

The Gantt Chart developed in Chapter 9 is similar to the Shift Schedule. It displays the positions and the overlap of shifts, plus the work details related to the flow of the day.

Communicating the Schedule

Needless to say, a schedule works only if communicated clearly to all employees. Once the schedule has been developed, post it in a highly visible location for review by all employees. The policy on posted schedules should make it clear to each employee that it is his or her responsibility to review the schedule and comply with it.

It is the manager's responsibility to post the schedule far enough in advance so employees can review it and adjust their personal activities to coordinate with their work times (typically one week before the new pay period). For example, you cannot post a schedule on Saturday if it takes effect on Monday, as many employees may not be at work, and would not know what their schedules are. Employees who are not at work before a new schedule goes into effect should be advised to call and confirm when they are working.

A schedule should be clear and specific:

- When two employees have the same first name, it's important to use a last name or initial to avoid confusion.
- Each schedule should clearly identify the dates, so that employees do not confuse the schedule for one pay period with that of another.
- Pencil or erasable versions of the schedule should not be posted.
- Only the supervisor or manager should have authority to edit a posted schedule, never the employees themselves.
- Any changes to a posted schedule should be entered in colored ink (red, green, purple, etc.) so each edit can be quickly seen.
  - > White-out® or Liquid Paper® should not be used on a schedule.

Finally, the manager should keep an extra copy of the schedule in a secure location, in case the posted schedule disappears or becomes damaged.

After use, the actual edited copy of the schedules should be retained. You may need them for several purposes, such as reviewing and completing the records for payroll at the end of a pay period, reviewing past actions in order to enforce scheduling policies, and responding to inquires or complaints that may arise in the future. The actual posted copy of the schedule records which employees were absent from work, the days they missed and any changes in other staff schedules to cover.

Scheduling Adjustments

As with all things, the best laid plans can go awry. The most common scheduling challenge concerns employee tardiness and absence. When a job needs to be covered, other employees may be called to see if they would be willing to come to work on short notice. (Due to privacy concerns, maintain a master list of employees with current contact information in a secure location available to managers. Your list may also identify what jobs each employee is trained to do.) Depending upon the policies and/or union contract, coverage for a missing staff member may be based on the most available employee or the most senior.

As part of the scheduling process, many managers maintain a call record posted in the office where all supervisors can access the information to plan their workflow for the day. The call record, see Figure 12.2, documents who has "called-out" and a general reason for the absence. In addition, it records who was contacted to cover the open shift and their response. This can be particularly important in a union-staffed department.

From here, adjustments may have to be made to the schedule to avoid incurring overtime for the employee who has just punched in. Or, overtime may be authorized for this employee. An alternative method of dealing with employee absence is the re-assignment of duties among existing staff. Sometimes, it is possible to divide the duties of an absent employee among staff members who are present. This requires careful planning, fairness and tact.

To minimize the disruption and difficulty associated with finding coverage for jobs or re-working assignments, every facility develops and enforces some basic policies regarding unscheduled absences and tardiness. Most likely, these policies will come from the human resources department of the facility.

For example, an attendance policy might specify that any employee should not exceed a total of six occurrences of unscheduled absence or tardiness over the past 12-month period. It may specify how far in advance a supervisor must be notified if an employee will be unable to come to work or will be late. It may specify that non-compliance with this policy is cause for corrective action.

Putting It Into Practice

2. What variables in a facility will affect scheduling in the foodservice department?

Figure 12.2 **Sample Call Record**

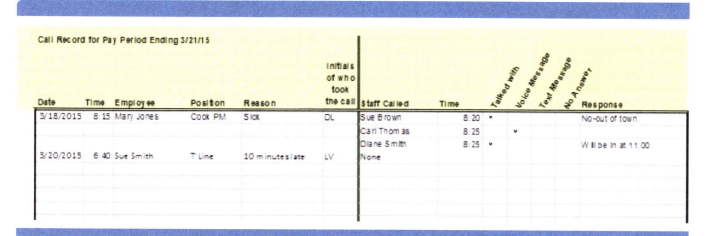

Call Record for Pay Period Ending 3/21/15

Date	Time	Employee	Position	Reason	Initials of who took the call	Staff Called	Time	Talked with	Voice Message	Text Message	No Answer	Response
3/18/2015	8:15	Mary Jones	Cook PM	Sick	DL	Sue Brown	8:20	✓				No-out of town
						Carl Thomas	8:25		✓			
						Diane Smith	8:25	✓				Will be in at 11:00
3/20/2015	6:40	Sue Smith	T Line	10 minutes late	LV	None						

A specific policy may also address what is known as no-call, no-show. In this situation, an employee does not come to work, and does not call to notify the manager. This is a serious situation that makes it especially difficult for a manager to direct and control the activities of the department. In some facilities, two occurrences of no-call, no-show may be considered job abandonment and grounds for immediate dismissal.

Reports and Documents

As a Certified Dietary Manager, you will most likely be responsible for ensuring that all documents and paperwork related to scheduling and payroll are maintained in a complete and accurate fashion. Typically, the manager is required to initial timesheets and authorize any overtime and check time records against the schedule to ensure there are no discrepancies.

Depending on the system in the organization, time records may be automated through an electronic timeclock or computer-generated payroll reports. Review of the payroll time and attendance records allows the manager to monitor employee timeclock patterns: Who clocks in early, who leaves a few minutes late resulting in overtime, who is frequently absent on Fridays, who picks up extra shifts and who never does.

Often an electronic scheduling program has the capability to notify the manager how many absences and tardies an employee has accumulated in the past 12 months. Within the department's personnel filing system, the manager should also maintain accurate and timely records indicating when employees have come to work tardy and/or had unscheduled absences. Routine monitoring can help provide timely feedback, and if need be, initiate disciplinary actions.

If budget information is contained in these reports, labor usage for each time period can be checked against the financials. This will verify good labor controls. Payroll reporting documents reflect the number of **productive hours** to be paid for time worked, training and education plus **non-productive hours** paid for holidays, sick, and vacation time (unpaid Leave of Absence may also be recorded). Hours paid should be monitored in addition to the dollar cost of the labor.

Often, the payroll reports include the pay scale and dollars paid to each employee for the pay period. This personal and sensitive information should be treated as confidential data.

Controlling Overtime

What is overtime? **Overtime** refers to time worked in excess of the allowable amount beyond which laws require payment of one-and-one-half times the hourly rate for every hour worked. There is more than one definition of when overtime must be paid.

- The most common guideline is the 40 hour work week.
  - > Based on the federal **Fair Labor Standards Act**: *"Under the FLSA, "overtime" means "time actually worked beyond a prescribed threshold." The normal FLSA work period is the work week—7 consecutive days—and the normal FLSA overtime threshold is 40 hours per work week." (http://www.flsa.com/overtime.html)*
  - > For example, an employee paid $8 per hour and working for 44 hours would receive an overtime payment of $48 (4 hours overtime at $12 per hour) in addition to the 40 hours' worth of regular pay.
  - > A 40-hour work week allows employees to be scheduled with variable hours, such as 10 hours on Tuesday and only 6 hours on Friday, but no more than 40 hours in the 7-day work week.

Glossary

Productive Hours
Time paid for time worked, training and education

Non-Productive Hours
Employee hours paid (or tracked) for not working: Vacation, Holiday, Sick Time, Leave of Absence

Overtime
Refers to time worked by nonexempt employees in excess of the allowable amount, typically 40 hours per week, resulting in one-and-one-half times the hourly rate

Fair Labor Standards Act
This Act of 1938, also referred to as the Wages and Hours Bill, is a federal statute of the United States

Putting It Into Practice

3. You have the biweekly schedule posted but the facility census has dropped and you have to cut 0.5 FTE. How would you handle this scheduling issue?

> If an employee works a consistent 8 hour shift they can work no more than 5 shifts a week.

- An alternative used in some medical care settings is called "8/ 80" or "8 and 80":

  > Based on the federal Fair Labor Standards Act: *"Nonexempt medical care providers working at medical care facilities may be paid based either on the standard 40 hour work week or on so-called "8/80" systems. If the medical employer chooses, it may pay these employees FLSA overtime for actual time worked in excess of 8 hours per day, or 80 hours every two weeks (whichever is better for the employee), instead of for hours worked in excess of 40 hours per work week."* (http://www.flsa.com/overtime.html)

  > Overtime is paid on anything over eight hours per day or over 80 hours in a two week period.

  > This allows employees to work six days in one week and four days in the second week, with every other weekend off.

  > This is not a common work status, but it is an option in some healthcare settings.

- States, union contracts and even individual employers may develop additional criteria for overtime:

  > Union contracts may specify anything over 8 hours within 24 consecutive hours.

    - 10:00-6:30 on Tuesday plus 8:00–4:30 on Wednesday equals two hours of overtime for the 8:00–10:00 time on Wednesday.

  > Nevada has a similar requirement for employees who earn less than one-and-one-half times the current minimum wage.

    - The state defined minimum wage in 2015 is $8.25 (with no employer paid health benefits).

    - If an employee is paid less than $12.37 an hour (1.5 x $8.25 = $12.37), then any time over 8.00 hours within 24 hours is paid overtime.

Clearly, overtime is very expensive and should be minimized to remain within budget. In some facilities, it may not be permitted at all. If overtime occurs frequently, look for factors that may be contributing to this situation, such as:

- Ineffective or unrealistic scheduling.

- Inaccurate estimation of the volume of work or failure to adjust staffing according to an increase in volume.

- Poor compliance with performance standards or poor work habits.

A Certified Dietary Manager can generally contain overtime through sound supervision. The key is to establish a policy of requiring advance authorization for overtime. Prior approval requires the employee to check with the manager or supervisor, who must approve the overtime. This gives the manager an opportunity to review why the need for overtime is arising and address any issues that require intervention. It also gives the manager a chance to use an alternate method of meeting the need, such as assigning another employee on a regular shift to pick up certain tasks.

Putting It Into Practice

4. How much would you pay in overtime for someone who earns $11.35 per hour and worked three additional hours?

Manage Department Personnel

Overview and Objectives

Healthcare, corrections, education and most large dining service departments are structured around documented policies and procedures. The regulations related to providing meals for the public and managing labor issues require written processes. Documentation of department activities, communication to staff and appropriate record keeping are the responsibility of the Certified Dietary Manager. After completing this chapter, you should be able to:

- ✓ Define the difference between policies and procedures
- ✓ Maintain personnel records
- ✓ Identify personnel management laws and practices (including union contracts)
- ✓ Identify promotion criteria
- ✓ Identify termination criteria
- ✓ Compile documentation for promotion and termination
- ✓ Conduct performance evaluations
- ✓ Recommend salary and wage adjustments
- ✓ Follow disciplinary procedures to correct problem (e.g., coaching, performance improvement plan)
- ✓ Ensure employee compliance with procedures

Policies and Procedures

In any organization, a set of documents called policies and procedures serve as an essential reference. A **policy** describes an organization's approach to a certain situation. A **procedure** details the steps in completing the task. The two are combined into a document called a "policy and procedure." (Chapter 14 provides more information on the structure, design and writing of policies.) For example, a policy and procedure for washing dishes may first state a policy that clean dishes are required for sanitation and for aesthetic reasons. Then, it would detail the steps involved in washing dishes.

Specific documented policies and procedures may be required by third-party entities such as OSHA, CMS, TJC, the local health department, or others. In addition to the required policies, which are typically related to safety and personnel issues, there are many other processes that should be documented in a policy. A written policy helps define both the expected outcome and the steps, when performed consistently by every employee needed to reach that outcome.

Without a policy and procedure manual, no one knows what is expected and it all becomes a matter of individual interpretation. "During orientation, Tommy said, 'This is the way to deliver the meals.'" With no policies you have no defined standards and no accountability for doing the job right or wrong.

When errors happen, and they will, how will the manager correct the issue without a policy? What basis is there to apply discipline for the employee? From a surveyor's perspective and a legal liability perspective, how will you verify that there is a defined process and the staff know what the policy is? (Remember, if it is not in writing, it did not happen.)

Most healthcare facilities use policies and procedures to describe how to carry out the facility's mission. **Standard operating procedures (SOP)** are also used. The SOP is separate from the **P&P Manual,** and more of a step-by-step detailed written instruction to; completing specific tasks accurately and consistently.

The policies and procedures tell what needs to be done and why, where the SOP defines how it is to be done. For example, the policy may state that nutritionally appropriate meals are served three times a day. The procedures might define the serving times, cut off times for diet order changes, and reference other policies for between meal snacks and supplements, etc. The SOP may get down to the details of how food is placed on the plates and where each meal part is located on the tray or client placesetting.

Standard operating procedures support the quality and performance standards. Like policies and procedures, all SOPs should be maintained in a notebook or manual, for easy reference by all employees, and should be kept up to date as procedures change.

Using job analysis and performance standards, develop standard operating procedures. **Performance standards** are specific statements describing the outcomes of the work performed. Performance standards specify what the task is, how it is to be done, and how well it has to be done.

A particular SOP may apply to several distinct job descriptions. While the Policy and Procedure Manual provides the overall guidelines for the functioning of the trayline, the SOP provides the details for the consistent operating of the trayline. For example, you may have four trayline positions with certain tasks that overlap. A single SOP for portioning food on trays may apply to all, while the SOP for placement of food items on the plate is more specific to the entrée server.

Policies and procedures SOPs, define the performance standards essential for managing the completion and quality of work.

Glossary

Policy
Describes an organization's approach to a certain situation

Procedure
Details the steps in carrying out a policy

P&P Manual
Printed or electronic documentation that describes almost every activity in the department

Standard Operating Procedures (SOP)
A step-by-step detailed written instruction for completing specific tasks accurately and consistently

Performance Standards

To ensure that work is "done well," you need to have a definition of what "well" means. This definition should be objective and very specific. It allows quality measurement in a definable manner.

One type of standard that serves as an essential management tool is a performance standard. Here are some simple examples:

- A trayline employee is responsible for portioning food on trays.
  - > Items served match the list of food ordered, as specified on each tray ticket. In this example,
    - the <u>what part</u> is *items served;*
    - the <u>how</u> is *match portions;*
    - the <u>how well</u> is as *specified on each tray ticket.*
  - > Food portions on tray match portions specified on each tray ticket. In this example:
    - the <u>what</u> is *food portions* on tray*;*
    - the <u>how</u> is *match portions;*
    - the <u>how well</u> is as *specified on each tray ticket.*

A performance standard for a food production job might specify that

- Employee prepares food in accordance with standardized recipes.
- Employee prepares food in the quantity specified on the daily food production schedule.
- Employee delivers food to the service area by the time stated on the daily food production schedule.
- Endpoint cooking temperatures meet the standards specified on each recipe, and are accurately documented on the temperature log.

To develop meaningful performance standards, include these three criteria:

- The standard addresses the outcome in specific, clear, complete, and accurate terms
  - > It should tell the employee exactly what is expected. There should be nothing that is confusing or could be misunderstood.
- The standard describes how the outcome will be measured through observable behavior.
  - > "Good" and "well" are subjective terms to avoid. The manager will use this standard to evaluate the employee's work performance, and the manager needs an objective standard to assure fairness.
- The standard explains the action verb used.
  - > For example, if the action verb is "document", the performance standard would require the employee to document.

An effective performance standard is within the physical and mental capabilities of the employees and is realistic in the working environment. Unrealistic expectations will result in employee failing to meet them. If a particular standard is not being met on a consistent basis, re-examine the validity of the standard before proceeding with other interventions.

When reasonable, involve employees in developing fair and realistic standards for their own work. Needless to say, each standard must adhere to company policies, company goals, and applicable legal and moral constraints.

Glossary

Performance Standards
Specific statements describing the outcomes of the work performed

While we all want performance to be perfect, we realize that this is not possible. It is not realistic to specify 100% compliance with every performance standard. What we can do, though, is specify a realistic and acceptable gauge of performance, often expressed in terms of numbers. It may be speed, quantity, or rate. For example:

- An accuracy rate is a number:
  > Food is portioned correctly, as specified on each tray ticket, at a rate of 99% accuracy.
- Another example might measure rate of output, or productivity, such as:
  > Employee accurately sets up the snack assembly station within a period of 15 minutes.

Developing Performance Standards. The steps for developing a performance standard are as follows:

Step 1: Using the organization chart or the staffing pattern, list all the job titles in the department. For example, the list may include buffet server, receiving clerk, morning cook, afternoon cook, pot washer, and others.

Step 2: Review the job analysis workflow (Gantt Chart) for each position and list the tasks or sets of tasks that need a performance standard. For example, the tasks of "sanitizing pots" will require a performance standard.

Step 3: Write a performance standard for each task. Seek employee input.

Step 4: Train employees.

Step 5: Evaluate performance (ongoing).

Performance standards as a communications tool. In the process of interviewing prospective employees, explain that the operation uses performance standards. This prepares a candidate for the commitment to quality that will be expected. You may choose to show a candidate a sample performance standard that relates to the position the candidate is applying for.

Training for employees follows from the job analysis, the job description and the performance standards. Whatever the procedures and standards specify must be included in both new employee orientation and ongoing employee training. For example, if performance standards have been developed on documenting information for HACCP records, then training must include the details of how to do this (the procedure), as well as the description of how an employee will know it has been done effectively (the performance standard).

Once training has been completed, ongoing evaluation and feedback of outcomes is based on the performance standards. If employees are consistently not meeting a standard, determine why not. They may need more or different training. The performance standard may need to be revised to be more clear and realistic. If one particular employee is not meeting the standard but others are, this may be a clue that the employee needs coaching and direction, or even disciplinary action.

It can be easy just to assume that all employees know what is expected of them. However, this simply is not true. It is not fair to evaluate employees based on unwritten rules or a judgment call of what constitutes good work. Instead, spell out the expectations through performance standards. Clear and fair performance standards improve consistency, accountability and quality because everyone knows what the outcome should to be.

Performance Review

Performance standards are an essential point of reference during a performance review. The process should account for how the quality and quantity of an employee's work compares with the performance standards that have already been established for the job.

As part of the ongoing responsibility to provide feedback to employees, a Certified Dietary Manager must comply with organizational policies and procedures. The **performance review** is a formal evaluation of an employee's work on the job. At times, a manager must also take corrective action to help improve performance. Both of these are documented activities and the documents become part of an employee's personnel file.

When a particular employee continues to have performance problems a manager must decide how to intervene. Unfortunately, termination occasionally becomes the only solution. On the flip side of the coin, when employee performance meets or exceeds established standards, the manager is charged with providing recognition to encourage excellent performance.

Purpose of a Performance Review

The **Performance Review** is a structured and scheduled component of nearly every organization. A performance review, performance appraisal or evaluation, is a formal, structured meeting between the employee and their supervisor/manager that encourages an exchange about the individual employee's performance on the job.

A performance review does several things:

- Ensures that the supervisor/manager talks with the employee about performance, and provides extensive feedback.
- Identifies needs for improvement and growth.
- Serves as a formal basis for wage increases related to performance.
- Provides an opportunity for an employee to set personal work objectives that relate to the departmental objectives.
- Provides an opportunity for the employee to raise needs related to the work, and for the supervisor/manager to help.
- Provides documentation for the employee's personnel record.
- May be used to help evaluate eligibility for promotion.

How often a performance review occurs is generally dictated by the policy of the facility. For example, one facility may conduct performance reviews for every employee at three months of employment, six months of employment, and annually thereafter. The review is typically documented on a form that is standardized for the facility, signed by both employee and supervisor, and retained as part of the personnel file. The department manager typically signs every performance review before forwarding them to Human Resources.

Employee performance review programs can benefit the employee, the Certified Dietary Manager, and the organization itself. For example, a manager who recognizes individual staff members through a formal review process may obtain ideas from employees about how work procedures can be improved. As strengths and weaknesses of each employee are identified, the employee and manager together can develop action plans to improve performance.

The groundwork for motivation can be laid during a performance review as well. This occurs when employees understand that the Certified Dietary Manager is concerned about them and is interested in learning about their needs. Coaching, counseling, training, orientation, and many other ongoing programs can be strengthened as the result of information learned during performance appraisal.

It also becomes easier to justify job actions such as promotions, transfers and demotions, when formalized evaluation sessions have been completed and documented. If the Certified Dietary Manager can show that performance is consistently inadequate and the employee has agreed that a problem exists, improvements are expected. However, employee failure to make these improvements may provide justification for disciplinary actions that are taken.

The performance evaluation can help improve the relationship between the Certified Dietary Manager and employee. An effective manager asks for feedback during a review and sometimes learns more about how to lead and motivate employees through this process. As the manager and employees work together as partners in the performance review process, a relationship can be built which helps each gain mutual understanding and respect.

Types of Performance Reviews

There are several basic types of performance reviews. Some of the options include a review that uses absolute standards, an open-ended summary, an objectives-based evaluation, and a 360 review. Performance reviews may be a printed form to be manually completed, or more often today, the form is an electronic version to be completed online.

Typically, performance reviews are designed to reference the general characteristics of a position without addressing the specific tasks of the job. The evaluation likely has questions about communication skills, safety, accountability, attendance, quality of work and other general performance terms. Specific job tasks are usually addressed in the comment section of the evaluation.

A Certified Dietary Manager may keep a catalog of commonly used evaluation comments for easy referral of appropriate commentary. The online versions of a performance review often include a drop-down list of relevant comments, both positive and negative, that can be added to an evaluation.

Absolute Standards Performance Review. In this type of performance review, work performance of an individual staff member is considered as a stand-alone function without comparison to others. One popular example of the absolute standard type of performance review is the **critical incident method.** Using this technique, the Certified Dietary Manager keeps a log of incidents that represent both effective and ineffective job performance. The log is then used to measure employee performance. The manager simply lists any activity observed on the job that he or she judges to be critical to job performance and compares the observations with established performance standards. This way an employee is receiving both reinforcement and coaching about observed behaviors.

Glossary

Critical Incident Method
A log of incidents that represent both effective and ineffective job performance

Absolute Standards Performance Review
A review to set standards with no comparison to others

Certain events are called critical because they illustrate the key behaviors that define (or violate) standards for performance. For example:

> A Certified Dietary Manager observes an employee arguing with a client. The manager may record this as a critical incident because it represents failure to meet a performance standard about providing friendly service.
>
> In another event, the same employee may check and record food temperatures of hot and cold foods before service with 100% accuracy. This may relate to another performance standard about documenting food temperatures accurately before serving trays. The manager may record this, too, as a critical incident on the performance review form.

In today's digital world, a Certified Dietary Manager may have an electronic file for each employee. An efficient way to record a critical incident is to send yourself a brief email with the details that provide the date and information regarding the incident. When time allows, move email into the employee's file.

Another type of absolute standards review is a checklist developed by the manager or the facility. The evaluation lists important performance items and provides a numeric rating scale. The supervisor/manager completing the evaluation selects a number to rate the performance of the employee related to each item. A sample checklist evaluation is shown in Figure 13.1.

Another example of the absolute standards approach is a forced-choice plan, which requires a Certified Dietary Manager to select a statement judged most accurate in describing how an employee performs on the job. A sample is shown in Figure 13.2. The manager first lists factors judged important to successful job performance in the left-hand column, then he or she must indicate how the work performance of the employee meets each of the criteria. In some facilities, both the employee and the manager mark separate forms and then compare their answers during the performance review.

Open-Ended Summary Performance Review. A review based on free text allows the supervisor to note strengths and weaknesses of the employee's performance and to indicate suggestions and support for improvement. A sample appears in Figure 13.3.

Objectives-Based Performance Review. This is based on individualized objectives; developed with input from both the Certified Dietary Manager and the employee. First, the two develop a mutually-defined set of job-related objectives. Later, during a performance review session, the two assess how well these objectives have been met. They also develop a new set of objectives. This system is also called **management by objectives (MBO)**.

Basic steps in an objectives-based evaluation plan include:

- The manager and employee set measurable behavioral objectives. The employee commits to attaining these objectives by the time of the next review.
- The employee is given assistance on the job through training, coaching, and/or other developmental activities.
- Employee and supervisor, separately, prepare a reflection on how each feels the employee met the objectives.

Glossary

Management By Objectives (MBO)
The process of setting objectives through participative goal setting by management and employee

Figure 13.1 Checklist Performance Review Form

Name of Supervisor _____ Department _____ Date _____

Circle one for each item: *Scale: 7 = the highest level of performance*

ADMINISTRATION

Knows and utilizes proper forms and procedures	7 6 5 4 3 2 1
Meets deadlines	7 6 5 4 3 2 1
Organizes personal workload	7 6 5 4 3 2 1
Organizes work of those supervised	7 6 5 4 3 2 1
Apprises immediate superior of all current developments	7 6 5 4 3 2 1

Explain where improvement is needed:

_____

LEADERSHIP

Sets goals and objectives for self	7 6 5 4 3 2 1
Sets goals and objectives for employees supervised	7 6 5 4 3 2 1
Meets goals and objectives for self	7 6 5 4 3 2 1
Helps employees meet goals and objectives	7 6 5 4 3 2 1
Supports employees supervised	7 6 5 4 3 2 1
Supports policies and procedures	7 6 5 4 3 2 1
Helps develop employee potential for advancement	7 6 5 4 3 2 1

Explain where improvement is needed:

_____

MOTIVATION

Displays high propensity to accomplish and achieve	7 6 5 4 3 2 1
Supports goals of hospital	7 6 5 4 3 2 1
Functions as part of a team	7 6 5 4 3 2 1
Attempts to help others understand the importance of their work	7 6 5 4 3 2 1
Urges others to excel	7 6 5 4 3 2 1
Gives competent professional image	7 6 5 4 3 2 1

Explain where improvement is needed:

_____

SUPERVISION

Gives continuous orientation and on-the-job training to employees supervised	7 6 5 4 3 2 1
Explains orders whenever possible	7 6 5 4 3 2 1
Answers questions fully or obtains answers for employees supervised	7 6 5 4 3 2 1
Administers and supports proper policy	7 6 5 4 3 2 1
Listens to and attempts to correct employee complaints	7 6 5 4 3 2 1
Holds periodic meetings with employees to pass on information	7 6 5 4 3 2 1
Provides effective feedback to employees	7 6 5 4 3 2 1

Explain where improvement is needed:

_____

COMMENTS—Describe the supervisor specifically in terms of the following:

Technical competence:_____

Creative ability:_____

Motivation and drive: _____

Human relations:_____

Overall performance: _____

Additional comments: _____

Signature and title of individual completing evaluation: _____

Signature of supervisor being evaluated: _____

Supervisor's comments: _____

Figure 13.2 Forced Choice Review Form

Employee Name _____ Job Title _____

Dept. Name_____ No._____ For Period_____ through _____

Reason for Evaluation: end of probation ○ wage increase ○ annual evaluation ○ termination ○ transfer ○ promotion ○ Other:

The purpose of this evaluation is to aid employees and their supervisors in determining the employee's strong points and shortcomings, if any, on the job. Asterisked (*) entries must be justified in the remarks section. All pre-written statements may be modified by adding or deleting words. Use additional paper if needed and indicate the total number of pages for this evaluation at the bottom of this page.

QUALITY

The accuracy or completeness of each unit of work or assigned task. Don't confuse with quantity.	* Superior, virtually every procedure is accomplished error-free.	Above average, each procedure is above standards normally expected.	Does job completely and thoroughly.	Sometimes inadequate, usually meets minimum standards.	* Careless, needs constant supervision and follow up.
	[ ]	[ ]	[ ]	[ ]	[ ]

QUANTITY

Volume of work produced in terms of assigned units or tasks.	* Top producer, exceptionally fast.	Very fast employee, produces more than expected.	Completes assignments on time.	Marginal producer, sometimes falls behind.	* Needs prodding, consistently produces less than is expected.
	[ ]	[ ]	[ ]	[ ]	[ ]

INITIATIVE

Desire to perform the job properly. Adherence to rules and regulations.	* Top producer, exceptionally fast.	Completes work and seeks additional tasks.	* Meets the requirements of the job.	Marginal producer, sometimes fails behind.	* Lacks initiative, seems to be lazy and/or uninterested.
	[ ]	[ ]	[ ]	[ ]	[ ]

PERSONAL GROOMING

Personal hygiene, grooming, use of makeup, appropriateness of dress.	* Exceptionally well groomed, demonstrates good taste in dress.	Better-than-average appearance.	Meets requirements of the job.	* Frequently careless in appearance.	* Wears inappropriate clothing, disregards departmental standards.
	[ ]	[ ]	[ ]	[ ]	[ ]

ATTENDANCE

Punctuality, absenteeism, tardiness.	Always dependable and on time.	Above average, seldom absent or tardy.	Demonstrates responsibility toward job requirements. Occasionally absent or tardy.	Needs improvement; is tardy or absent several times per month.	* Chronically absent or late.
	[ ]	[ ]	[ ]	[ ]	[ ]

DEPENDABILITY

Judgment demonstrated in conserving confidential information, performing on the job, following instructions.	* Demonstrates exceptional judgment, learns quickly, needs little supervision.	Efficient, demonstrates discretion, good professional attitude.	Usually reliable, carries out instructions with normal supervision.	Inconsistent, requires follow-up and/or monitoring.	* Violates policy, fails to follow instructions.
	[ ]	[ ]	[ ]	[ ]	[ ]

RELATIONSHIP WITH OTHERS

Patients, co-workers, public. General courtesies and attitudes.	Goes out of way to promote good will.	Gets along well with others, good attitude.	Satisfactory relationship with others, generally adapts to persons and situations, pleasant.	* Defensive, sometimes rigid to change, not always cooperative	* Antagonistic toward others, inconsiderate.
	[ ]	[ ]	[ ]	[ ]	[ ]

Date of Evaluation _____ Evaluator (print) _____ Page 1 of _____ (total # of pages)

Evaluator's (supervisor's) remarks: _____

Evaluator's Signature _____

Employee's remarks;_____

Employee's signature _____

Note: The employee's signature in no way shows that he or she agrees with this evaluation. It merely indicates that the employee has seen the evaluation and understands the contents.

Figure 13.3 Open-Ended Performance Review Form

Employee's Name: _____ Assignment: _____ Date: _____

List areas of strength:

List areas of weakness:

List help provided:

List disciplinary action if no improvement is shown:

General comments:

Comments by employee:

Signature of employee: _____ Date: _____

Signature of evaluator: _____ Date: _____

- At the time of the performance review, the actual level of performance is measured against the level defined by the objectives and progress is discussed.
- The supervisor and staff member work together to develop new objectives and plan strategies for attaining the objectives before the next performance review session.

The **360 Review** has been gaining acceptance at the manager and professional level. In a traditional evaluation, the performance review tends to focus on how well the employee performs their assigned tasks. While the manager may seek input from co-workers, their comments are not the basis of the evaluation. In a 360 Review, the emphasis is more on how the employee contributes to the organization.

Peer review of the employee's leadership skills, work habits, accountability, effective communication and level of teamwork make up the core of a 360 Review. Managers seek feedback from the employee's peers and representatives from the other departments that the employee regularly interacts with, such as nursing directors and administrative or medical staff. The objective is to provide the employee with both positive and constructive feedback based on how well they function within the organization.

Performance Review Process

The exact type of performance review forms used will likely depend on the facility. Using the form and method defined by administration or Human Resources, you may need to customize the feedback somewhat for a food production or dining services employee. For example, if the standard form lists "quality of work" as a factor for evaluation, the manager needs to edit the indicators to reflect the specific tasks related to the employee's position.

Glossary

360 Review
In a 360 Review, the emphasis is more on how the employee contributes to the organization. Peer review of the employee's leadership skills and work habits

As with any feedback, a performance review should be specific. The more an employee knows what the criteria are for evaluation, the more readily an employee can meet these criteria. Some Certified Dietary Managers provide a blank copy of the evaluation form to a new employee during orientation. This is a way to define expectations for the employee and makes clear what the employee needs to do to succeed.

Before conducting a review, take the time to complete the form and give the review some thought. If multiple supervisors work with one employee, talk to each of them about the performance review and obtain specific feedback and comments to include.

To conduct a performance review schedule time with the employee. Find a time when both you and the employee will not feel rushed, to allow a meaningful discussion. Then set aside a private place to talk. A performance review should not be held in a high-traffic area or in any place where others are likely to overhear the conversation. A performance review is a confidential exchange between the manager and the employee.

During a review explain each item—what it is measuring, what standard is being used, and what specific observations have been made about the employee's performance. Throughout the review give the employee time to react, respond, and ask questions. As with other types of feedback, a performance review gives the Certified Dietary Manager time to listen to employees.

Often, the manager can learn how to remove obstacles on the job, provide training and support, and help the employee solve problems. Let this be an exploration in which both parties walk away with greater understanding. As the review concludes, design a plan for development on the job. It may include items such as additional training for the employee, practice of certain skills, and more.

Both the employee and the manager should sign and date the form. Signing the form indicates that the employee has received this feedback (not that the employee agrees with everything it says). If the employee disagrees with points in the evaluation, these should be discussed. A typical procedure allows an employee to add comments. If an employee refuses to sign the form, write "refused to sign," and date and initial the note.

A performance review is often a time when an employee shares personal development needs in more detail. One employee may state that he would really like to train for a cook's position, or another may share that she wants to sign up for the CDM education program. These aspirations are important and should be considered for the staff development plans. By encouraging staff to expand their skills, advance their education or even pursue a different job opportunity, you raise the quality of staff in the department and become an employer of choice.

Finally, the paperwork should follow the procedure defined for the facility to assure that a pay raise, if indicated, is processed, and that the form is filed in the employee's personnel record.

Several common pitfalls can occur during the employee performance review process. Some include:

- Surprising employees with negative feedback:
  - > If there has been an ongoing problem, the employee should know well before a performance review. The manager should be giving feedback on a regular basis so that there are no surprises.
  - > The same is true for positive feedback.
  - > Thus, an effective performance review becomes a summary of items that have already been discussed.

- Using reviews for corrective action:
  - > Sometimes performance reviews are used only to reprimand employees rather than to assess where, if at all, employees can improve.

- Using ineffective review forms:
  - > If review forms do not correctly summarize factors important for effective job performance, the evaluation process will suffer. A Certified Dietary Manager should identify the specific, job-related criteria for review.

- Failing to use or keep up with performance reviews:
  - > Some managers may procrastinate due to busy schedules. Although it can be difficult to schedule time, a manager must give this process high priority.
  - > On occasion, an employee whose review has been postponed or overlooked begins to experience poor morale. If a pay raise is associated with the review, the situation becomes compounded.
  - > The employee needs to know that their performance is important to the organization.

- Comparing employees:
  - > The objective of performance reviews should be to compare an employee's performance with defined performance standards, not with that of other employees.

- Failing to use performance review information:
  - > Some managers may perform reviews—but then fail to make use of information gained, or neglect to follow through with commitments to support an employee's development.
  - > The best action is to follow through with plans and commitments.

- Failure to be thoroughly familiar with the union contract:
  - > If employees are represented by a union, the contract will outline the performance review process.
  - > Make sure, as the manager, that you know it and follow it.

The basic elements of a functioning employee review program are shown in Figure 13.4. Be familiar with, and follow, the specific procedures established for the facility.

Figure 13.4 Elements for a Performance Review System

- Objectives for conducting performance reviews are defined.

- Performance standards are in place and have been communicated to employees.

- Employees are aware of the performance review process, criteria, and timetable from the time of initial employment.

- Employees have received relevant training.

- The schedule for completing performance reviews has been established and is being followed.

- The manager applies a consistent and fair review process to all employees.

- The manager provides objective, specific feedback during the review process, describing observed behaviors.

- The manager uses methods to solicit employee participation and comments during a review.

- The manager listens attentively.

- The manager and employee work together during a review to solve performance-related problems, as appropriate.

- The manager seeks to resolve any misunderstandings and clarify expectations as needed during a review.

- The manager and employee agree upon areas for improvement and growth.

- If needed, the manager and employee create follow-up plans.

- The manager asks for the employee's commitment to achieving objectives.

- The manager completes required documentation and obtains the employee's signature as well. Documentation is placed in the personnel file.

Legal Implications

If you work with a union contract that covers transfers, promotions, and discharges, make sure you read and follow the union contract when disciplining, transferring, or promoting staff. Many of the government regulations from Chapter 8 also impact performance reviews such as the Civil Rights Act of 1991 and the Americans with Disabilities Act (ADA). If there is a human resource office, they can help navigate the legal implications of employee relations. If not, be aware of legislation that will impact performance reviews.

Diversity In the Workplace

According to the Bureau of Labor Statistics, (2014), at least 16.5% of the U.S. workforce is foreign-born. In some states and in certain industries—such as foodservice—the proportion of foreign born employees is higher (BLS reports 24.1% in 2014). This alone tells us that the cultural backgrounds of foodservice employees can be highly diverse. Beyond national origin, U.S. society is a melting pot in many different respects. People come to the workplace of a dining services department with different languages and levels of literacy in written English. Differences in customs, values, lifestyles, sexual preferences, religious beliefs, style of dress, age and communication styles impact their interactions with co-workers and clients.

Diversity is a term that describes the many ways in which people differ from each other. Diversity means that Certified Dietary Managers cannot assume all employees respond to the same style of communication, coaching or reward. Managing diversity is essential for promoting teamwork and accomplishing department objectives.

Every facility should have a clearly stated diversity policy which may say, for example, that the organization is committed to respecting the diversity of the work team. A policy may also explicitly prohibit derogatory comments about cultural groups. As a manager, you need to communicate this policy clearly, make it part of the employee orientation, and enforce it.

When recruiting employees, some recruitment avenues may, in themselves, seek out various groups. For example, consider recruiting through neighborhood newspapers in addition to the traditional ads to include members of the local community in an equitable manner. During the interview process, ensure that you are not filtering the applicant's responses through you own cultural history. Instead, appreciate how individuals may be different and seek to hire people who represent the community in which the facility resides.

Multicultural management does not mean that there are no rules. Be alert to differences in nonverbal behavior and how it is interpreted, which varies greatly among cultures. For example, if a male employee comes from a cultural background in which men do not accept orders from women—and the employee has a female supervisor—it is not the employer's job to give the employee a male supervisor. Conflicts that result in behavioral or performance issues need to be addressed. Discussion of cultural differences may help improve the employee interaction. Ultimately, an agreement of the job expectations is essential for the department to accomplish its mission. By recognizing the cultural differences, you can make the process much easier than it would be otherwise.

Diversity In the Workforce

There is more than one application of the term diversity in the workplace. The above discussion refers to the characteristics commonly associated with Human Resources and diversity. Additionally, diversity is based on areas of education, experience and "life lessons" which all define one's perspective of an issue. As a matter of fact, diversity is often the key resource that helps a work team meet its objectives. Why? Because each member of the team has something unique to contribute. Diversity means having multiple perspectives and many points of view. Managers need to recognize and appreciate what is unique in every person on the team, including themselves. While this takes effort, it is very much worthwhile.

Today, many facilities offer diversity training, to help Certified Dietary Managers uncover their own internal biases and teach skills for managing diversity. This can be a great resource. In all, a non-judgmental attitude of openness and acceptance can go a long way towards managing a diverse work team.

Within your department, it is not enough to examine only yourself and your own practices. As a Certified Dietary Manager, you need to observe behaviors within your work team, listen to employees, and express an interest in others. A manager can encourage employees to share their backgrounds through involvement in cultural theme days, for example.

Disputes and Consensus

A work team is comprised of many individuals. Each has a unique cultural background, and a unique set of values, which can lead to occasional disputes. To maintain an effective work team, a manager needs to be alert to conflict situations and intervene in a timely manner to resolve disputes.

To be successful as a group, employees must be encouraged to share one critical value: respect for themselves and each other. Based on a respectful relationship, many disputes and conflicts can be resolved. Often, the steps are as simple as hearing the issue from everyone's perspective and helping everyone involved reach an understanding or consensus. A **consensus** is a general agreement within a group. It may not reflect the first choice of every individual member of the group. However, it reflects a plan that has been developed through some type of group process to represent the best, acceptable middle ground for everyone.

A process, such as this, can help resolve conflicts between or among employees; conflicts between a union and an employer; conflicts that arise from the presence of a diverse workforce, and many other situations. The steps are as follows:

1. Base the process on respect, and do not let anything change this.

2. Recognize the importance of relationships among people and protect these relationships.

3. Establish what the outcome of the process must be, such as a policy everyone will honor, or an agreement to which everyone will commit.

4. Discuss and clarify the issues from multiple perspectives.

5. Assure that every member of the group participates.

6. Work creatively and fairly as a group to come up with solutions.

7. Select a solution that meets the defined needs of everyone involved as closely as possible. Apply a sense of fairness and balance during this process.

8. Ask each member of the group to commit to this solution.

Corrective Action

Corrective Action is action taken by a manager to correct an employee performance problem. The goal is always to correct or improve performance. Despite how it sometimes may be viewed, corrective action is neither negative nor punitive. It is one of the basic tasks of management required to control the activities of the department.

As defined by the human resources policies of the facility, corrective action is generally a formal, documented process. A corrective action becomes part of an employee's personnel record. The form, like a performance review, is dated and signed by both manager and employee. Also, as in a performance review, the employee's signature represents acknowledgment that the employee has seen it, not that the employee agrees with the action. The corrective action form shows that an employee has been asked to make a specific behavioral change. In some organizations, this may be called a written warning or something similar. An example of a corrective action form appears in Figure 13.5.

Glossary

Consensus
A general agreement within a group

Corrective Action
An action taken by a manager to correct an employee performance problem

Figure 13.5 Sample Corrective Action Form

Employee's Name: _____ Position:_____

Department: _____ Supervisor's Name:_____

○ Check if Violation of a Critical Rule   ○ First Written Warning   ○ Second Written Warning   ○ Suspension Notice

Describe the performance to be corrected:

How to correct performance:

Follow-up plan and timetable:

Employee's comments:

Employee's signature (acknowledges receipt only) _____

Union representative's signature (if applicable) _____

Supervisor's signature _____ Date _____

As a Certified Dietary Manager, when you become aware of a performance problem, there are a few questions to be asked right away. These are:

- Have the relevant expectations and performance standards been previously communicated to the employee?
- Has appropriate training to support the employee's success been provided?
- Has constructive feedback been previously given to the employee?

When the answers to these three questions are "YES," it is generally time to take corrective action.

Formal corrective action, which may also be called discipline or disciplinary action, is a serious matter. In the extreme situation, it may provide documentation for termination of employment. Here are some examples of continued behavior that may require a formal, documented corrective action.

- Absenteeism/tardiness:

  > An employee who is habitually late or absent disrupts operations. Feedback regarding attendance should be based upon clearly established standards and policies that are uniformly administered. For example, a facility may have a policy that states an employee may not be absent or late to work more than six times in a 12-month period. In some facilities, an event of "no-call, no-show" (not calling in and not showing up for work) may be cause for immediate suspension or discharge.

- Violation of timeclock policies:

  > Punching in too early, leaving early, not clocking out for lunch, or incurring unauthorized overtime can all be examples in this category.

- Repeated failure to meet work standards:

  > If an employee's performance does not improve with ongoing feedback and provision of all required support, a manager may need to take formal corrective action.

- Violation of critical rules:

  > Most facilities have defined a set of higher level rules, the violation of which may be cause for immediate corrective action, suspension from work, or even termination. As a manager, become familiar with the policies in the facility. In some facilities, any of the following might be considered cause for serious disciplinary action or immediate termination:

  - » Theft
  - » Violation of confidentiality policies
  - » Sleeping on duty
  - » Violating safety rules or willfully endangering others
  - » Willful injury to another person (employee or client)
  - » **Insubordination**, direct refusal to do what the supervisor asks.

Most facilities also have specific policies governing corrective action related to using drugs, drinking on duty, sexual harassment, possession of weapons on facility property, immoral, indecent conduct on duty, falsification of records, and punching someone else's time card. In some cases, such as drug use, a facility policy may define a series of steps for helping the employee address the problem, rather than dismissing the employee.

An **Employee Assistance Program (EAP)** may be designed for this purpose. An employee assistance program provides support to employees in solving personal problems that may be interfering with work. These may include drug use, alcohol abuse, family problems, and others. Some EAPs may provide assistance in identifying those who have, or are at risk of, alcohol and drug problems.

To take the appropriate course of action, a Certified Dietary Manager needs to know the facility's policy and the proper corrective action procedure. Particularly in serious situations, the manager needs to secure input from human resources and/or other managers. Gather the facts and impose action only after a fair hearing of all sides from all persons involved. When practical, action should occur as soon as possible after a problem has occurred.

Glossary

Insubordination
A direct refusal to do what the supervisor asks

Employee Assistance Program (EAP)
Provides support to employees in solving personal problems that may be interfering with work such as drug and alcohol abuse, family problems, teamwork problems

To prepare for a corrective action meeting with an employee, the Certified Dietary Manager should:

- Carefully investigate and gather facts.

- Prepare a corrective action document, writing out the description of the problem and steps for improvement. Write in factual, objective terms. (Avoid using "hearsay" or behavior described only by others.)

- Set aside a private time and location and ask the employee to meet.

- Request the presence of a supervisor or representative from Human Resources to avoid a one-on-one meeting with the employee (and provide a third party witness).

- Explain to the employee the reason for the meeting, and explain that this is a corrective action that will become part of the employee's record.

- Explain the corrective action process and the policies related to it.

  > For example, tell the employee that documentation of this meeting will become part of the personnel record.

  > Outline the flow and timeframe of the corrective action process, as defined by the facility.

- State the objective, e.g., "I would like you to know that your performance is not acceptable and I want to support you in correcting it immediately."

- Describe the performance problem to the employee. Be calm, objective, and matter-of-fact. Using the document as a reference, describe what you have observed.

- Firmly and clearly state why this behavior is not acceptable. Describe the established standard or policy that applies.

- Give a reason why this is a concern.

- Ask the employee for input. Ask why this behavior is happening.

- Ask the employee what he or she can do to correct this situation. As warranted, discuss with the employee and seek to problem-solve together.

- Agree on a plan of action, which may be very simple. If the plan requires action on the manager's part, identify how to follow through.

- Specifically ask for the employee's commitment to improving performance.

- Sign and ask the employee to sign the document and add comments, if desired. Provide a copy to the employee.

- File the document according to the policies and procedures.

- If the manager anticipates that the employee may disagree with the written documentation, meet with senior staff first and review the write up.

- Work with Human Resources when corrective actions result in suspension or termination of employment.

- Advise security of pending terminations.

Putting It Into Practice

1. You have the opportunity to provide input into a new employee discipline process. What basic principles should be included in the new process?

While Certified Dietary Managers may feel stressed and anxious about corrective action, it is helpful to keep in mind that performance comes from the employee. As a manager, provide the proper direction and support. Ultimately, the manager does not control the employee's behavior. During a corrective action meeting, keep responsibility for action where it rightfully belongs—in the employee's realm. When an employee is asked, "What can you do to correct this situation?" the manager is asking the employee to accept responsibility and take action. Managers who do this find that this question removes a lot of pressure, and also builds a framework for successful performance improvement.

After taking corrective action, continue to be positive and upbeat in your interactions with the employee. Recognize that the employee may feel embarrassed or even angry. As follow-up, continue to observe performance. As soon as corrected behavior is demonstrated, be sure to call it to the employee's attention and provide positive reinforcement. This helps an employee make a positive change in behavior.

Human resources policies and procedures should also specify a process for appealing a corrective action. In other words, if an employee feels the action is not justified, the employee can go to a union steward, a department or division head, or another person higher in the organization chart, as designated in the policy and procedure. See Figure 13.6 for basic prerequisites in a corrective action form.

Figure 13.6 Basic Prerequisites for Effective Corrective Action

- Policies, rules, and procedures must be developed for all areas in the facility.

- Rules and policies must be explained to employees—and also provided in written form. For example, they can be included in employee handbooks and can be explained during orientation, training, and other activities.

- Policies, rules, and procedures must be reasonable, fair, and just from the perspective of both employees and the Certified Dietary Manager.

- Policies, rules, and procedures must be enforced in a consistent, fair, and honest manner. Thus, if one employee receives a formal written warning for missing three days of work during the past month, another employee who has the same attendance record should receive a written warning as well.

- Specific situations must be taken into account. The supervisor must determine whether observed problems were within or beyond the employee's control.

- The manager must use objective judgment.

- Supervisors must prepare for corrective action and make an effort to understand why the behavior is occurring and how the employee is motivated.

- Affected employees must be informed of any changes in policies, rules, and procedures before they are implemented.

- Corrective action programs should be administered objectively, without bias.

- The supervisor should not threaten, argue, and/or display anger.

- Corrective action should be done in private.

- A manager must keep corrective action a confidential exchange and refrain from discussing it with other employees. (A manager may need to discuss the action confidentially with an immediate supervisor, a human resources staff member, or others who also commit to this confidentiality.)

- The corrective action should spell out exactly what the employee needs to do to improve behavior on the job. Both the manager and the employee must discuss this.

- A manager who is newly promoted or new to an organization needs to begin applying consistent performance standards from the start. Waiting and letting things slide becomes a set up for poor success of corrective action in the future.

Glossary

Progressive Discipline
A series of defined steps taken to correct ongoing employee performance problems

Corrective action falls within the realm of **progressive discipline**, which is a series of defined steps a Certified Dietary Manager takes to correct ongoing employee performance problems. The exact set of steps is defined by the human resources policies and procedures. Generally, each step in the progressive disciplinary process becomes more severe. For example, one progressive discipline policy might state the following:

Step 1: The initial step is a verbal warning resulting in a dated note in the file.

Step 2: The first time a manager takes documented corrective action, it references the prior verbal warning, such as "on June 19th we discussed..." and is reviewed with the employee, signed, and placed in the personnel file as a "first written warning."

Step 3: If the problem continues, a second corrective action is taken and classified as a "second written warning."

Step 4: If the problem continues, the employee is suspended without pay, (e.g., for three days).

Step 5: If the problem continues, the employee is terminated.

Why Don't Employees Perform?

The toughest problem that can arise is the situation in which an employee simply does not perform well. An employee is asked to comply with performance standards and it does not happen. An employee is directed to follow a specific procedure, but he does not. Why does this occur?

Needless to say, there is no easy answer to this troubling question. A Certified Dietary Manager needs to understand that certain aspects of employee performance are beyond immediate control. A good leader motivates and influences employees. However, excellent performance comes from within the employee. Some individuals are more able or ready to perform than others, even the first day on the job.

In research about client service issues, for example, experts have concluded that a portion of service skills can be trained. Yet another portion must come from the employee's unique personality. Thus, the advice is: hire someone who will do well. This advice probably extends to most employment situations. From the beginning, some individuals possess the drive and talent to perform well, given the proper supportive environment. So a Certified Dietary Manager should seek to identify these characteristics in the recruitment process.

What can you do when events are past this point? Re-evaluate the Performance Standards, are they realistic for this employee? Is there a supervisory problem or personality clash? Is there an alternative approach that could be used? In addition, seek the advice of other managers, their experience and observations may help. Figure 13.7 identifies some questions to pinpoint areas that may be a target for action.

Sometimes employees appear to have all of the trained skills and experience to perform a job well, but still struggle to meet expectations. Their performance may not be a direct violation of the job but more a chronic problem of not measuring up. A **Performance Improvement Plan (PIP)** is a way to assist an employee through additional training and clarification of expectations.

Glossary

Performance Improvement Plan (PIP)
A method to assist an employee through additional training and clarification of expectations

Putting It Into Practice

2. Your most experienced cashier arrives at work apparently drunk. What steps do you take to address this behavior?

Figure 13.7 What to Check When Employees Don't Perform Well

- Does the employee know what you expect? How can you be sure?

- Are your expectations and standards attainable? Measurable?

- Does the employee know how to do the work to the established standards of quality/quantity?

- Are there any obstacles to the employee's performance that relate to systems, procedures, resources, or interference? If so, identify them and intervene.

- What social relationships in the workplace may be affecting the employee's work? (For example, is the employee following an informal leader whose direction conflicts with yours?)

- Have you provided feedback to the employee? If so, how many times? How close to the event? How specific has your feedback been?

- Are you interacting with the employee on a fair and objective basis?

- What does the employee say is causing the problem you have identified?

- Is the employee capable of doing this particular job? If not, is there an alternate job in the organization that might be a better fit?

- What is the employee's attitude towards the job, and where is this attitude coming from? Can you influence it?

- Have you examined the employee's needs and sources of motivation?

The intent of a PIP is not to document poor performance for termination, although that is how it is frequently used, but rather to provide the employee with a developmental plan for them to succeed in their job. A PIP should include the following components:

1. Statement of the observed problem or concern.

2. Action plan:

   a. What needs to be done, by when, and to what reasonable level of expectation

3. Interim follow-up steps:

   a. Scheduled meetings, review dates, defined points of progress.

4. Conclusion:

   a. If the employee is successful close the PIP,

   b. Partial success may lead to extended time for completion or adjustment of the action plan.

   c. Failure to meet expectations should result in termination or re-assignment to an alternative position.

Termination

The questions listed in Figure 13.7 will not solve every problem. In the final analysis, a few situations may come to a dead end, when there appears to be nothing further that will change the situation. First of all, it is important to acknowledge that there are no reasonable alternatives. Here are some examples of situations that may, not be resolvable:

- The employee's performance issue relates to an attitude that you are not able to influence.

- The employee simply lacks the ability to perform the job as defined, even with training. The employee is in the wrong job.

A situation such as this may have two options. If the employee is willing and motivated but simply not suited to the job, the supervisor may explore whether a transfer to a different position and/or different department may be a positive resolution.

If the employee is essentially unwilling to improve, **termination** of employment may be the best course of action. Before terminating an employee, review the facts of the situation with human resources and/or senior management, as defined by the policy. Ensure that each step of a progressive disciplinary process with an employee has been completed, and the termination is the next step.

Finally, meet with the employee to complete a termination. This does not have to be a hostile interaction and should not be a surprise. If progressive disciplinary actions have been taken. It is best to approach it matter-of-factly, reviewing the events that led to this decision. If a union represents the employee, invite the union steward to this meeting. As with a formal corrective action, avoid conducting a termination without a third party witness present. Termination can generate anger and unexpected responses. Assess the situation before beginning a termination meeting, and be prepared with assistance should it be required.

A termination must be documented according to established policies. Like other paperwork, it becomes part of the employee's record. If the employee files for unemployment compensation, or a grievance with the Equal Employment Opportunity Commission, the documentation becomes an essential paper trail. Accurate and complete employment records will determine the outcome.

Following a termination, some members of the workteam may feel distressed. Verify that the employee is no longer with the organization, however, do not violate confidentiality by discussing the termination and the factors that led up to it. Many employees will understand the action through their own observations. Sometimes, termination of an employee who has been disruptive to the work of the team brings about an unexpected, positive shift in morale.

An exception to the above discussion of progressive discipline is the probationary period for new employees, such as three months. During a probationary period, unique policies may apply. An employee may be working on a trial basis, and termination during this time period may not require all steps outlined in progressive discipline.

Employee Turnover

Employee turnover is common in foodservice operations. Many of the employees view their position as a transition to their "real" job. The turnover rate for hospitality was over 29% in 2013 (www.compensationforce.com/2014/02/2013-turnover-rates-by-industry.html). Some employees leave the job for explainable reasons such as relocation, graduation, and retirement. Some leave for better pay.

Often, turnover results in significant expense for a foodservice operation. The cost of turnover to replace an employee is about 16% of the annual wages for the position (www.americanprogress.org/wp-content/uploads/2012/11/CostofTurnover.pdf) This expense takes the form of:

- Managerial time required to recruit, interview, and select new employees.
- Advertising expenses related to recruitment.
- Managerial time required to orient and train new employees.
- Temporary setbacks in productivity and/or quality during transitional phases.
- The stress of adjustment for existing staff.

Glossary

Termination
The dismissal of an employee by the employer

Putting It Into Practice

3. You have been the Certified Dietary Manager in a large county nursing home for six months. You observe that the long-term evening cook consistently exceeds the needed production levels resulting in excessive leftovers and is often late bringing food to the supper line. What are your options?

Turnover rates can and should be calculated by the manager. **Turnover Rate** is used as a measure of stability in the foodservice department. Turnover is equal to the number of employees who leave in a defined period of time divided by the average total number of employees in the department during the same time period (multiplied by 100 to convert to a percentage).

To calculate the average number of employees, add the number of employees at the beginning of the year to the number of employees at the end of the year and divide the total by 2. For example:

- There were 15 employees who left the organization in the last 12 months.
- At the beginning of the year there were 52 employees.
- At the end of the year there were 50 employees.
- The calculation would be:
  - Turnover = (15 / ((52 + 50) / 2)) *100 OR
  - Turnover = (15 / ((102) / 2)) *100 OR
  - Turnover = (15 / (51) *100 OR
  - Turnover = (0.294) *100 OR 29.4%

Clearly, a wise Certified Dietary Manager strives to retain valuable employees in order to minimize the burden and expense of ongoing recruitment. Why do employees leave? Several factors can contribute to turnover. These include:

- Lack of opportunities for professional growth and development
- Lack of effective supervision
- Inadequate levels of trust between the employee and the supervisor
- Lack of participative opportunities
- Perceived inequality regarding how employees are treated
- Poor compensation, such as wages and/or benefits
- Lack of rewards
- Competitive offers elsewhere
- Personal reasons.

Surprisingly, when surveyed about what makes them want to stay on the job, many employees rate pay as relatively unimportant. Some employees in the service industry stay because of the rewards of working with others and serving people. Good relationships with peers, supervisors, and even clients—along with a positive work climate—also rank very high.

One approach that is very helpful in retention is participative management. This can take many forms, but the basic idea is to involve employees in the facility. Empowerment provides a form of participative management. Employee teams assigned to develop improvements, standards, procedures, or systems can be another form of participative management. These actions all encourage employees to be more engaged in their jobs and the workplace.

Exit Interview

When an employee does leave, it is important to conduct an **exit interview**. Depending on organizational policy, it may be conducted for employees who voluntarily leave or for all departing employees, including those who are terminated. It may be conducted by the Certified Dietary Manager, or by a designated member of the Human Resources staff.

Glossary

Turnover Rate
The number of employees who left the department divided by the number of positions in the department

Exit Interview
An interview with an employee who is leaving the organization

An exit interview often provides valuable information which the organization can use to improve employee retention. Sometimes an exit interview yields surprises, and it becomes apparent that without this process, managers may never have learned something they really needed to know. Questions that are typically asked during an exit interview appear in Figure 13.8.

As a matter of policy, information gathered through exit interviews should be routinely reviewed and assessed by human resources staff. The manager should also review this information and seek to learn from it to improving retention.

Figure 13.8 Sample Exit Interview Questions

- Why are you leaving the organization?*
- What did you enjoy most about working here?
- What did you enjoy least about working here?
- How would you describe your relationship with your supervisor?
- How would you describe the working environment?
- Is there anything that would have changed your decision to leave?*

* Omit these questions if the employee is not leaving voluntarily.

Labor Unions

It is not uncommon to work as a Certified Dietary Manager in an environment where food production and dining services staff belongs to a labor union (an organization representing employees and designed to advance the needs and interests of its members). The union's focus generally relates to wages, benefits, working conditions, employee safety and other aspects of human resources management. Unionization provides certain advantages to employees. It also defines certain guidelines for the manager related to employee scheduling and assignments.

Once employees are represented by a union, the policies and procedures related to those employees need to agree with the contract. Some union guidelines, such as seniority, may become a factor in matters affecting personnel-related decisions. While all employees should be treated fairly and equally, a union contract may identify fair and equal differently.

A Certified Dietary Manager should be familiar with the provisions of any existing agreement between a union and the facility. When the union representatives and senior management (Certified Dietary Manager to Chief Executive Officer) work together, through effective management practices, it can benefit both the employees and the organization.

Employee Recognition

Many studies have been conducted to determine why employees leave their place of employment. Managers frequently believe it is because the employees want higher pay. In reality, it is often because employees want recognition for what they do and they want to feel appreciated. There are three management strategies that will help retain your employees:

- Treat employees like clients—with respect and dignity.
- Provide an atmosphere of trust and support.
- Reward employees for a good job and deal fairly with those who don't.

Treat Your Employees Like Your Clients

One of the main reasons clients leave is because their needs are not being met. The same can be said for employees; they most often leave because their needs are not being met. Treating employees with respect and dignity is demonstrated by:

- Treating each employee fairly regardless of the type of decisions made or required.

- Demonstrating integrity by doing what you say you are going to do.

- Providing regular feedback to each employee.

  > Communicate to each employee what is required of them, what the rewards are, and how they are doing.

  > Remember that communication goes two ways, so make sure you ask them for feedback about what is required of them, what the rewards are, and how they think they are doing.

Provide an Atmosphere of Trust and Support

Communication is also the key to providing an atmosphere of trust and support. Communicate with employees about the direction of the department. Develop a consistent habit of communicating with each employee in person. Get to know about their lives outside of work by listening to them. Encourage and support their growth. Establish a relationship of trust and respect, both outside the workplace and inside. Keep your relationship friendly, but always professional.

Reward Employees for a Good Job

Rewarding employees for a good job doesn't mean waiting until performance evaluation time. When you "catch them in the act of doing a good job," let them know it right then. One manager carried bite-sized candy bars with her, and any time she caught an employee doing a good job, she would toss them a candy bar.

Rewards don't have to be monetary. In fact in today's economy, it probably won't be. Employees appreciate a simple thank you or a personal note. Ask during a staff meeting, "What went well this week?" then acknowledge the successes. There are many resources available to get ideas about rewarding employees. Don't forget to ask the employees how they want to be rewarded.

The Association of Nutrition & Foodservice Professionals (ANFP) promotes Pride in Foodservice Week in early February. This can be an opportunity to call attention to the contribution foodservice employees make to the facility.

Along with rewarding employees is treating each person fairly. There will be some employees who are liked better than others, but that should not interfere with fair treatment for all employees. For example, if there are staff lay-offs due to a declining census, make sure the layoff decisions are based on the job duties, not the employee. Treating each person fairly also means taking the responsibility to address those who are not carrying their load. When this is not addressed, the positive performers are penalized with more work.

Employee Satisfaction Surveys

One way to gather feedback from staff is through formal or informal employee satisfaction surveys. Some facilities have satisfaction surveys for the staff of the entire facility. Satisfied staff usually means satisfied clients.

The satisfaction surveys help identify areas where employees are motivated, and encourages all staff to become more engaged in the workplace. A motivated employee works to reach a goal and the related reward, where, the **Engaged Employee** works to complete the task because it "is the right thing to do" to improve the organization. The engaged employees bring new ideas, ownership and commitment to the mission.

If employees have an opportunity to express their feelings and beliefs about their job, they may be more engaged in the workplace. There are a number of corporate programs, such as Gallup and Press-Ganey, that conduct formal employee satisfaction surveys. Figure 13.9 on page 233 shows a sample informal employee satisfaction survey.

Promotion, Development and Succession Planning

An often overlooked role of the Certified Dietary Manager is the importance of training and developing staff for the future. Part of the performance appraisal process is identifying staff members with aspirations and capabilities for promotion. It is short-sighted to keep the best employees in their current positions. Investing in their training through actively assigning them to new tasks or formally supporting their educational training has long-term benefits for the department and the organization.

Cross-training staff gives the facility a multifaceted employee with skills in many areas. Exposing employees to new areas of service prepares them for a lateral move to a different position, promotion or even transfer to other departments. Encouraging staff to complete their education, become a CDM or pursue a college degree builds bench strength for the department.

Transfer to other departments, resignation to take another job or even promotion within create short-term staffing issues with lasting employee benefit. Providing access to a career path for their growth and development motivates the best of employees and positions the manager as the employer of choice, improving the quality of future job candidates. When you support and champion for the staff, they commit and support you as their manager.

The promotion and development of staff members also aides in **succession planning**, the identification and grooming of potential leaders of the department. Succession planning is a way for the organization to plan for replacement of leadership through training, goal setting, and progressive management experience. The planned training of potential leaders ensures a smooth transition when a leadership role becomes open.

Putting It Into Practice

4. You have two employees who are interested in a new position you are creating to implement a culture change in your facility. One employee is pregnant and you know she will miss an important time in the training for this position, but she is better qualified the other applicant. Who should you choose for this position and why?

Figure 13.9 **Job Satisfaction Survey for Employees**

Please note that answers to this survey are anonymous and confidential, and participation is voluntary. If you choose to complete the survey, it is due on (enter date here). We plan to use the results to improve job satisfaction and address any problems deemed necessary. When formulating your responses, please answer honestly and thoroughly. Thank you for your time!

Sincerely,
The Management Team

1. How satisfied are you with the overall management of the department?
   a. Very satisfied
   b. Mostly satisfied
   c. Mostly unsatisfied
   d. Very unsatisfied

Comments:

2. Are you provided with the tools and materials necessary to complete your job duties?
   a. Yes
   b. Sometimes
   c. No

Comments:

3. Are you encouraged to share your thoughts, ideas, and feelings about the department?
   a. Yes
   b. Sometimes
   c. No

Comments:

4. Do you believe that employees of the department are treated equally and that the management team does not demonstrate favoritism?
   a. Yes
   b. Sometimes
   c. No

Comments:

5. Do the job duties that you complete on a regular basis (not including special events or during emergencies) match the job description that you were provided with when you were hired?
   a. Yes
   b. Sometimes
   c. No

Comments:

Additional Comments and Suggestions:

6. Are you valued as a person by management?
   a. Yes
   b. Sometimes
   c. No

Comments:

7. Does management encourage teamwork?
   a. Yes
   b. Sometimes
   c. No

Comments:

8. Are meetings held appropriately (when needed, in a timely and organized manner, etc)?
   a. Yes
   b. Sometimes
   c. No

Comments:

9. Is management willing to make changes and improvements to the department when necessary?
   a. Yes
   b. Sometimes
   c. No

Comments:

10. Do you feel hopeful about the future of the department?
    a. Yes
    b. Sometimes
    c. No

Comments:

Review Date 3/09

G-0969

Source: Nutrition411.com, used with permission.

Plan and Implement Department Goals

Overview and Objectives

Certified Dietary Managers are expected to meet department goals. Communicating the goals, responsibilities and plans of action helps motivate employees to accomplish the end results. This communication will be important in helping motivate employees to accomplish department goals and objectives. Policy and procedures and performance standards represent an essential tool for presenting work procedures. After completing this chapter, you should be able to:

✓ Participate in developing policies and procedures

✓ Develop short term and long term goals for the department

✓ Identify expectations to establish priorities

✓ Compare department goals against resources available

✓ Identify opportunities for staff motivation

Policies and Procedures

As discussed in Chapter 13, Policies and Procedures define both the expected outcome and the steps needed to reach that conclusion. There are several reasons for maintaining a set of written department policies and procedures. They are to:

• Serve as reference for anyone unfamiliar with the task.

• Serve as a communication tool within the department when presenting procedural plans.

• Serve as a communication tool for people external to the department.

• May be required by inspectors or surveyors examining the practices.

• Serve as reference for those who may succeed the manager.

• And ultimately, "if it isn't written down, then it did not happen," and no one is accountable.

When surveyors and reviewers come into the facility for license or accreditation renewal, they are evaluating the performance and compliance of the organization to their regulatory set of standards. If they observe events outside of the expected, they reference the facility's or department's Policy and Procedure Manual against what they have observed to verify that processes are being followed correctly. The regulatory guidelines are often the basis of written policies for dining services.

Figure 14.1 Policy and Procedure Manual Relationships

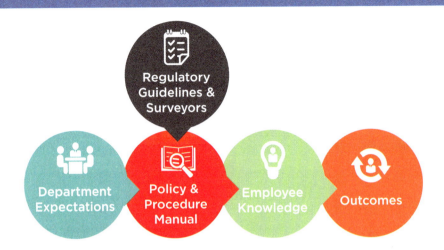

For the employees, policies and procedures also define what the department expects them to do, and often details how the task is to be performed. For your employees, the policies and procedures also define what the department expects them to do and often details how the task is to be performed.

Many organizations have a policy template set by administration with defined content and format guidelines. Often departments have revised and maintained a **P&P Manual** that describes almost every activity of the department, who is responsible, and what the expected outcomes are. A printed, paper version of the P&P Manual, or an electronic version on the facility server, may have more than 100 different policies.

To make policies and procedures easy to understand, present each one in a consistent, organized format. For example, the Certified Dietary Manager may maintain a notebook divided into sections with policies and procedures for:

- Departmental organization (including an organization chart)
- Menu planning
- Purchasing and inventory
- Food production
- Customer/client service
- Special services and catering
- Clinical services
- Client rights
- HIPAA compliance and confidentiality
- Scheduling and staffing
- Personnel issues
- Emergency contact information
- Disaster management

If the facility is part of a network or healthcare system, surveyors expect to find that the Policies and Procedure manual is consistent across the system with variations specific to the facility. The Diet Manual (discussed in the companion textbook Nutrition

Fundamentals and Medical Nutrition Therapy) is approved by medical staff and serves as clinical support for the policies and procedures.

Each policy and procedure should have a clear identifier. Some facilities use both numbers and titles. Any time a procedure is changed, date it and update the document in each location it is filed: a notebook in the department, the facility administrative offices, or the corporate shared filed network. Include other departments that the policy may affect. For example: A procedure addressing how to order in-house catering services, may be an essential reference in other departments. If this is the case, make sure that revised procedures are distributed to those concerned.

The manager is responsible for maintaining the policies on a regular basis, so the P&P accurately reflects the activity of the department. Typically, policies are reviewed on an annual basis with a review or revision date and the signature of the department manager.

If there is no P&P Manual for the department, or if new policies need to be written, the manager is responsible for developing them. Writing a new policy to document a change in service is not difficult when you have a well-documented P&P Manual to use as a guideline. However, developing a comprehensive manual from scratch is a massive undertaking.

There is an old saying "Don't reinvent the wheel. We already know that it is round." Instead of trying to develop all of the appropriate policies on your own, access what is already out there. Several electronic manuals are available for healthcare and school foodservices. An internet search for "healthcare foodservice policy manual" or "school foodservice policy manual" will pull in a number of options.

If you purchase a P&P Manual, verify that it has an editable electronic version that can be adapted to the facility without having to re-type the whole policy. Review each policy and determine if it applies to your operation. Skip any policies that do not apply, for example, if Home Delivered Meals is not a service provided, then the policies related to satellite meal services may not be relevant.

Figure 14.2 Sample Policy and Procedure: Social Networking

Policy Number: 684   Refixed: 3/1/xx   Approved by: _____

POLICY

[Facility Name] will be viewed by the public as a professional organization. This professional image extends to all types of media including but not limited to: blogs, social networking sites (e.g., Facebook, Twitter), professional networks (e.g., LinkedIn), photo sharing, video sharing, microblogging and podcasts.

PROCEDURE

1. Use personal email when engaging in any social media or professional social networking such as LinkedIn.
2. If you choose to list work affiliation in your personal profile such as on Facebook, then all posts to that network should be professional and respectful in nature. Your online presence reflects the facility.
3. If you choose to list work affiliation in your personal profile, do not "friend" anyone that you do not personally know.
4. Refer to IT policies and procedures regarding using personal email and social networking at work.
5. Keep client information confidential. Never use a client's information in any form of online media.
6. Personal blogs should have a disclosure statement so that readers know the content is personal.

Refer to Figure 14.2 for a sample policy and procedure on social networking. (Even if this is not a corporate or organization-wide policy, it should be a department policy, as employees utilize social media to communicate with friends and family about their work experience.)

How should you communicate new or revised procedures? While maintaining complete documentation is important, written policies alone are not the best means of communicating. As procedures change, think about everyone who may be affected. This includes employees in the dining services department, as well as in others. Procedures do not change until people do things differently. The basic principles of communication and managing change apply to making new procedures take effect.

In designing policies, and managing daily activity in a foodservice department, consider some of the guidelines you must follow and use them as tools. For example, policies and procedures may need to support compliance with CMS regulations, OSHA requirements, health department codes, and other standards. Adapting these guidelines into policies for the organization is up to the manager. Base decisions on how systems actually function in the facility, the flow of work, the responsibility and accountability detailed in the organization chart, and other practical factors.

Without a Policy and Procedure Manual no one *knows* what is expected, and it all becomes a matter of individual interpretation. "During orientation, this is the way that Tommy showed me how to deliver the meals to the unit." With no policies, there are no defined standards and no accountability for doing the job right or wrong.

When errors happen, and they will, how will the manager correct the issue without a policy? Based on what will you discipline the employee? From a surveyor's perspective and a legal liability perspective, how will you verify that there is a defined process and the staff know what the policy is? (Remember, if it is not in writing, it did not happen.)

P&P, SOPs, and the performance standards (discussed in Chapter 13) define the basis upon which the department functions. These documents establish where the department is. Going beyond the standards and required activities are the department goals. Typically, new goals for the organization and for the department are written every year.

Goals Versus Objectives

Goals and objectives are closely related. Both describe purpose. However, a **goal** is a statement that outlines a broad direction or intention. An **objective** is a specific step that will help in accomplishing a goal. Here are some other comparisons:

- A goal is broad in focus while an objective is narrow.
- A goal is the aim. The objectives are how you get there.
- A goal may be abstract, but an objective is concrete and measurable.
- A goal is more long term, while an objective is short- to medium-term.
- A goal is the result we want; objectives are the actions to get there.

Many facilities create master plans for growth that may describe goals for the coming year, as well as long range goals for a five-year or even 10-year period. This kind of forward thinking helps to focus the direction a facility takes and keep it moving forward in a meaningful and effective manner. For example, an organization that operates skilled nursing facilities may establish a goal of expanding most of its properties into senior living communities, with assisted living and other services, over a period of five years. Or, a school system may establish a goal of centralizing most of its services, including foodservice operations, over the coming two years.

Glossary

Goal
A statement that outlines an outcome or result

Objective
The steps to achieve the goal or the actions that lead to the goal

Organizations set goals by looking into the future and predicting what will be necessary for success. Factors that may influence goal-setting include: financial constraints, regulatory changes, staffing needs, challenges faced by the industry, new opportunities, a review of available and needed resources, and client feedback. Goals align with the vision and mission of the organization, helping to fulfill them.

Setting Objectives

Once broad goals have been established in any facility, a number of related objectives must be developed. Every branch, department, and individual plays a role in helping the facility define its goals and achieve its objectives. A Certified Dietary Manager may play several key roles in managing objectives.

In some facilities, managers are involved in setting the objectives for the facility. In others, it may be less direct. Recognize that as the manager of a service oriented department, you will have information and insights that can contribute to the formation of actionable objectives for the department and others.

Before customizing the goals and objectives to the department, first understand the big picture. Talk with your supervisor and peers to clarify the scope and intent. Then, extend these organizational objectives to be more specific to food production and dining services. For example, if a goal is to improve client satisfaction, an objective may be to improve satisfaction with food temperatures.

Look for ways to make each objective clear and measurable. A meal satisfaction objective may be measured with ratings or percent change. Here is a measurable objective: *Client ratings about the temperature of food will improve by at least 10 percentage points by December.*

There are a number of different goal setting systems used in business today. The S.M.A.R.T. goal method is a structured process to help identify the direction and plan the mid-point guideposts to achieve the intended goals. The use of the S.M.A.R.T. goal system process adds discipline to goal setting. Criteria for goals and objectives are summarized in Figure 14.3.

Plan of Action

Goals and objectives are good management techniques but accomplish little without an **action plan**. As a Certified Dietary Manager, use the work team as a resource for developing a plan of action. Break the process down into parts: What objectives are needed to reach the goal? What steps are needed to accomplish the objective? In a plan of action, there may be a series of steps associated with each objective. Figure 14.4 provides an example of a sample action plan.

Glossary

Action Plan
A plan of action to accomplish specific goals and objectives

Figure 14.3 Criteria for Goals and Objectives

S.M.A.R.T. Goals Are:

S SPECIFIC	Answer questions, such as: What precisely will happen (describe the outcome)?
M MEANINGFUL	Answer questions, such as: How does this relate to the mission?
A ACHIEVABLE	Answer questions, such as: How can this be achieved with the resources available?
R REASONABLE	Answer questions, such as: What makes this possible to achieve?
T TIMELY	Answer questions, such as: When will this be accomplished?

Effective Objectives Are:

SPECIFIC	They describe what will be done and by whom.
CHALLENGING	They represent growth rather than status quo, but are nevertheless practical.
OBSERVABLE	They describe a change that you as a Certified Dietary Manager can objectively observe.
MEASURABLE	They provide a form of a measure you can use to evaluate achievement.
SIMPLE	They each cover one clear action item.

For goals and objectives to be most successful, involvement of supervisors and employees is needed. Creating special teams focused on individual objectives, or even specific action plans, will improve staff "buy-in" to the steps being taken. Participation of staff in the planning process and building the action plan increases their level of engagement in department. Essentially, the manager's role becomes one of final approval, oversight and coordination of the different activities. (See an example of a plan of action to implement Hazard Analysis & Critical Control Points (HACCP) in the online *Supplement Textbook Material—Foodservice*).

In virtually any facility, change is inevitable when carrying out goals, objectives and a plan of action. It may come from external sources such as regulations and standards as they are revised, from within as a facility seeks to improve itself, or from personnel changes. Setting priorities, assessing available resources and determining the timeline often define whether the manager will be able to successfully reach the goals.

Putting it into Practice

1. Write a S.M.A.R.T. goal for replacing the dishware in the dining room.

Figure 14.4 Sample Goal With Action Plan

GOAL SETTING AND ACTION TASKS WORKSHEET

Writing an Effective Goal Statement

Rules for writing goal statements:

1. Use clear, specific language.
2. Start your goal statement with TO + a verb.
3. Write your goal statement using S.M.A.R.T. goal criteria.
4. Avoid using negative language. Think positive.

S.M.A.R.T. GOALS

S	Specific
M	Measurable
A	Achievable
R	Reasonable
T	Timely

Goal	Tasks	Target Date for Completion	Who's Responsible	Completed Date
Example: To review and revise the current menu to reflect the new or revised dining venue by (state the date.):	1. Meet with Resident Food Council to brainstorm menu items.	Date	FSD	
	2. Prepare new menu for the new venue.	Date	FSD, Supervisor, Dietitian, and Consultants	
	3. Evaluate recipes and costing.	Date	Supervisor and Cooks	
	4. Create production sheets, including recipes.	Date	Supervisor	
	5. Educate staff on new menu.	Date	FSD and Supervisors	

Meeting Goals and Priorities for the Department

Once the organization's goals have been developed and communicated to all the directors, often at the annual planning meeting, it is now time to relate them to the department goals. Start by listing the overall facility goals and a second list of the goals you think could or should be the focus of your department. How many of the potential department goals fit into one or more of the organizational goals? Some goals may fit in perfectly while others, although good ideas, just do not fit with the direction the organization is taking. Typically, those goals that best align with the facility goals take on a higher priority.

Assess the availability of resources to accomplish the goals. Some goals may be procedural and require little or no funding to be highly successful. Other goals need major capital investment or the addition of labor hours, which may not be available. Resources can refer to dollars for investment, labor for completing implementation, or equipment and space to accommodate the planned changes. Demands on resources often determines whether the goal is a high or a low priority.

Determining department goals is the result of coordinating organizational goals and priorities, resources available, regulations and appropriate fit with the services being provided. If the highest priority department goals do not align with the organizational goals, the manager has to be prepared to advocate for his or her goals.

Departmental and facility goals may have a very high priority due to regulatory requirements. Implementation of ICD-10 for medical record coding has consumed financial and labor resources for many facilities at the expense of completing other goals that would be nice, but are not required. Likewise, a failing meal delivery system may need replacement within the next nine months, making it the department goal priority even when it does not match the organizational goals.

Once the goals and resources have been aligned, continue the planning process with a list of the tasks to be accomplished in the action plan. Assign staff members to the various tasks and identify measurable outcomes for each step. Schedule interim dates for progress reports to keep all staff on track with the goals. Working with and through staff members takes more effort on the part of the manager to support and mentor the work teams without taking over the process. The best planning will not succeed unless the manager motivates employees to help carry out the plan, then directs and coaches employees in their actions.

Motivation

Motivation is an internal force that makes people do something in order to reach a goal. Motivation comes from within a person. A Certified Dietary Manager cannot force motivation upon an employee but can encourage it. A manager can provide job conditions that help employees to attain their goals.

When a manager can match the employees' goals with those of the department, both benefit. Matching employee goals begins during the hiring interview process. Managers strive to hire people capable of doing the jobs that are assigned to them. If employees are not capable of doing the jobs, no amount of training or motivational support will make them effective.

Employees also need to be willing to do the job. They can have the ability to do the job, but if they don't really want to do it, they probably will not be effective. Finally, employees can be willing to do the job and perfectly capable, but if they are not shown how to do the job correctly they still may not be effective. In-services and on-the-job training are useful techniques for developing employees skills and aide in motivating staff.

Theories of Motivation

Several theories of motivation address the question of why people do things. Some approaches take the stance that most people strive to reach their full potential. How far they have advanced toward reaching their full potential will determine what motivates them. The idea here is that if a manager knows what motivates employees, and they can provide the appropriate incentives, performance improvement will follow.

The best-known theory in this arena is psychologist Abraham Maslow's hierarchy of needs. He states that individuals' specific needs drive behavior. **Maslow's Hierarchy of Needs** represents the order in which these needs become motivators of human behavior. These are illustrated in Figure 14.5.

Maslow says that the physiological needs of survival, such as food and water, come first. When these needs are being met, an individual moves from focusing on survival to the second level of needs: Security and safety, such as stability, protection, and freedom from

Glossary

Motivation
An internal force that makes people do something in order to reach a goal

Maslow's Hierarchy of Needs
The best known theory of human-motivation

Figure 14.5 Maslow's Hierarchy of Needs, With Job Context Examples

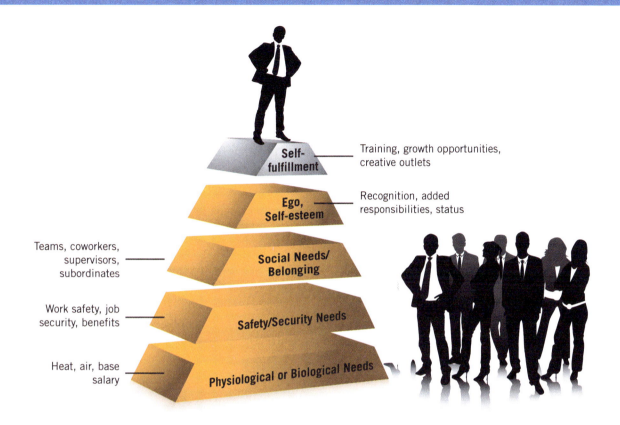

Training, growth opportunities, creative outlets

Self-fulfillment

Recognition, added responsibilities, status

Ego, Self-esteem

Teams, coworkers, supervisors, subordinates

Social Needs/ Belonging

Work safety, job security, benefits

Safety/Security Needs

Heat, air, base salary

Physiological or Biological Needs

Source: Adapted Maslow, 1954

fear and chaos. The third level motivating behavior is social needs. These revolve around friendship, love, and the need to belong.

Esteem comprises the fourth level within the hierarchy. Starting with recognition and respect by others, esteem progresses to self-respect and self-worth. Public recognition and pride in a job well done or humiliation and personal shame in poor performance are powerful motivators. The need for esteem gives rise in some people to the need for power as a way of commanding the esteem of others. Satisfaction of the need for self-esteem leads to feelings of self-confidence, strength, and worth. When these needs go unsatisfied, they produce feelings of inferiority, weakness, and helplessness.

The final level in Maslow's hierarchy is that of self-actualization or self-fulfillment. The drive to be all that we can be is a balance between meeting our other needs first and coming to accept "What a man can be, he must be." (Maslow, A. (1954). *Motivation and personality*. New York, NY: Harper. pp. 91.) Maslow believed that to reach self-fulfillment, the person needed to not only meet the prior levels of needs but they needed to master them. Creative outlets might be as simple as a garden or painting. Or, creativity might be the fulfillment of a dream to teach as a second career in retirement.

It is important to recognize that not everyone is motivated by the same thing. A Certified Dietary Manager can use these ideas to help an employee meet their needs of performance and commitment at work. Employee needs can be met, or supported on the job in a variety of ways:

- Physiological Needs: rest breaks, pay checks, bonuses.
- Safety/Security Needs: consistent application of work rules, policies, evaluation and performance feedback, non-threatening environment, proper working equipment, effective safety management programs.
- Social Needs: committee assignments, teamwork, friendship with fellow employees, sponsoring social activities such as bowling teams, employee picnics, newsletters.
- Esteem Needs: awards (e.g., employee of the month), attendance at seminars, recognition, promotions.
- Self-fulfillment Needs: support of personal development and/or tuition reimbursement; participation in planning of work area goals and objectives; encouraging creative projects.

It is generally true that:

- The staff member who is interested in the work is more likely to have internal motivation, which will benefit the employee, the dining services department, and the organization itself.
- The staff member who can identify with the organization and believe in it will be more willing to help the organization than will one motivated only by punishment and reward.
- Few people make an effort to analyze themselves objectively. The Certified Dietary Manager is challenged to recognize aspects of motivation that the employee may not be able to verbalize.
- Money is not a primary and important motivator for many employees. In fact, money is often a maintenance factor, not a motivation factor.
- Competition among employees or groups of staff members within the same organization generally does not motivate staff.

The Certified Dietary Manager needs to pay attention to what motivates different employees. By providing for basic needs and supporting the development and advancement of staff members, the manager can help employees want to perform on the job. For most employees, the desire to succeed and perform well, is a more constructive and effective motivator than the fear or humiliation of losing the job.

Strong workplace motivators include a positive work climate, empowered employees, building a team, meaningful feedback, and providing consistent, honest recognition. How do these points apply?

Work Climate

Work climate refers to how it feels to work in a given environment. It is the tone or attitude set by the Certified Dietary Managers, and is often closely intertwined with the facility's philosophy. However, it is also greatly influenced by the attitudes and actions of all the staff.

A constructive work climate supports employee development and workplace participation. Essentially, work climate becomes the state of mind employees have on the job which, in turn, affects how they perform that job.

Clients are also affected by the work climate, employees who feel positive about their jobs tend to treat them with more respect. Employees who are unhappy on the job may complain to clients, or perform their work grudgingly. All of this affects customer/client service and the image of the department.

Glossary

Work Climate
Tone or attitude of how it feels to work in a given environment

Putting it into Practice

2. During an interview a potential employee explains that she left her previous job because there was no teamwork or camaraderie among the employees. What level of motivation does this clue you to?

Some of the factors that help promote a positive work climate include:

- A role model of respect and support.
- A belief in the value and talents of every individual in the organization.
- Support for employees' needs, especially training and development.
- Listening to others.
- Managerial attention to problems that create stress among employees.
- Encouragement of teamwork and enthusiasm.
- A sense of calm, even when there are deadlines and time pressures.
- Frequently expressed praise for the value of employees' accomplishments.
- Emphasize team work whenever possible.

Empowerment

Another idea that relates very closely to work climate is called **empowerment**. In contrast with old management theories that were highly autocratic, empowerment means that a Certified Dietary Manager gives the power to an employee to take action and an opportunity to achieve. As such, it is strongly motivating.

How does it work? Clearly, a manager cannot just say to employees, "Do whatever you want." A manager has to provide direction to this process. To empower employees, consider the following steps:

1. **Define objectives very clearly**: Tell employees what the department is trying to achieve and keep these objectives in the forefront by discussing them often.

2. **Clarify policies so that employees have a solid framework for decisions they will make on their own**: For example, if you have a policy of always providing a substitution for a client who is unhappy with the food, make sure employees know this and follow the policy.

3. **Define the limits**: Tell employees what situations you support them in handling on their own, and what situations you wish to become involved. For example, employees might be empowered to accept a complaint, but are expected to involve management if a complaining client becomes abusive or violent.

4. **Communicate and coach**: As employees take power into their own hands, be accessible to coach employees. Be willing to provide support at any time, and to discuss actions after the fact to help an employee develop a greater range of skills. Ask to be informed, at least after the fact, about information that is important to you as a manager.

Consider this example of using empowerment to achieve a department goal of improving customer/client service:

> A waitstaff takes a complaint from a client in the dining room. The client says the roast beef was too tough. The waitstaff does not have to call a supervisor. He knows, through policies that have been established, that he has the power to do what he thinks will help the client feel satisfied. He immediately offers an alternative, which the client graciously accepts. He brings the client a new plate of food. He also passes along the concern about the roast beef to his supervisor and documents the substitute.
>
> In checking further, the food production supervisor may bring the problem to the cook who prepared the beef, asking for help in solving the quality issue, and now empowering the cook as well.

Glossary

Empowerment
When management gives power to the employees to take action and resolve issues

Putting it into Practice

3. One of your department goals is to reduce food costs. What could you do to empower your chef to help achieve this goal?

Team Building

Yet another technique that is critical to the success of every dining services operation is team building. A team approach recognizes that each employee is not working alone. Instead, all employees are working together to accomplish defined objectives. The parallel is a sports team. On a football team, the action of each player critically affects the bottom line—who wins the game. Players have to work together cohesively in order to win.

Actually, the same ideas hold true in a dining services department, as well as in a facility itself. The systems approach to management says that all the parts work together to accomplish the job. Serving a meal, for example, requires the coordinated efforts of people who purchase, receive, store, withdraw, prepare and serve food. When the meal is successful, it is because everyone on the team performed well and worked together. Recognize that every position contributes to the success of the team: The cooks cannot prepare the meal if the pots have not been washed.

When a sense of teamwork does not exist, efforts can become disjointed and the work flow within systems can deteriorate. The result is poor performance and poor quality. To encourage teamwork, you can take a number of actions:

- **Communicate objectives.** Keep the objective in front of all staff members: "We are going to serve these clients the best food they have ever eaten!" or "We are going to re-define the meaning of excellent service." A common objective draws people together.

- **Believe in your team.** Your belief that the team can perform has a tremendous impact on what happens. Employees who are not sure what they can do will respond to your belief in their capabilities. Instilling confidence is a great motivator.

- **Use enthusiasm**. Enthusiasm is contagious and is a key factor in getting the team truly excited about meeting objectives. It also contributes to a very positive work climate.

- **Give team members roles and responsibilities.** Make the contribution of each team member clear.

- **Use informal leaders.** While a formal leader may have a position on the organization chart that defines authority over someone else, every business also has informal leaders. An informal leader is one who, through personality factors, tends to gain the cooperation of others. Informal leaders can help support the objectives of the team and help support each player.

- **Provide the resources needed.** The manager needs to equip the employee team with everything they need to do their work and meet their objectives.

- **Provide opportunities for fun.** Letting off steam from a tiring day, enjoying an appropriate joke, or attending a departmental picnic are all examples of how members of a team can have fun together. When work is finished and employees are relaxing, more team building takes place.

- **Resolve conflicts.** Conflicts naturally arise among employees from time to time. An effective manager recognizes conflict and works openly toward a resolution to keep the team together.

- **Celebrate successes.** Meeting a goal, completing a project or earning recognition sometimes is by just getting through the meal.

- **Reward and recognize the team.** As the team meets objectives, this should become cause for cheering, celebration, and public recognition. These actions reinforce the efforts of the team and provide fulfillment to each team member.

Through effective teamwork, a Certified Dietary Manager finds that a group accomplishes more, employees gain satisfaction and systems function better. Thus, a manager often needs to function as a coach and build each employee's identity as part of the team.

Tools for Meeting Goals and Objectives

Meeting goals takes tools as well as motivation. There are several options to help: the organization chart, delegation, performance standards, policies and procedures, and communicating results.

Note the word "organization" in organization chart. Remember, in the first part of this chapter on planning, you created a list of tasks that will be required to accomplish your goals. As you group these tasks and decide which staff members will be assigned to them, you are organizing. Use this chart to help with this task. The organization chart illustrates division of, and helps determine to which employee the tasks should be delegated.

Delegation is assigning tasks to the appropriate employee within the department. Delegation is one way to develop the potential of employees. Remember, some employees may be motivated by the opportunity to take on added responsibility. As you delegate, consider the following:

- Tasks must be communicated clearly and effectively.
- Employees must be empowered with the authority to accomplish these tasks.

It is not delegation if you assign the responsibility for a task but do not convey the authority to complete the task.

Policies and procedures, along with performance standards, help identify employees who are directly involved in the goals affected activities. Who knows the current process better than those who currently do the tasks? The policies and performance standards define what is supposed to be done while the employees can clarify what is actually being done. Bridging the gap between what should be and what is will help you develop more realistic goals and action plans. With the input and buy-in of the staff, ownership of the outcomes is increased.

Goal Reporting

To monitor progress and ensure completion of the goal, many organizations utilize a quarterly or monthly reporting process. Typically the formal quarterly report sent to administration is a follow-up to the Goal and Action Plan form in Figure 14.4. In addition, the manager is also frequently responsible with updating the department staff on **key performance indicators (KPI)** for the facility and the department. The KPI are benchmark performance points tracked on a monthly basis and often relate to the department goals for improvement. (See Figure 14.6 for a sample KPI report.)

An Excel template for tracking the KPI for a facility is available online in the *Supplemental Textbook Material—Foodservice.*

Summary

In healthcare, education, corrections, senior living and corporate settings, the Dining Services Department is highly structured and built upon written documentation of all activities. We are monitored, tracked, certified and evaluated based upon our performance to those documents. You can choose to be "buried" by the paperwork of this process or you can leverage the guidelines to help you provide a consistently better service to your clientele.

Glossary

Delegation
Passing authority for tasks or assigning duties downward through the organization chart

Key Performance Indicators (KPI)
Benchmark performance points tracked over time

Putting it into Practice

4. Your department goal is to ensure the health and safety of the clients. One objective is: Provide annual sanitation and safety training. Write one performance standard for the objective that would tell the employee **what** you want, **how** to do it, and **how well** it should be done.

Figure 14.6 Sample Key Performance Indicator Score Card

DINING SERVICES CARE SCORE CARD—MAY 2016

	Annual	Target Budget	Met or Not Met Target	Comments
Operational Efficiency Strategy				
Facility Finance-Reductions	$230,000	$525,000	▼	Our work needs to continue in reducing expenses to meet this budget.
Average Daily Census	106	116	▼	Continues to be below budget, it is better than last month.
Nutrition Care Expenses	$112,605	$114,436	▲	We are under budget year-to-date but need to continue looking for more reductions including: disposables, food and tube feedings and salaries.
Nutrition Care Revenue (Income)	$28,476	$26,528	▲	We are running 3.33% above our budget. These numbers are helping with offsetting our expenses—Good Job.
Number Meals Served	19,149	18,731	▲	Hours per meal: 0.168 budget 0.18. Target to reach 0.164.
Employee Strategy				
Employee Engagement—First Choice—Department	3.89	4.08	▼	Work is being done on equipment needs and opinions count. **Are you using the sugesstion box?** Exceeded 2015 goal of 3.66 work towards a goal of 4.08 for 2016.
Consumer Strategy				
Courtesy of person serving food	46%	50%	▼	March: Temp: 38%; Quality: 41% Courtesy: 46%. Thanks for working so hard to please our patients. It's making a difference.
Special/Restricted diet explained	21%	100%	▼	Implement visit cards starting in June
Food temperature at time of meal delivery	60%	90%	▼	Implementing new meals on-demand in TCU in July: 20% points YTD. Stay focused on prompt delivery of meals.

 Favorable and on track   Unfavorable and needs more work

Manage Professional Communications

Overview and Objectives

In every foodservice department, meetings are an important method of communicating. Successful meetings require communication before, during, and after. Likewise, you can expect to become involved in interdepartmental teams, committees, and task forces. The obligation is to effectively represent the department by being prepared, professional, and ensuring that department activities are coordinated with overall facility systems. After completing this chapter, you should be able to:

✓ Manage department meetings

✓ Participate in meetings outside the department

✓ Participate in regulatory agency surveys

In many respects, a Certified Dietary Manager functions as a communicator and facilitator. This role is especially true when representing the department at meetings. Understanding both the facility needs and expectations will help determine how the department team can carry them through. Ensuring that department activities are coordinated with those of the system, requires cooperation and consistent ongoing communication at meetings.

Department Meetings

Monthly department staff meetings are the norm in many facilities. A department manager holds meetings to update staff on facility and department activities, introduce new procedures, recognize the work of the department, clarify policies, gather feedback, and present ongoing training. Meetings help generate common understandings, stimulate creative problem-solving, and bring everyone onto the "same page" to promote teamwork.

Many Certified Dietary Managers face time pressures with their work. It is important to take the broad view, recognizing that time spent organizing, planning, and communicating in meetings can often improve productivity and effectiveness throughout the operation.

When scheduling meetings, a manager may need to hold the same meeting, such as a training session, at several different times/days in order to reach all employee groups. Staggering meetings or meeting in small groups can be a good way to accommodate a meeting without impacting the department's activities.

Types of Meetings

There are five basic types of meetings within the Dining Services department for which you may be responsible:

- Production meeting—Daily and Weekly
- Pre-Meal Line Meeting
- Training meeting, such as an in-service
- Monthly department and goal progress meeting
- Teamwork meetings

Each of these meetings will have different guidelines, require different preparation, and will have a positive impact on the department. See Figure 15.1 for the details in conducting these meetings.

Figure 15.1 Types of Department Meetings

TYPE OF MEETING	PURPOSE	PREPARATION
Daily Production Meeting **Weekly Production Meeting**	• Review production, catering and cafeteria needs	• Quick 15 minute stand-up meeting for updates • Held in kitchen • Review problems or concerns from day before • Plan for needs in coming days
Pre-Meal Line Meeting	• Review meal to be served, presentation of the meal, special needs	• Quick 15 minute stand-up meeting for updates • Held at the serving line • Discuss the display plate • Identify clients with concerns • Review problems or concerns from day/meal before
Training Meeting	• O-J-T (on-the-job training) and planned in-service meetings • Review sanitation and safety regulations	• 30-45 minute education meeting • Typically required attendance • May use outside trainer
Monthly Department and Goal Progress Meeting	• Review progress toward facility and department goals	• Formal 30-60 minute meeting • Review of department activities • Review of financial performance • Update on Goals
Teamwork Meeting	• Work on department initiatives and performance goals • Work on Interdepartmental goals	• Formal meeting • Team reports on task assignments • Progress Reports • Action Planning

Techniques for Effective Meetings

Planning is essential for effective meetings. The meeting leader needs to identify the specific purpose of the meeting, gather any necessary background information and plan an agenda and time limit for the meeting.

During the planning, consider who should attend, specific objectives for the discussion, and the best approach to involve group members in discussion.

- Select a time and day for the meeting that is most convenient for everyone.
- List the materials and equipment needed, such as audio-visuals, handouts or equipment.
- Choose a place for the meeting that is quiet, comfortable, well lit, and large enough to provide ample space for all attendees.
- Notify all participants in advance.

How best to notify participants depends on the usual communication methods with the group involved. For example, for the organization's safety committee, meeting announcements are probably sent to each participant as a memo or an email. However, a training meeting for foodservice employees may be more effective posted as a prominent notice over the timeclock, or added as a meeting notice to employees' paychecks.

Depending upon the type of meeting, consult with key personnel prior to the meeting to plan additional content and objectives. For instance, if the meeting is to review progress of department goals, you may want to meet with other interdisciplinary team leaders to collect information from them. Discuss with them how they presented the organizational goals or perhaps any training needs for use during in-service training.

When appropriate, distribute an agenda for the meeting to each member in advance. An **agenda** is a planned outline and timetable for what will happen during a meeting. It should also be reviewed verbally at the start of a meeting. A time limit should be established for each topic but this limit should not be so rigid that it cannot be adjusted. The agenda serves as an outline for the meeting and can help keep it on track. In planning an agenda, be sure to work with small, achievable objectives that can be accomplished within the established time-frame for a meeting.

If this is the first meeting of a new work group, introductions are very important. "Icebreaker" questions, such as, "What is your favorite home-cooked meal?" or "Where did you go for your last vacation?" can help acquaint new members to the group. At the beginning of the meeting, clearly state the objective(s) of the meeting and state the expected outcomes. Present all relevant tasks and encourage all attendees to participate actively in the meeting. The leader should encourage a friendly team spirit and discuss the meeting's importance.

The group leader has several responsibilities as the meeting evolves. On occasion, use a pre-meeting assignment to generate interest and discussion when the meeting actually happens. Keep the group on track, keep the discussion moving forward, and draw in unresponsive members of the group. The leader may have to actively ask for the views and experiences of all attendees, to ensure that one or a few speakers do not overpower the discussion.

If disagreement arises among group members, explore the reason for the disagreement and try to seek consensus. Clarify comments made by the attendees to ensure that their viewpoint is understood by everyone. Summarize progress and monitor that time is spent

Glossary

Agenda
Planned objectives, outline and timetable for a meeting

Putting It Into Practice

1. Your objective is to create a new system for receiving and storing food. What type of meeting would work best for this objective?

effectively and addresses the meeting objectives. If necessary, bring the group back by reviewing the problem, goals and progress achieved.

As a group leader, watch the agenda as the meeting goes on, and take firm, polite action as required to conform to the timetable and objectives. Managing time during a meeting is easiest if you state the time allotted for each part of the meeting as it begins. For example, before discussing ideas for improving food temperatures on trayline, say: *We have 10 minutes for discussion on this. What are your ideas?* About eight minutes into the discussion, you can say: *We have two more minutes for discussion about this. Is there anyone who hasn't spoken yet who would like to offer an idea?*

In a special technique called **brainstorming**, participants are asked to list ideas for solving a problem. Explain that no idea is out of bounds, no idea is "good" or "bad," and discussion and judgment of ideas will be held until brainstorming is complete. Even an idea that immediately proves ineffective can spark additional ideas.

During any meeting, each individual should be allowed to state opinions. As a group leader, make sure that all points made are considered fairly and openly. When establishing ground rules for a meeting, make it clear that all ideas will be respected and that each attendee should participate.

As a group leader, observe participants and look for feedback, including nonverbal communication. Identify and resolve any resistance or conflicts that occur. If the discussion during a meeting brings out a conflict or a problem that is not part of the meeting's purpose, recognize it as important and set aside a separate time for it to be addressed. You may say: *Thanks for bringing this up. This sounds like an important issue for us to review. Since it's not related to our objectives in this meeting, we will need to set aside time to focus on this separately. Would you please talk to me after the meeting and tell me more about your concern?*

Sometimes, members of a group need special attention as a meeting evolves. Figure 15.2 suggests some basic strategies that can be used in troublesome situations.

At the end of the meeting, summarize the progress made. Identify the next actions to be taken, and see that everyone understands the those steps. Review tasks assigned to individuals that may result from the meeting. When possible, identify the time and location of the next meeting.

Glossary

Brainstorming
Asking all participants to suggest ideas for solving a problem

Figure 15.2 Strategies for Handling Group Problems

THE GROUP MEMBER WHO:	STRATEGY TO USE:
Wants to argue	Do not get involved. State/summarize the member's ideas and let the group decide upon their values.
Wants to help	Encourage the member to give ideas, especially when the discussion is veering off course.
Wants to discuss details	Acknowledge the member's points, but also remind the member of the meeting's objective and the time limit that has been set.
Will not stop talking	Interrupt the group member tactfully, then ask a question to bring the participant back to the topic.
Is afraid to speak	Ask the group member easy questions, recognize earlier contributions, and make the person feel important.
Wants to be recognized	Recognize the individual and ask the person for unique solutions to the problems at hand.
Is not interested	Ask the group member how the discussion will impact him/her.
Acts superior	Recognize this person's ability and ask this person the most difficult and challenging questions.
Wants to show cleverness	Identify any trick questions and give them to the group for response.

Meeting Documentation

Documenting meetings is essential. The **meeting minutes**, a summary of what has been discussed and decided, provides reference to everyone who has attended. Minutes can be used as reference for the next meeting on an ongoing project. They should include a summary of the action plan, assignments, and deadlines, as applicable. If appropriate, a recorder should be appointed to maintain a record of the meeting. This record should include at least:

- Name of meeting
- Date
- Time the meeting started and ended
- Name of the leader and recorder
- Names of those present
- Key points and discussion topics (brief)
- Action to take
- Who is responsible to take the action and related deadlines

Glossary

Meeting Minutes
A summary of what was discussed and decided during a meeting

All participants should be provided a copy of the minutes. Corrections, if needed, should occur at the next meeting.

In meetings conducted for training purposes, documentation is important for proving that employees have received training. This documentation may be requested by inspectors and surveyors to verify that established standards are being met. A training meeting typically includes an attendance roster and a summary of the presentation.

Effective Speaking

Although we have been doing it since we were toddlers, each of us has more to learn about speaking. In a business environment, we routinely speak with employees, supervisors, clients, team members, suppliers, and many more people. Some spoken communications are one-on-one and informal. Others are group presentations and may be very formal.

A number of basic tips can help with speaking:

- Know what you are going to say and develop a plan or outline, if needed.
- Identify the most important points of the message and organize what you are going to say around these points.
- Deliver your most important point(s) first. This is when the receiver's attention is likely to be at its peak. It also helps the receiver focus on the remainder of your message.
- Concentrate on the listener. Speak to listeners' perspectives, and notice feedback.
- Make eye contact.
- Share pride or compliments with employees when appropriate.

Figure 15.3 lists some of the traits and qualities that promote effective speaking.

Figure 15.3 Elements of Effective Speaking

• Confidence	• Understanding
• Knowledge	• Humility
• Organization	• Concern for Listener
• Pleasing Voice	• Responsiveness
• Concern	• Awareness of Situation
• Control of Emotion	• Humor
• Language Command	• Forcefulness
• Friendliness	• Sensitivity
• Objectivity	• Charisma
• Empathy	• Concentration
• Open-Mindedness	• Spontaneity
• Trustworthiness	• Tact
• Acceptable Appearance	• Intelligence
• Honest	• Enthusiasm

In spoken communications, remember the value of silence and attention. Allow yourself to relax and listen to others. A manager who is a good listener can obtain work-related information, be more effective in interpersonal relationships, and generate information necessary to make good decisions. There are several basic principles helpful in effective listening:

- Think about the central idea the speaker is trying to convey.
- Focus attention on what the speaker is saying rather than on distracting factors.
- Listen objectively to what is being said, without trying to make an immediate judgment.
- Listen for more than facts. There may be a hidden agenda or a subtle message the speaker is hesitant to convey.
- Understand the speaker's basic ideas before discussing or disagreeing.

What about situations in which spoken communication is a public presentation or a more formal event? Use presentations for a number of purposes, such as training or defending a budget or sharing information with colleagues, or asking for resources to implement a new idea.

Formal Presentations

In presentations, a lecture alone can become boring. A wide variety of techniques make presentations more effective. These include:

- Demonstration: In this mode, show people how to do something. For example, demonstrate methods for garnishing plates or taking an order for a meal.
- Discussion: This is a planned approach that uses group participation. For example, present basic information to a group and then permit the exchange of information through discussion.
- Panel presentation: With this method, the Certified Dietary Manager may serve as a member of a small group. Frequently, panel members make a presentation, share discussion with each other, and then open up the floor for questions and further discussion from the audience.
- Role playing: A technique in which participants assume the role of someone else in a defined situation and act it out. Role playing is often effective in training because it gives participants a chance to try and practice new skills in a safe environment.
- Case studies: A description of a specific situation, either real or imaginary. Events are reported without explanation and attendees then use the experiences illustrated in the case as a basis for discussion.

When giving a presentation, it is not unnatural to feel nervous in front of a group. This feeling can be managed, practice and experience can make a big difference. Several tips are included in a Presentation Tips Page available online in the *Supplemental Textbook Material—Foodservice*.

Meeting Follow-Up

If the meeting includes delegating staff members to accomplish a task after the meeting is over, it will be important to follow up with them before the next meeting. Depending on the task, it may be helpful to work with the staff members to develop a timeline to complete the tasks. Then, check with them to make sure they are following their timeline. The manager's role is to check progress and ensure that tasks are being completed.

Meeting follow-up also includes publishing meeting minutes. Some recommend that minutes should be distributed within twenty-four hours of the meeting. Correct any errors in a timely manner rather than waiting weeks to review the proceedings.

External Meetings

There are at least two categories of external meetings where the manager needs to represent the department: interdepartmental meetings and professional association meetings. On an interdepartmental basis, the manager may need to hold or participate in meetings that help ensure organization-wide problem-solving, quality management, and/or systems revision.

Interdepartmental Meetings

Interdisciplinary Care Team. In healthcare facilities, there is usually a team approach to the care of clients. The team may be composed of a Certified Dietary Manager, a Registered Dietitian Nutritionist, a diet technician, a nurse, a physical therapist, an occupational therapist, a speech therapist, a social worker, a clinical pharmacist, a physician, and/or many others. How a team is structured and the roles of each team member are governed by healthcare standards as well as the policies and practices of each facility. The role of the Certified Dietary Manager in Care Team Meetings is discussed in Chapter 14 of the *Nutrition Fundamentals and Medical Nutrition Therapy* textbook.

Task Forces and Committees. As a Certified Dietary Manager, you may be asked to represent the foodservice department on a number of facility committees and task forces led by an appointed chairperson. Meetings are regularly scheduled. In meetings such as these, attendance and minutes typically are recorded and distributed to all members. Committees and task forces are established to:

- Coordinate activities within the organization.
- Solve problems.
- Evaluate or revise systems.
- Devise plans for meeting objectives.

As a Certified Dietary Manager, you may be asked to serve on facility-wide committees, such as:

- **Infection Control.** This committee's usual purpose is to develop policies and procedures for sanitation techniques, isolation procedures, reporting of infectious diseases, and educating and training all personnel.
- **Safety Committee.** A typical purpose of this committee is to review all unsafe acts within the facility both for clients and others. Establishing fire safety and disaster preparedness, the implementation, OSHA and other regulatory standards are also the concern of a safety committee, along with providing education and training materials to all personnel.
- **Cost Control.** The purpose of this committee may be to provide, develop, and implement cost-effectiveness procedures and plans.
- **Quality Assessment and Improvement.** The purpose of this committee is to monitor, evaluate, and document actions for the provision of quality service and products for all clients.
- **Customer/Client Service.** A committee such as this may focus on ways to improve customer/client service and satisfaction in all areas.
- **Marketing Committee.** Be involved, particularly if the facility is expanding services related to dining services.

There may be other committees to which the manager belongs. The number and types of committees vary from one facility to the next.

In a committee, a group of persons work together to solve problems and perform assigned administrative activities. Committees may be temporary or permanent. Committees are usually appointed for ongoing activities, and may be mandated by regulatory agencies.

Task forces are usually appointed to deal with specific problems. Members of a task force analyze a problem, complete research, and make recommendations for action. Once the problem is solved, the task force is usually disbanded.

Survey and Agency Meetings

As the author and/or reviewer of the Policy and Procedure Manual, SOPs, and personnel documentation, the manager has the most direct knowledge of the department. The manager is the primary contact point for accreditation surveyors, healthcare inspectors, unemployment officers, lawyers, risk management coordinators and other official boards of inquiry.

The best preparation for any governmental or legal meeting is knowledge of your own documents. When the written department guidelines comply with the regulations, or consistently document personnel actions (both positive and negative), then answering a surveyor's question can be complete and professional.

Clinical Care Meetings

Participation in the clinical activities that many Certified Dietary Managers are responsible for is addressed in Chapter 14 of the *Nutrition Fundamentals and Medical Nutrition Therapy* textbook.

Professional Association Meetings

As a Certified Dietary Manager, what could be next? Consider joining one or more professional associations of like professionals. This allows growth, both professionally and personally. The following are some examples of the benefits of membership:

- **Networking opportunities.** Networking, or interacting with others in the profession, can be an excellent source of support, resources, ideas, and friendship. By networking with others, you usually discover that management challenges are not unique and that colleagues can help each other advance the practice of foodservice management. Some professional associations, such as Association of Nutrition & Foodservice Professionals, offer web-based discussion areas or chat rooms, where members can meet with others from diverse locations to discuss professional issues. These associations may also offer local meetings to become involved in.

- **Educational opportunities.** Professional associations are one of the best resources for educational sessions, meetings, and materials that help develop skills and continue professional growth.

- **Research.** A professional association typically conducts research on matters of interest to its members, such as salaries, professional practices, and other issues. This research is shared with members.

- **Publications.** A professional association issues publications that address the unique needs and interests of its members.

- **Employment services.** Many professional associations operate job boards on the internet. Here, find information about employment opportunities that relate to your qualifications.

- **Contact with suppliers.** Through trade events and vendor relationships, professional associations become a conduit for information about suppliers and vendors.

• **Legislative activity.** A professional association may lobby for the interests of its members in state and regional governments, supporting legislation that supports the interests of the profession and the industry.

Joining a professional association presents many opportunities. Most professionals agree that you can benefit from contributing time and energy to an association. Joining in activities, serving on committees, or becoming a leader can advance professional development. Whatever the role, remember that you represent your facility and the department.

Certified Dietary Manager Role

To work well in a team, it is important to understand the role of the Certified Dietary Manager. The Academy of Nutrition and Dietetics (Academy) and the Association of Foodservice & Nutrition Professionals (ANFP) have defined the roles of the food production and dining services team members through delineation studies by both associations. Together, Academy and ANFP are responsible for setting educational requirements, program approvals and continuing education standards for their accredited members.

In addition, each of these organizations provides the **standards of practice** for professional members as the basis for quality in professional activities. As a Certified Dietary Manager, use the standards of practice to help clarify your role and scope of responsibility, and the work of other professionals to whom the standards apply. Figure 15.4 provides an example of a ANFP standard of practice.

Additional Tips for Personal Professionalism

As a professional, the manager has many responsibilities. There are four tips for personal professionalism that will help when representing the profession or your department at meetings and other settings: professional ethics, time management, stress management, and lifelong learning.

Professional Ethics

The concept of ethics refers to views, attitudes, and practices about what is right or wrong. It describes moral standards. This is subjective information. There are no absolute and uniform standards from which to devise a set of ethics. Professional ethics take into account many basic values such as integrity, honesty, fairness, responsibility, and trust.

In addition to personal values, many professional organizations have their own codes of professional ethics for members. For example, Association of Nutrition & Foodservice Professionals presents a **code of ethics** for its members, illustrated in Figure 15.5.

Some ethical issues are fairly straightforward. For example, a policy about client confidentiality specifies that you should not disclose information about clients to others (family, friends, co-workers, etc.) who are not directly involved in their clinical care. From time to time, ethical choices as a professional may be less clear. For example, ethical practices in purchasing usually prohibit accepting gifts from a supplier or potential supplier.

Now, what happens when you attend a food show and are invited to register for a free drawing? Are you accepting a gift? Are you violating sound ethical practices? This question, recently discussed by Certified Dietary Managers in an online forum, can bring on a range of answers. One manager says that this is clearly unethical. Another says the intent of the no-gift practice is to avoid influencing purchasing decisions and this drawing

Figure 15.4 AFNP Standard of Practice: Menu Planning, Calories, and Portion Sizes

The Certified Dietary Manager (CDM) shall ensure that a menu planning process is in place in the facility. Menus shall meet the needs of the clientele as well as the facility.

Criteria

1.1 The menu will include a variety of foods from day to day

1.2 The general menu will meet a government food guide such as Choose MyPlate or the Recommended Dietary Allowances (e.g., Menu will include a food from Vitamin A group every other day and from Vitamin C group daily).

1.3 The menu will avoid repeating the same food on the same day of the week. Cycle menus should be set up so they are not divisible by seven to help avoid this (e.g., a cycle menu that is five days long).

1.4 New food will be introduced regularly; selective menus will include a familiar food with a new food.

1.5 The menu will include a variety of preparation methods and offer a contrast in texture and flavor.

1.6 The menu should be planned for eye appeal and include at least one or two colorful foods on each menu.

1.7 The menu includes foods that can be prepared with available personnel and equipment.

1.8 Menu planning guides such as those from vendors or books such as *Food for Fifty* or *Menu Solutions—Quantity Recipes for Regular and Special Diets* are available in the foodservice department.

1.9 Food preferences of clientele are periodically assessed or when complaints warrant (e.g., resident council meetings, quarterly assessments, individual complaints, or surveys).

1.10 Staff uses a checklist with criteria such as 1.3-1.5 above when serving meals.

1.11 Staff receives training on how to add eye appeal, prepare foods with a contrast in texture and flavor, and keep food costs within the budget allowance.

1.12 Staff receives training on the proper substitutions for food groups (e.g., What to serve to replace a vitamin A group).

Assessment

1.1 Checklists used by staff are evaluated weekly and menus corrected as needed.

1.2 Training records are evaluated to make sure all cooking staff has received training in food preparation, sanitation, meal service, etc.: training records are maintained in the foodservice department.

1.3 Data from food preference surveys are used for menu planning purposes.

has no impact. Yet another manager says that her superior goes to the shows with her and they both register for the drawing.

When faced with an ethical dilemma, what should you do? A few steps can help reach a resolution. First, check the codes of ethics for the professional association(s) and the facility. Sometimes, the codes of ethics of other related associations can provided added insight.

Next, talk the situation over with peers and colleagues. Ask whether they have faced a similar dilemma. If so, ask how they considered the issue and what resolution they reached. Of course, think about the situation from your own perspective. What feels right—and why?

Furthermore, discuss a job-related ethical dilemma with your supervisor. When making a difficult decision: 1) drawing from additional experiences, your supervisor may be able to help, and 2) they should be alerted to the issues and concerns, so there will be no surprises or questions down the line. Enlisting approval and support ahead of time protects you, your supervisor, and the facility.

Figure 15.5 ANFP Code of Ethics

The Code of Ethics for members of the Association of Nutrition & Foodservice Professionals (ANFP) has been adopted to promote and maintain the highest standards of foodservice and personal conduct among its members. Adherence to this code is required for membership and serves to assure public confidence in the integrity and service of ANFP.

As a member of ANFP, I pledge myself to:

- Reflect my pride in my competence as a dietary manager by wearing my pin and emblem and displaying my certificate.
- Use only legal and ethical means in the practice of my profession.
- Use every opportunity to improve public understanding of the role of the dietary manager.
- Promote and encourage the highest level of ethics within the industry.
- Refuse to engage in, or countenance, activities for personal gain at the expense of my employer, the industry, or the profession.
- Maintain the confidentiality of privileged information entrusted or known to me by virtue of my position.
- Maintain loyalty to my employer and pursue their objectives in ways that are consistent with the public interest.

- Always communicate administrative decisions of my employer in a truthful and accurate manner.
- Communicate to proper authorities, but disclose to no one else, any evidence of infraction of established rules and regulations.
- Strive for excellence in all aspects of management and nutritional practices with constant attention to self-improvement.
- Maintain the highest standard of personal conduct.

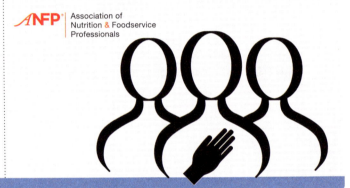

In most respects, ethical practices come naturally to individuals with well-developed personal value systems. Nevertheless, an occasional challenge does arise.

Time Management

Time is, like many resources, limited. How can critical needs be managed? What's the technique? Often, the easy answer is to work longer hours to get things done. Managers in foodservice are especially vulnerable to this problem, as foodservice facilities tend to operate for long hours each day. To manage the day from breakfast preparation through supper clean-up is usually a 15 hour day. Additional information on time management is available in the online *Supplemental Textbook Material—Foodservice*.

Certified Dietary Managers use various tools to assist with time management. A simple calendar, posted on the wall or on a phone and carried in the pocket, is a start. Personal calendar systems also help organize and track to-do items. When making to-do lists, set priorities for each item to help stay focused as interruptions or surprises occur throughout the day. If you cannot accomplish everything on the list, at least focus on the most important tasks in order. A sample to-do list appears in Figure 15.6.

To track commitments further in the future and follow up on action items, and/or the time-related responsibilities of others who report to you, also use a tickler list. A tickler list is designed to "jog" your memory about selected items or tasks. Figure 15.7 illustrates a tickler list.

Figure 15.6 To-Do List

WEEK OF 2/3-2/10	PRIORITY
Attend safety meeting (2/6)	1
Rewrite job description (due 2/11)	1
Work on budget (due 3/10	2
Go to Sally's luncheon	3
Review CQ1 (due 2/17)	2
Attend staff meeting	1
Call John in New Orleans	3
Answer mail	2
Meeting with Manager	1

Figure 15.7 Tickler List

March 1	• Quality Improvement Plan due
	• Employee Recognition Dinner
April 10	• Quarterly QA Reports due
	• Annual P&P Updates due
April 20	• Quarter 1 Financial Variance Report due

Today, access to a wide variety of computer-based tools helps with time management. Some Certified Dietary Managers use email to manage a calendar, track recurring events, and manage to-do and tickler lists. The calendar may also issue an audible alarm or reminder for an upcoming deadline or appointment. Today's cell phones provide excellent tools with the additional advantage of portability. In some facilities, a project management software application is used throughout the facility to help track and coordinate work. Through email and voice mail, messages and instructions can be quickly passed and acknowledged.

Stress Management

Stress is a condition that arises from physical or mental strain, anxiety, and overwork. It is a familiar word not only to Certified Dietary Managers, but to most employees in the workplace. The demands and schedules of the job can be strenuous. Client interactions can be satisfying but draining. Along with work-related stress, you may experience stress from factors outside the workplace.

Stress is a natural experience and it is not unique to Certified Dietary Managers. A few ideas can help manage stress in the everyday work life:

- **Take breaks.** Physical breaks, emotional breaks, and mental breaks are all important. Examples include: talking a walk, stopping to enjoy a joke, or switching tasks for a while. Each of these helps to restore energy.

Putting It Into Practice

3. You are always busy but your work this morning seems overwhelming. Here are the items on your to-do list at 7:30 AM:

- Cooler temperature was too high this morning as reported by a.m. cook

- Weekly production meeting at 8:30 AM

- Care planning meeting at 10:00 AM for a client who is losing weight

- New employee orientation, third session, meeting at 9:00 AM to go over typical work day

- First draft of next year's budget is due to administrator by noon today.

How would you prioritize these tasks to better manage your time?

- Accept what you cannot change. It takes a lot of emotional energy to worry about things you cannot control, or feeling angry about something you cannot influence.

- Use relaxation exercises. Physical and mental relaxation exercises can help loosen tense muscles or release negative thoughts.

- Take things one at a time. Focus on one task at a time to concentrate your energy. Thinking about other tasks at the same time only creates more stress.

- Focus on the positive results of your efforts. In addition to hard work and job-related pressure, you can usually see results and satisfaction in the outcomes. Good food and satisfied clients help balance out the stress.

- Be realistic. Setting goals and expectations that are out of reach is very stressful.

- Keep a positive outlook. A healthy perspective is one in which you remember the big picture and focus on the things that can be accomplished. Keep the details in mind but do not get caught in the fine print.

- Seek help when needed. Request assistance and tap into available resources when the tasks call for it. If stress is taking a greater toll, do not hesitate to seek professional help.

Lifelong Learning

It is not uncommon for a Certified Dietary Manager to pursue additional training at some point during a career to develop new skills.

- One may choose to go to culinary school.
- Another may choose to obtain an associate or bachelor's degree.
- Another may pursue a degree in business management.
- Yet another may seek additional credentials.

When planning your own development, give some thought to both short-term and long-range goals. In the short term, learn more about standards, or labor unions, or another specific topic. Use results-oriented objectives for something you need to do—or will need to do soon, and work backward to identify resources for training or acquiring training.

Resources for development may come from a professional association, in-house training department, community resources, local schools, business seminars, the Internet, and self-study courses. An online or advanced study course is one way a Certified Dietary Manager can pursue additional education while still holding down a full-time job with variable hours. Along with formal class-room training, develop knowledge through DVDs, videotapes, food books, trade magazines, and websites.

Putting It Into Practice

4. You and your staff have had a very hectic week in the foodservice department. It's the first week of May and you had extra catering duties to celebrate National Older American's Month and Mother's Day. What might you do to reduce your stress and your employee stress at the same time?

Change Management

Overview and Objectives

A Certified Dietary Manager's job is to manage people to work in every part of the food production and dining services department. The best planning will not work unless the manager is able to motivate employees to help carry out the plan and to direct and coach employees in their actions. In addition to supervising employees, providing direction, managing service issues, and implementing change, a manager must be able to communicate effectively. After completing this chapter, you should be able to:

✓ Identify existing problems and needs

✓ Prepare justification for changes

✓ Implement the plan of action

Identify Existing Problems and Needs

The day-to-day activities of a Certified Dietary Manager are largely influenced by a bigger picture—how you are doing relative to the department and the facility's goals and objectives. As discussed in Chapter 14, goals and objectives are critical components of managerial planning and should help address existing problems and identify opportunities for change. Goals and objectives can help measure progress, evaluate work, and set priorities.

The Quality Process, discussed in Chapter 8, also identifies opportunities for change. Self-audits, system monitors and survey results highlight both processes that are successful and areas for improvement. The basis for the Quality Improvement Committee or Performance Improvement Plan, is the belief that every organization has opportunities for improvement in performance or outcomes.

Sometimes, the need for change is identified through an unexpected Risk Management Event (also known as an Incident or Unusual Occurrence Report), a worker injury or product/equipment loss. Often the immediate response does provide a temporary relief, however, to fix the problem may require a process change.

For example, imagine you have a department goal to reduce food costs by one-percent this year. An objective to meet that goal is to monitor inventory costs every week. Over the first six weeks of the year, inventory costs have gone up. Is the problem an issue with the goal (look back at the writing of a S.M.A.R.T. goal)? Is the problem an issue with the objectives to reach that goal? Or is the problem an issue with the implementation of the planned changes?

Change

Change is anything that requires revisions in the roles and routines of a workforce. Sometimes change is made voluntarily, as when employee groups generate ideas about performing work more effectively. At other times, change may be forced upon the department from higher levels in the facility or from external agencies, such as CMS, or TJC, or the local health department.

Change is a continuing process, not an activity with a distinct start and finish. The facility in general and the dining services department specifically, are evolving at all times. In fact, experts in organizational behavior agree that change is a sign of a healthy, successful organization. An organization that is not able to change also is not able to adapt and excel. Change can generate excitement, commitment, and pride, but it should be managed in a way that helps employees feel positively about it.

All elements in the dining services department and within the organization itself, are closely related. Therefore, a change made in one area is likely to have an impact on other areas as well.

For change to be effective, the Certified Dietary Manager should to first show employees why there is a need for change. It is important to be honest and provide the facts. Whenever possible employees should be involved in the earliest planning phases of change.

While dining services employees may not have the option of rejecting change, they should have the option of participating in decisions about how to implement a change. Certified Dietary Managers can use participative management approaches to involve employees in planning. As employees are trained, coached, and counseled about changes being proposed, their involvement will, ideally, reduce their resistance to the change. Typically, employee ownership and commitment will grow in direct relation to the amount of input they have into the entire process.

Examples of impending change include: mergers, new software, new dining services equipment, remodeling, menu revisions, new regulations, budget cuts, census variations, new administrative staff and/or philosophies, and evolution of professional practice.

Resistance to Change

Resistance to change makes it difficult for Certified Dietary Managers to implement change. It is human nature to be anxious and hesitant about the uncertainty of a change. Reasons for resisting can include the following:

- Economic concerns: Sometimes change has a negative economic impact upon employees.
- Inconvenience: Some changes will require employees to learn new operating procedures or become responsible for extra duties.
- Anxiety: Fear of the unknown makes people feel threatened or insecure about their own work situations.
- Changing relationships: Some new work assignments and reporting structures can alter working relationships.
- Increased control by others: Some changes take away employees' independence. For example, increased supervision may be part of implementing a new procedure.
- Low trust: A sense of mistrust or fear of what will happen next. Concern that the company, supervisors or fellow workers cannot competently manage the change.

- Concerns about performance: Some changes generate fear no longer doing a good job. A dedicated employee may be troubled by change, and worry about their ability to performance the new tasks, new procedures, or work with new tools.

An organizational change, such as a move to a better office can be warmly accepted, simply because it is seen to have obvious advantages. But not all changes fit into this category. Where changes create ambiguity and uncertainty, then resistance to change is likely to emerge.

Change is inevitable in every organization. Sometimes the change is a carefully planned transition from one process to another. In healthcare, change is often the result of evolving regulations or decreasing re-imbursements. All too often, change is the result of a crisis or unexpected event.

If you can accept that change is a normal part of the workplace, then planning for and implementing change becomes a way of doing business. It becomes part of the culture. Successful implementation of change leads to a willingness to try more.

Involvement of all levels of staff early on helps develop a better plan. Too often the changes are planned with little input by frontline staff. Yet, who knows more about how the job is done, and how it could be done faster, than those who actually do the tasks? This begins with involving them in planning goals, objectives and action plans. Early participation of frontline staff in the planning and evaluation stages of implementing change also increases their buy-in to the new processes, location or structure.

Your credibility as a manager, and in turn your ability to implement major changes, is established through a history of open communications, honesty, and a concern for the welfare of staff members. Frequent communication of the plan, progress and outcomes is invaluable. Fear of hidden agendas and unknown goals increases resistance to change.

It is best to use the tools of communication, participation, and negotiation to help employees accept change. If necessary, a manager may use authority as a tool in implementing change. It is helpful to involve both formal and informal employee groups and their leaders in the change process. Training programs are often necessary as changes are implemented. To help overcome resistance, employees need an opportunity to learn new procedures and gain confidence.

Commitment of senior leadership, visible support by administration and celebration of successes all start at the top. Senior leadership can encourage cooperation of multiple departments to ensure participation, which in turn, improves the likelihood of success.

After change has been implemented, it must be evaluated. It is important to see whether the change has been beneficial and whether any additional changes are needed to further improve the effectiveness of the dining services department. The Certified Dietary Manager should also assess whether there have been any unexpected spin-off effects of the change.

An extensive checklist for planning a change is available in the online *Supplemental Textbook Material—Foodservice*. Additional information and extensive resources on managing change are available through online search tools.

Putting It Into Practice

1. Your administrative team has just told you that they want you to open a new cafeteria. How would you introduce this idea to your staff?

Communication

Effective, frequent communication is key to successful change management. Communication is an exchange of information. Even when we say nothing, we are still communicating through our actions. Most people talk; few people communicate.

As a Certified Dietary Manager, you will need different communication skills as you interact with administrators, physicians, clients, employees, and families. Miscommunication leads to dissatisfaction, misunderstanding, misinterpretation, and, in some cases, anger and resentment. There are basic principles of communication that can help every manager be more effective.

Communications of all types share a few basic components. There is always a sender, a receiver, a message, and feedback. Figure 16.1 illustrates these elements.

Figure 16.1 Elements of Basic Communication

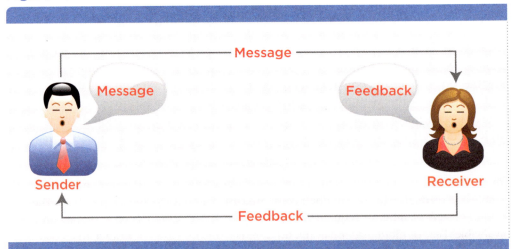

If you are the sender, you have a message to transmit. Consider the receiver's perspective as you put the message together. The message, verbal and/or nonverbal, is transmitted through formal and/or informal channels of communication. Examples of formal channels are: meetings, memos, and rules. Informal communication channels include the grapevine, rumors, and general conversations. Finally, the message is received and the receiver attempts to understand it based upon his or her own perceptions.

Feedback is the reaction that the receiver has to the sender's message. Feedback tells the sender how the message is being received. To be an effective communicator, you need to process the feedback. The receiver may be saying anything from: *I agree with you*, to, *I have no idea what you are talking about*, to, *I think your idea is off the wall!*

How to read feedback? By listening and watching. Just like the original message may take many forms: such as oral, written, email, and body movements, (such as a shrug of the shoulders), so can feedback. The ability to read feedback and respond accordingly, builds trust, fosters problem-solving, and provides effective communication.

Another aspect of communication is called interference. Sometimes, certain factors disrupt the flow of information between sender and receiver. Here are some examples of factors that can cause interference:

- Differences in perception
- Lack of knowledge
- Emotions
- Lack of interest
- Personality
- Distractions
- Disorganization
- Language
- Indirect access—the telephone game

To communicate well, particularly when discussing events related to major change, keep in mind a few basic tips:

- Analyze the receiver: As a sender, consider the receiver's position. What is the best form of communication for this person?
  - > Are they visual—an email may be best?
  - > Are they auditory—a voice message or face to face discussion would be better?
  - > Are they kinesthetic (they need to see & touch)—a demonstration or sample would work well?
- Use feedback: Watch and listen as you communicate.
- Make messages meaningful: It is important to consider the perceptions and prior knowledge of the receiver as the message is developed.
- Use face-to-face communications: Whenever possible, talk directly to others, so that you can ensure your message is not distorted and to read feedback and respond accordingly.
- Communicate nonverbally: Your nonverbal communication affects the message. In fact, the majority of what you communicate in person comes from your nonverbal language, rather than from your words. Be alert to the message sent with body language. At the same time, you can read the receiver's body language to obtain valuable feedback that you otherwise might not hear. Figure 16.2 lists a number of nonverbal clues. Note that cultural influences make a difference in the interpretation of body language.
- Cultural influences make a difference in interpretation of body language.
- Respect personal space: For most North Americans, a distance of about 19″ between people is comfortable. Moving in closer can create distress.
- Use clear language: Use words you know the receiver will understand. Recognize that specific words do not mean the same thing to everyone. Choose words carefully and watch for responses.
- Repeat the message: In both oral and written communications, a common method is to: tell the listener what you're about to tell them, tell them your message, and then explain what you just told them.
- Empathize: Seek to understand and respect the receiver's opinions, ideas, attitudes, and perceptions.
- Timing: Pick the timing to avoid distractions and ensure the receiver is in a listening mode.

Putting It Into Practice

2. You want to meet privately with an employee to listen to a concern. The noise from the kitchen is interfering. What should you do?

- Consider the environment: It should be comfortable and impose minimal disruptions.
- Listen: This is perhaps the most critical aspect of communication. It helps you become a receiver, not just a sender. If you work as both a sender and a receiver, communication becomes a two-way process.

Figure 16.2 Nonverbal Communications

Using nonverbal communications can help you both send your message and understand feedback from the receiver.

BODY LANGUAGE	WHAT IT MEANS
Leaning slightly towards a person	I'm interested
Relaxed posture	I'm open to what you are saying
Eye contact	I think you are important
Nodding	I'm listening
Pulling or touching ear	I want to listen to you
Looking away	I'm not interested
Touching nose	I don't like what you're saying
Rubbing nose and breaking eye contact	I'm lying
Touching cheek	I'm evaluating what you are saying
Hand over mouth	I disapprove, or I'm trying not to say anything
Hands clasped behind head	I'm arrogant
Tapping fingers	I'm feeling impatient
Fidgeting	I'm ready to go
Smile	I feel good about you and about myself
Clutching an object tightly	I'm nervous or afraid
Clasping hands behind back	I'm angry or frustrated
Crossed arms	I'm protecting myself
Open palms	I'm sincere and open
Looking at watch	I'm ready to end this conversation

Effective communication with department staff, other managers and senior leadership is a critical piece of managing change. However, communication can be confusing sometimes when it needs to go in so many different directions.

Flow of Communications In an Organization

In a facility, there is communication flowing in many directions. Some messages flows downwards, from superiors to managers, or from manager to the line staff. Others may flow upwards, from manager to supervisor, or from subordinates to manager. Some communication flows laterally, between and among peers.

In most organizations **downward communication** is frequently used to convey policies, procedures, directives, objectives, and other information to subordinate personnel. It may be written or spoken. When a Certified Dietary Manager uses downward communication, it is often to give instructions, explain information or procedures, train employees, or communicate information that may have a bearing on employees' jobs.

Downward communication may be the only contact subordinates have with upper management. It usually follows the chain of command, meaning that you would receive the information from your supervisor who received it from his/her director or from the CEO. As a result, administration needs to:

• Be honest, accurate, and factual, whether the information is good or bad news.

• Use words and phrases that subordinates can understand.

• Make the message specific; explain what effect it will have on the employee.

Your job, as the manager, is to continue communicating down the chain of command with accurate, reliable, relevant information.

Employees also will communicate ideas, requests, and opinions to their supervisor. **Upward communication** is usually reporting and questioning. The Certified Dietary Manager is responsible for keeping a superior informed on concerns and comments expressed by the staff.

In many facilities, upward communication is limited. Subordinates know the supervisor has the authority to fire, block promotions or salary increases, and give unpleasant assignments. So a reluctance to communicate upward is common. The supervisor must find ways to work with subordinates to maintain face-to-face communication that is free-flowing, open, honest, and respectful of differences in opinions.

Effective Certified Dietary Managers help to invite this flow of communications by establishing an explicit open door policy. This policy says: *My door is always open. Come talk to me any time about anything.* Stating this to employees helps to ease reluctance. This policy can be challenging to honor, as a manager is busy. If you establish this policy and an employee asks to speak with you at an inopportune time, it is fair to say: *I really want to hear what you have to say. At the moment, there are some distractions. May we sit down together at 4:00 so that I can give you my full attention?*

If you have an open door policy, be sure to honor it. Nothing can be more disruptive to communication than to go back on your promise and violate trust.

Lateral communication among peers may involve discussions and meetings to solve problems and accomplish tasks that cross department or functional lines. This communication is critical in coordination, teamwork, and cooperation. Peers can be very effective at solving problems through discussion.

Informally, lateral communication can also involve the channel called the grapevine or the rumor mill. These exists in all organizations. The grapevine is a major communication tool in any organization, whether or not you recognize it. A savvy manager keeps in touch with the

Glossary

Downward Communication
Used to convey policies, procedures, directives, objectives and other information to subordinate personnel and follows the chain of command

Upward Communication
Used to communicate ideas, requests and opinions to supervisors

Lateral Communication
Occurs among peers and may involve discussion and meetings to solve problems and/or accomplish tasks

grapevine, where the most uninhibited communications take place among employees. It is not realistic, or even wise, to attempt to close off the grapevine and prevent communications among employees. However, a manager should be aware that the grapevine can lead to distortion of messages, communication of rumors, and other problems.

How do you prevent problems on the grapevine? The best answer is to communicate openly with all employees. For example, if employees have reason to guess that a change is coming—such as a layoff or a major system overhaul—give them information. When you don't, they guess. Guesses become rumors. Anxiety and ill feelings can snowball. What if you don't have all the information yourself? Then, simply be honest. Tell employees what you know, what you don't know, and when you expect to know more.

Keep in mind that effective change involves:

* Planning and communication
* Staff participation and communication
* Implementation and oh yeah, communication

In Chapter 15, key points of conducting a meeting and public speaking as a means of communicating were discussed. Written memos and emails are also a common daily form of communication for the Certified Dietary Manager.

Effective Writing

Whether you enjoy it or not, count on the periodic need to express yourself in writing. Written communications may include business correspondence, memos, reports, policies and procedures, email, posted notices, and more. When writing, always consider the reader. The message will be understood according to the receiver's perceptions and the ability to understand your choice of words.

Compared with interpersonal communication, formal writing can be challenging. You cannot "see" how the receiver is reacting to the information you are presenting. In a business environment, many feel a need to use obscure words, long sentences, and other techniques to impress the reader.

In fact, the most effective business communication sounds like a professional speaking to you face-to-face. Try to keep it clear without over-simplifying the information (dumbing-down) or assuming knowledge the receiver may not have. There are a few cautions, though.

Written business communications should do a few things that are not always necessary in casual conversation, such as:

* Follow grammatical rules.
* Use complete sentences.
* Use proper terminology to describe things, rather than slang.
* Present ideas in a logically organized flow.

Figure 16.3 lists some tips for effective writing in a business environment.

Putting It Into Practice

3. The following are types of communication in the workplace. Label them as to the correct flow of communication (upward, downward, lateral):

* Policy statement posted on the bulletin board
* Suggestion box
* E-mail to other department heads
* Loudspeaker announcements
* Focus group
* Inservice

Figure 16.3 Effective Writing Tips

Be concise	**Ineffective:** It is necessary to implement a unique and innovative mechanism for acquiring and obtaining required supplies and accoutrements through the established food procurement system.
	Improved: We would like to try a new method of purchasing.
Use business terminology	**Ineffective:** Let's rock.
	Improved: We are eager to proceed.
Use "I" and "me" correctly	**Ineffective:** You and me need to discuss this.
	Improved: You and I need to discuss this.
	Ineffective: Perhaps she could share her thoughts with you and I.
	Improved: Perhaps she could share her thoughts with you and me.
Avoid run-on sentences	**Ineffective:** We will evaluate this, you and I can meet next week.
	Improved: We will evaluate this. Then, let's meet next week.
Be specific	**Ineffective:** Certain individuals have raised a number of complaints regarding temperature of foods.
	Improved: Last week, Mrs. Wiley said her mashed potatoes were too cold. Mr. Jones did too.
Address people directly	**Ineffective:** One can see from this report that the foodservice department has improved client satisfaction scores.
	Improved: As you can see, the foodservice department has improved client satisfaction scores.
Use simple words when possible	**Ineffective:** We would like to utilize the budgetary monies.
	Improved: We would like to use budget funds.

As you organize written documents, make sure the content flows in a logical manner. Present facts a reader needs to know before drawing a conclusion. Present steps in sequence. Provide a brief introduction at the beginning of a document and a summary at the end. For a long document, include page numbers and a table of contents for easier reference. Use simple charts, graphs, or other appropriate images to illustrate information that is difficult to comprehend through words alone.

After writing anything, take the time to read it through and proof-read carefully. This is especially true of email. It helps to leave the "to" line blank until you have proofed the entire message. Check for errors in spelling, punctuation, or grammar—all of which can create interference in communication. Check whether the sentences are concise and clear. Check whether any thoughts may be vague or easily misunderstood. Often, it is easiest to proofread by reading a piece out loud exactly as it is written – this is where you will hear what you intended to say.

Finally, if the content of a communication is likely to startle, surprise, or upset the receiver, consider a face-to-face conversation instead. For example, you would not use email to tell your supervisor that you have accepted a new job, or that the department is in crisis. If necessary, follow up with written communication.

Writing a Memo

A memo is a specific type of written business communication that is used frequently. A memo is a brief document that provides a message about new information, such as a new procedure, or requests a reader to take an action, such as approving a plan or attending a meeting. To make a memo effective, direct it specifically to the reader(s), and spell out the action being requested.

A memo has five parts: a heading, an opening, a background, a brief discussion, and a summary. The heading includes these components: **to**, **from**, **date** and **subject**. The opening should state the purpose of the memo. The background gives the context of the information or request. A simple discussion section provides more detail about the plan or request. The summary is a short statement that ties in with the opening, reminding the reader what should happen next. Figure 16.4 is an example of a memo in which these parts are labeled.

Figure 16.4 Memo Example

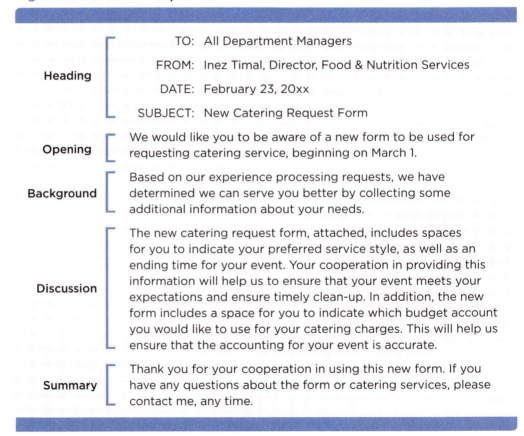

Heading	TO: All Department Managers
	FROM: Inez Timal, Director, Food & Nutrition Services
	DATE: February 23, 20xx
	SUBJECT: New Catering Request Form

Opening
We would like you to be aware of a new form to be used for requesting catering service, beginning on March 1.

Background
Based on our experience processing requests, we have determined we can serve you better by collecting some additional information about your needs.

Discussion
The new catering request form, attached, includes spaces for you to indicate your preferred service style, as well as an ending time for your event. Your cooperation in providing this information will help us to ensure that your event meets your expectations and ensure timely clean-up. In addition, the new form includes a space for you to indicate which budget account you would like to use for your catering charges. This will help us ensure that the accounting for your event is accurate.

Summary
Thank you for your cooperation in using this new form. If you have any questions about the form or catering services, please contact me, any time.

As a business communication, a memo should be well organized and concise. It should always leave the reader with a definite understanding of what to do next. As a Certified Dietary Manager, do not use a memo to substitute for face-to-face communications or to make major requests that may require meetings, presentations, and discussion. However, use it to relate straightforward information. A typical memo does not exceed one or two pages. Sometimes, an attachment may be needed.

E-mail Etiquette

Much of today's business communication occurs through email. Consider these simple rules if you communicate through email.

- It is no different than writing a letter so use a greeting, a closing and a signature line with contact information.
- Always reread the email (out loud) before you send it to make sure there are no errors and the tone of the email is friendly and professional.
- Do not use emoticons and refrain from using "texting" abbreviations.
- Refrain from sending an email if you are angry; communicate in person.
- Respond in a timely manner or at least let the person know when you can respond. Timely is generally within 24 hours.

Summary

Change is an ongoing process in today's business world. Some have said that the concept of managing change is unnecessary when you just simply accept change as a normal function of business. Identifying the opportunity for change, and developing an action plan, is part of the quality process and culture in the workplace. Effective communication, up and down the reporting structure, will improve both the action plan and the likelihood of success. Through attention to communication basics, a Certified Dietary Manager can implement required changes in the department.

Safe Food Handling: Personnel

Overview and Objectives

Every employer has a responsibility to protect the safety and well-being of employees and clients. Safety considerations when organizing work flow and the use of equipment is essential in the riskmanagement of employees; it can also have financial and regulatory ramifications. In this chapter, we examine the role of the Certified Dietary Manager in risk management, ensuring safety in the use of equipment, and work flow. After completing this chapter, you should be able to:

✓ Instruct employees in safety and sanitation

✓ Enforce employee compliance with safety and sanitation regulations

✓ Identify federal safety laws/regulations

✓ Write cleaning procedures for utensils, equipment, and work areas

✓ Evaluate equipment in terms of maintenance needs and costs

✓ Interpret safety data sheets

✓ Inspect all areas of department for sanitary conditions

Dining Services Managers

The Food Code provides special definitions for Certified Dietary Managers. The **permit holder** is the entity that is legally responsible for the operation of the food facility and possesses the valid permit to operate the facility. For example, a permit holder might be a school system or a nursing facility. A manager who oversees the dining services operation is typically defined as the **person in charge**. More specifically, the person in charge is accountable for developing, carrying out, and enforcing procedures aimed at preventing food-borne illness. The Certified Dietary Manager may be the person in charge or may designate a staff member to ensure that a person in charge should be on the premises at all times during operations.

Key changes to the 2013 Food Code include requiring that dining services operations have a certified food protection manager on staff.

2-102.12 Certified Food Protection Manager

(A) At least one *employee* that has supervisory and management responsibility and the authority to direct and control *food* preparation and service shall be a certified *food* protection manager who has shown proficiency of required information through passing a tcst that is part of an *accredited program*.

Glossary

Permit Holder
The entity that is legally responsible for the operation of the food facility such as the hospital, nursing facility, school district, or restaurant owner

Person in Charge
The manager of the dining services operation who is responsible for developing, carrying out and enforcing procedures aimed at preventing foodborne illness

The responsibilities of the person in charge are many and equally important. They must demonstrate knowledge in:

- Preventing foodborne illness
- HACCP and critical control points
- The impact of personal hygiene on food safety
- Symptoms of foodborne illness
- Time and temperature control standards for cooking PHF/TCS foods
- The hazards of consuming undercooked meat, poultry, eggs, and fish
- Temperatures for hot holding, storing, cooling, and reheating PHF/TCS food
- Prevention of cross-contamination
- Standards for avoiding bare hand contact with food
- Adequate and effective handwashing
- Cleaning and sanitation
- Food-safe equipment
- Safe water
- Safe use of chemicals
- Employee health restrictions/exclusions
- Food allergy awareness
- Proper training of employees in food safety, including food allergy awareness.

In addition to demonstrating this knowledge, the person in charge has additional duties to ensure food safety. Read Section 2.1 in the most current FDA Food Code, which has been included in the *Supplemental Textbook Material—Foodservice*. The designated person in charge works, work with the staff and administration to develop policies and procedures for carrying out these duties.

Dining Services Staff

Dining services staff must observe personal hygiene practices to reduce the likelihood of contaminating food and must also observe safe work practices. It is the responsibility of the Certified Dietary Manager to develop and implement policies for dining services employee hygiene. It is the obligation of every dining services employee to observe standards of personal hygiene in order to ensure food safety. Personal hygiene and handwashing are critical controls for food safety. Many foodborne illnesses travel from people to food and then to clients, who become ill. Dining services employees should observe the following standards for personal hygiene:

- Bathe daily.
- Cover mouth when coughing or sneezing and then wash hands.
- Do not eat, drink, or use tobacco or gum while preparing food. Wash hands after doing these activities on break.
- Restrain and cover hair.
- Frequently wash hands following established procedures.

Lavatory Facilities and Supplies

Dining services personnel must be provided with a sink specifically intended for washing hands. It is not acceptable to wash hands in sinks intended for food preparation or to perform food preparation activities in hand sinks. At least one sink must be provided and more may be required to ensure convenient use by employees. The sinks should be easily accessible to employees. Handwashing sinks should be available in food preparation, dining services,and warewashing areas, as well as in restrooms. A handwashing lavatory must provide water at a temperature of at least 100°F through a mixing valve or faucet. Some models of hand sinks are equipped with infrared sensors or flow control devices, which eliminate the need for staff to touch sink faucets (see Figure 17.1).

Figure 17.1 **Hand Sink With Infrared Sensor**

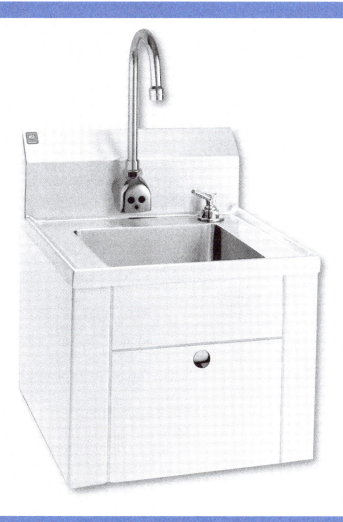

The lavatory must be supplied with a hand cleanser and materials for hand drying such as individual, disposable towels, a heated-air drying device, or a non-heated pressurized air device. When food exposure is limited and handwashing lavatories are not conveniently available—such as in some mobile or temporary food operations or at some vending machine locations—employees may use chemically treated towelettes for handwashing. Towelettes are not as effective as handwashing and are not accepted by all local food codes.

Handwashing and Hand Care

Preparing and serving foods with hands is a common way to transfer pathogens and other food hazards from people to food. Handwashing is the most important step that all dining services employees can take to protect food. All employees should be trained in proper handwashing procedures. To reinforce this important practice, post reminder signs at

Putting It Into Practice

1. Your cook is breading chicken for the evening meal when the dining services staff member requests more rolls for the lunch meal. The cook picks up a basket of Rolls and takes it to the staff member and then she returns to breading the chicken. Is this a concern? Why or why not?

every handwashing sink employees might use. The most effective way to determine employee compliance with handwashing standards is to observe on-the-job practices. Hands must be kept clean before, during, and after preparing foods. According to the FDA Food Code, hands should be washed:

- After touching bare human body parts.
- After using the restroom.
- After coughing, sneezing, using a tissue, using tobacco, eating, or drinking.
- After handling soiled equipment or utensils.
- Before food preparation.
- During food preparation, as often as necessary to remove soil and avoid cross-contamination.
- When switching between raw foods and ready-to-eat foods.
- After engaging in any activity that might contaminate hands.

Dining services personnel must clean their hands, wrists, forearms, and other exposed parts of their body with a cleaning compound (antibacterial soap is recommended). As shown in Figure 17.2, proper handwashing requires application of the cleaning compound and vigorously rubbing the hands for at least 10-15 seconds, followed by a rinse with potable water.

Ensuring the cleanliness of areas underneath fingernails and in between fingers is particularly important. A nail brush may be used to clean under fingernails, particularly after handling raw food which may be trapped under the fingernails, or after using the restroom. Recommendations about whether to use nail brushes vary. If used, sanitize it on a regular basis.

Dining services staff must keep their fingernails trimmed, filed, and maintained so the edges and surfaces are cleanable and not rough. Fingernail polish or artificial nails are not allowed for employees working with food, unless covered by a sanitary, disposable glove in good condition.

Hand Antiseptics

Hand antiseptics (previously called hand sanitizers) are permitted, according to the FDA Food Code. A hand antiseptic solution should be either approved by the FDA or contain antimicrobial ingredients listed by the FDA. A hand antiseptic may be used only after an employee has washed hands, following established procedure. In other words, *using a hand antiseptic is not a substitute for washing hands*. It is only a supplementary option.

Jewelry

Dining services staff should limit hand and arm jewelry to one single band ring. Jewelry can trap microorganisms and is difficult to keep clean.

The Food Code clarifies use of medical alert jewelry, such as a band indicating a drug allergy or medical condition. Medical information jewelry is not an exception to the "no-jewelry" guideline. It is not permitted on hands or arms. The Food Code guidance explains that an employee can wear an alert bracelet as a necklace or on the ankle.

Glossary

Hand Antiseptic
A solution with a FDA approved drug or antimicrobial ingredients used after an employee has washed hands

Figure 17.2 Handwashing Procedures

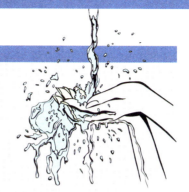

STEP 1
Rinse under clean, running warm water.

STEP 2
Apply an amount of cleaning compund recommended by the cleaning compound manufacturer.

STEP 3
Rub together vigorously for at least 10-15 seconds while:
a. Paying particular attention to removing soil from underneath the fingernails during the cleaning procedure.
b. Creating friction on the surfaces of the hands and arms or surrogate prosthetic devices for hands and arms, fingertips, and areas between the fingers.

STEP 4
If using antimicrobial soap, 15 seconds of vigorous washing is required.

STEP 5
Thoroughly rinse under clean, running, warm water.

STEP 6 MEAS-URA-BLE
Immediately follow the cleaning procedure with a thorough drying method. Such methods include individual, disposable towels, a continuous towel system that supplies the user with a clean towel; or a heated-air device.

NOTE: To avoid re-contaminating hands, food employees may use disposable clean towels or similar clean barriers when touching surfaces such as manually operated faucet handles or the handle of a restroom door.

Adapted from 2013 FDA Food Code, sections 2-301.12 to 2-301.16

Disposable Glove Usage

The use of disposable gloves/single-use gloves in dining services operations is increasingly common. It is important to note that wearing gloves is not a substitute for appropriate, effective, thorough and frequent handwashing. Single-use gloves should be stored and dispensed in a manner that prevents contamination. Gloves should be intact and free of tears or other imperfections. Before putting on a glove, wash hands, following the established procedure. Replace gloves at least hourly; when changing food preparation tasks; or after sneezing, coughing, touching hair, face, or non-disinfected surfaces. Skin lesions, cuts on the hands, wrists, or exposed portions of the arm must be covered with an impermeable cover such as a finger cot or stall. If on the hands or wrists, a disposable glove should be worn over the impermeable cover.

Putting It Into Practice

2. You observe a dining services staff member replacing ready-to-eat items in the cafeteria. She is wearing disposable gloves. At that moment, a client is waiting at the cash register. Your cook quickly removes her gloves, wipes her hands and helps the client at the cash register. She then returns to replacing the ready-to-eat items after putting on new gloves. Is this a concern? Why or why not?

Clothing

Dining services employees should always wear clean clothing to prevent contamination of food, equipment, utensils, and linens. If employees are expected to change into a uniform after reporting to work, provide a suitable changing area separate from food preparation and storage areas. Employees should not bring personal items such as coats, hats, and purses into food preparation areas.

To further minimize the risk of foodborne illness transmission from employees or employee work habits, protective clothing should be worn to keep body parts from coming in contact with exposed foods. Hair restraints and beard restraints should be worn to reduce contact with human hair. Aprons and disposable gloves may also be used to reduce the transfer of microorganisms to an exposed food. Aprons and disposable gloves should be changed frequently.

Avoid Hand Contact With Food

In addition to handwashing, the risk of foodborne illness can be reduced by eliminating direct contact of hands with ready-to-eat food. Except when washing fruits and vegetables, dining services employees should not contact exposed, ready-to-eat food with their bare hands. Instead, they should use suitable utensils such as deli tissue, spatulas, tongs, single-use gloves, or dispensing equipment. Dining services personnel should also minimize bare hand and arm contact with exposed food that is not in a ready-to-eat form.

Tasting Food

Dining services personnel should be trained in proper tasting techniques. To prevent contamination, employees should not taste food while standing over it. A dining services employee may not use a utensil more than once to taste food that is to be sold or served. A utensil used to taste food cannot be returned to the pot. It is a good idea to have a container of tasting spoons/forks close to the food prep area to avoid using the prep utensil for tasting.

Handling Sanitary Surfaces

Employees should avoid touching the eating ends of the utensils, the tops or insides of drinking glasses, the surfaces of plates, or any other utensil or serviceware in a manner that might allow hands to contaminate the item.

Employee Health

Dining services personnel who are suffering from illnesses that can be transmitted through food can present a major risk for any dining services operation. For example, many pathogens travel through what is called a fecal-oral route. This means an employee who does not wash hands after using the restroom may have pathogens on the hands and can later contaminate food with these pathogens. Clients who consume the food may become ill. In addition, some employees may themselves be ill with a pathogen that can be foodborne such as Norovirus or Hepatitis A. Those employees carry the pathogens on their hands and can contaminate food. Key changes to the Food Code (Section 2-501) stipulate that "food establishments have a plan for responding to and properly cleaning up after an employee or client becomes physically ill in areas where food is prepared, stored, or served."

Furthermore, some people can carry pathogens without actually having symptoms. Certain foodborne illnesses are primarily the result of **carrier**s contaminating food. A carrier may "carry" and transmit pathogens without having any symptoms of illness. For

Glossary

Carrier
A person who "carries" and may transmit a disease without symptoms of the illness

example, a person with Hepatitis A may pass along the virus for weeks before actually becoming ill. Some people carry Salmonella bacteria and foodborne illness outbreaks have been traced to this problem.

Staphylococcus aureus and other bacteria may thrive on skin and in infected wounds. These bacteria can cause foodborne illness. By scratching an infected cut or pimple and then touching food, employees can pass the bacteria to food, where it can multiply to numbers sufficient to produce illness in a person consuming the food. Also, pus in an infected wound can ooze into food or onto food contact surfaces and contaminate food.

With these risks in mind, a Certified Dietary Manager must take special precautions to identify any employee who may be capable of transmitting foodborne pathogens at any point in time and to limit the possibility of transmitting illness. The Food Code describes two categories of employees for whom the manager must enforce special policies to prevent transmission of illness: dining services employees and conditional employees.

A **dining services employee** is a person working with food, food equipment, utensils and/or food-contact surfaces.

A **conditional employee** is one who has been offered a job in dining services. The offer is considered conditional on responses to medical questions, examination, or health screening. The objective of health screening is to identify anyone who may have an illness that can be transmitted through food. According to the FDA Food Code, a conditional employee who reports specific symptoms that could indicate foodborne illness, a current diagnosis of a foodborne illness, past foodborne illness, or a history of exposure to foodborne pathogens must meet certain criteria before becoming employed. Generally, they must be cleared by a qualified medical practitioner, in writing. A conditional employee who cannot meet the criteria should not be hired. Figure 17.3 is a sample interview form that can be used for screening a conditional employee.

During health screening, a Certified Dietary Manager needs to be aware of conditional employees' rights. The Equal Employment Opportunity Commission (EEOC) offers advice about how to conduct screening and manage other health-related personnel activities without violating rights specified under Title I of the Americans with Disabilities Act (ADA). See Figure 17.4.

Reportable Health Information

The Food Code lists a number of health conditions that food employees must report to the person in charge. Each employee bears responsibility for reporting information that may have an impact on food safety. The FDA Food Code draws special attention to five pathogens that may be transmitted by dining services employees: Norovirus, Shigella, hepatitis A, Salmonella Typhi, and Shiga toxin-producing E. coli (STEC). An employee diagnosed with one of these illnesses should report this to the person in charge who is responsible for taking action to prevent disease transmission.

In addition, the Food Code says that even if employees have only symptoms—such as diarrhea, fever, vomiting, jaundice (yellowing of the skin, which can be a symptom of Hepatitis), sore throat with fever, or an infected wound that is open, draining, and/or contains pus—this is cause for action. Each of these may potentially indicate that a foodborne pathogen is at play. Thus, each of these must be reported to the person in charge.

As a Certified Dietary Manager, what should you do when an employee reports a diagnosis or symptom? For some symptoms or diagnoses, the answer depends upon what

Glossary

Dining Services Employee Employee
Per the FDA Food Code: An individual working with unpackaged food, food equipment, utensils, or food contact surfaces

Conditional Employee
Per the FDA Food Code: A potential foodservice employee to whom a job offer is made conditional on responses to subsequent medical questions or examination

type of client group being served. If it is a highly susceptible population, such as nursing home clients, young children, or hospitalized patients with compromised immune systems, action must be taken to protect clients. This is to excludes the employee (e.g., except for an infected wound). See Figure 17.5 for a summary of requirements for symptomatic employees.

Exclude simply means to prohibit employees from coming to work. A medical clearance is required for the employee to return to work. Also, note that if an employee is actually diagnosed with a foodborne illness, they should be excluded and notify the health department. Guidelines offered by the Food Code may be considered minimum standards, based on commonly-cited culprits in actual foodborne illness outbreaks. Local authorities and/or the facility's health policy may dictate further restrictions.

If the employee has an infected wound, the employee can come to work but must cover the wound with an impermeable cover.

Guidelines for responding to symptoms or illness are more liberal if serving a general, healthy population. Rather than exclude employees, restrict employees who have Norovirus with no symptoms, STEC with no symptoms, or sore throat with fever, for example. **Restrict** means to limit an employee's activities, so that there is no risk of transmitting foodborne illness. For example, a restricted employee should not work with food, clean equipment, clean dishes or utensils, or clean linens. An infected cut or wound must be bandaged and covered with an impermeable cover. If the wound is on the hand or wrist, this must also be covered with a clean, disposable glove.

The Food Code also addresses the concern of an employee who suffers sneezing, coughing, or a runny nose. Any employee who has a discharge from eyes, nose, or mouth should not work with exposed food, clean equipment, utensils, or linens; they also should not unwrap single serve items. This means that if an employee has a common cold, the manager may need to restrict the employee.

Viruses cannot multiply in food but can be transmitted through food. Examples of such viruses include Hepatitis A and Norovirus. Other viruses, such as the HIV virus, are very fragile outside of the human body and cannot be transmitted through food. Dining services employees with HIV or AIDS should not be excluded unless they are suffering from another illness or infectious disease.

For questions regarding who to restrict or not, review the current Food Code or contact local regulatory authority.

Health Policies and Documentation

One of the stipulations introduced in the 2005 Food Code is the concept of an employee health reporting agreement. The Food Code requires that both conditional and regular food employees acknowledge, in writing, their responsibility for reporting certain symptoms, diagnoses, and health conditions to the Certified Dietary Manager. Employees must also acknowledge their responsibility to comply with restriction or exclusion, when applicable. At the same time, the person in charge must acknowledge in writing, the responsibilities outlined in the Food Code for managing employee health. This means, that when the facility offers a dining services job to someone, they should ask that person to sign a reporting agreement. The FDA provides a sample form (see Figure 17.3).

Glossary

Exclude
Prohibit employees from coming to work

Restrict
To limit an employee's activities so there is no risk of transmitting foodborne illness (such as re-assign the employee to a non-food related position)

Putting It Into Practice

3. It is a hectic day in the dining services department because two employees are off sick. Your cook explains that he isn't feeling well and has visited the bathroom several times in the past two hours. What should you do?

Figure 17.3 Health Screening Sample Questionnaire

FORM 1-A: Conditional Employee and Food Employee Interview

Preventing Transmission of Diseases through Food by infected Food Employees or Conditional Employees with Emphasis on illness due to Norovirus, Salmonella Typhi, Shigella spp., Enterohemorrhagic (EHEC) or Shiga toxin-producing Escherichia coli (STEC), or Hepatitis A Virus

The purpose of this interview is to inform conditional employees and food employees to advise the person in charge of past and current conditions described so that the person in charge can take appropriate steps to preclude the transmission of foodborne illness.

Conditional employee name *(print)*_____

Food employee name *(print)* _____

Address _____

Telephone *(Daytime)* _____ *(Evening)* _____

Are you suffering from any of the following symptoms? (Check one)	YES	NO	If YES, Date of Onset
Diarrhea			
Vomiting			
Jaundice			
Sore Throat with Fever			
OR			
Infected cut or wound that is open and draining, or lesions containing pus on the hand, wrist, an exposed body part, or other body part and the cut, wound, or lesion not properly covered *(Examples: boils and infected wounds, however small)*			

In the Past:	YES	NO	
1. Have you ever been diagnosed as being ill with typhoid fever *(Salmonella Typhi)*. If YES, what was the date of the diagnosis?			
2. If within the past 3 months, did you take antibiotics for S. Typhi? 　> If YES, how many days did you take antibiotics?			
3. If you took antibiotics, did you finish the prescription?			

History of Exposure:	YES	NO	
1. Have you been suspected of causing or have you been exposed to a confirmed foodborne disease outbreak recently? If YES, date of outbreak:			

a. If YES, what was the cause of the illness and did it meet the following criteria:

Cause: **Date of Illness Outbreak**

  i.　Norovirus *(last exposure within the past 48 hours)*

  ii.　E. coli O157:H7 infection *(last exposure within the past 3 days)*

  iii. Hepatitis A virus *(last exposure within the past 30 days)*

  iv. Typhoid fever *(last exposure within the past 14 days)*

  v. Shigellosis *(last exposure within the past 3 days)*

Figure 17.3 **Health Screening Sample Questionnaire** *Continued...*

	YES	NO
b. If YES, did you:		
i. Consume food implicated in the outbreak?		
ii. Work in a food establishment that was the source of the outbreak?		
iii. Consume food at an event that was prepared by person who is ill?		
	YES	**NO**
2. Did you recently attend an event or work in a setting, where there was a confirmed disease outbreak?		
If YES, what was the cause of the confirmed disease outbreak?		
a. Norovirus *(last exposure within the past 48 hours)*		
b. E. coli O157:H7 or other EHEC/STEC *(last exposure within the past 3 days)*		
c. Shigella spp. *(last exposure within the past 3 days)*		
d. S. Typhi *(last exposure within the past 14 days)*		
e. Hepatitis A virus *(last exposure within the past 30 days)*		
3. Do you live in the same household as a person diagnosed with Norovirus, Shigellosis, typhoid fever, Hepatitis A, or illness due to E. coli O157:H7 or other EHEC/STEC? If YES, Date of onset of illness:		
4. Do you have a household member attending or working in a setting where there is a confirmed disease outbreak of Norovirus, typhoid fever, Shigellosis, EHEC/STEC infection, or Hepatitis A? If YES, Date of onset of illness:		

Health Practitioner Information

Name _____

Address _____

Telephone *(Daytime)* _____ *(Evening)* _____

Signature of Conditional Employee _____ Date _____

Signature of Food Employee _____ Date _____

Signature of Permit Holder or Representative _____ Date _____

2013 FDA Food Code Annex 7

Figure 17.4 ADA and Employee Health

ADA regulations protect persons with disabilities. They prohibit discrimination in employment decisions. They also stipulate that an employer must make reasonable accommodations for an employee who has a disability. As defined by the law, a disability is a medical condition or disorder that substantially limits a person in doing basic life activities. According to EEOC guidance, an employee who suffers key symptoms that could indicate foodborne illness is NOT disabled. Because a foodborne illness is generally a short-term condition, the ADA regulations do not apply. In other words, a manager can restrict or exclude an employee, following Food Code guidance.

However, a foodborne illness occasionally leads to long-term disability, such as chronic liver failure following Hepatitis A. If this occurs, ADA regulations do apply. In this case, you must follow the steps outlined by the ADA. First, determine whether there is a reasonable accommodation that would eliminate the risk of the employee transmitting illness. If not, or if accommodations would create undue hardship on your business, you should next investigate reassignment to a non food-handling position. According to the EEOC guidance, even when the Food Code says to exclude the employee, you still have an obligation to follow a thinking process and plan of action outlined by the ADA. Furthermore, you must handle health issues carefully when making hiring decisions. Here are some do's and don'ts as spelled out by the EEOC:

DON'T	Ask a job candidate about health status (including foodborne illness) before making a conditional job offer.
DO	Ask about health status (including foodborne illness) after offering a job, as part of a procedure that you apply uniformity to everyone.)
DON'T	Hire an employee whose pre-employment medical review indicates the applicant is diagnosed with one of the five illnesses listed in the Food Code (Norovirus, Hepatitis A, Shigella, STEC, or Salmonella typhi). If the applicant has a disability because of this illness, the position is a food handling job, and there is no reasonable accommodation that prevents the risk, you have a right to cancel the job offer.
DO	Require current employees to report symptoms, diagnosis, or past history of illness with the five illnesses described above.
DON'T	Dismiss an employee who has a foodborne illness without following all the steps outlined by the ADA.
DO	Hold a job open for an excluded employee with a foodborne illness and a disability, unless this causes undue hardship for your organization.
DON'T	Allow an employee who does NOT qualify as having a disability to work in a foodservice establishment serving high-risk clients (e.g., a nursing home) if the employee has symptoms or diagnosis of foodborne illness.
DO	Require an employee who has qualifying symptoms or diagnosis to obtain a medical clearance to return to work before you lift a restriction or exclusion.
DON'T	Mention the name of an employee who has a symptom or diagnosis of foodborne illness to other employees or allow access to this information on your computer.
DO	Keep employee medical information confidential as part of your HIPAA compliance.
DON'T	Discriminate against an employee who has AIDS or an HIV positive diagnosis.
DO	Allow an employee who is HIV positive to work in a foodservice department, because HIV is not transmitted through food.
DON'T	Allow a service animal in food preparation areas.
DO	Allow an employee to use a service animal at work if this does not create significant risk or harm. (This is a reasonable accommodation.) Do require the employee to wash hands after touching the animal.
DON'T	Allow co-workers to harass an employee who has a disability.

Reprinted from Food Protection Connection, Dietary Manager Magazine, May 2005; updated to reflect 2005 Food Code standards. Reference: EEOC. How to Comply with the ADA: A Guide for Restaurants and Other Food Service Employers, 2005.

Figure 17.5 Summary of Requirements for Symptomatic Food Employees

SYMPTOM	EXCLUSION OR RESTRICTION		Removing Symptomatic Food Employees from Exclusion or Restriction	RA Approval Needed to Return to Work?
	Facilities Serving an HSP	Facilities Not Serving an HSP		
Vomiting	EXCLUDE 2-201.12(A)(1)	EXCLUDE 2-201.12(A)(1)	When the excluded food employee has been asymptomatic for at least 24 hours or provides medical documentation 2-201.13(A)(1). *Exceptions:* If diagnosed with Norovirus, Shigella spp., E. coli O157:H7 or other EHEC/STEC, HAV, or typhoid fever (S. Typhi) (see Tables 1b & 2).	No, if not diagnosed
Diarrhea	EXCLUDE 2-201.12(A)(1)	EXCLUDE 2-201.12(A)(1)	When the excluded food employee has been asymptomatic for at least 24 hours or provides medical documentation 2-201.13(A). *Exceptions:* If Diagnosed with Norovirus, E. coli O157:H7 or other EHEC/STEC, HAV, or S. Typhi (see Tables 1b & 2).	No, if not diagnosed
Jaundice	EXCLUDE 2-201.12(B)(1) if the onset occurred within the last 7 days	EXCLUDE 2-201.12(B)(1) if the onset occurred within the last 7 days	When approval is obtained from the RA 2-201.13 (B), and: • Food employee has been jaundiced for more than 7 calendar days 2-201.13(B)(1), *OR* • Food employee provides medical documentation 2-201.13(B)(3).	Yes
Sore Throat with Fever	EXCLUDE 2-201.12(G)(1)	RESTRICT 2-201.12(G)(2)	When food employee provides written medical documentation 201.13(G) (1)-(3).	No
Infected Wound or Pustular Boil	RESTRICT 2-201.12(H)	RESTRICT 2-201.12(H)	When the infected wound or boil is properly covered 2-201.13(H)(1)-(3).	No

NOTES:

- Food employees and condition employees shall report symptoms immediately to the person in charge.
- The person in charge shall prohibit a conditional employee who reports a listed symptom from becoming a food employee until meeting the criteria listed in section 2-201.13 of the Food Code, for reinstatement of a symptomatic food employee.

Key for Tables 1, 2, 3, and 4:

RA = Regulatory Authority

EHEC/STEC = Enterohemorrhagic, or Shiga toxin-producing Escherichia coli

HAV = Hepatitis A virus

HSP = Highly Susceptible Population

Source: FDA 2013 Food Code Annex 3 – Public Health Reasons/Administrative Guidance, pg. 347
Additional Exclusions and Restrictions can be located on pages 348-355

In addition, the Food Code stipulates that a dining services operation must have a written employee health policy. The policy must address, at a minimum, how the operation complies with the rules for reporting illness/symptoms and managing restrictions or exclusion.

In addition to employee wellness and contact with food products, is the management of the work environment. Maintaining a safe workplace, equipment andmanaging risk is a daily activity.

Risk Management

In a food production and dining services environment, risks confront both management and employees. Managing these risks can lead to lower employee injury rates and higher productivity. **Risks** are the possibility of injury. **Risk management** is the practice of managing the possibility of injury to employees and clients or harm to the organization.

A food production department presents many risks. There are open flames, steam-releasing machines, sharp knives, hot liquids, wet or slippery floors, and heavy objects to move. Employees often move fairly quickly in efforts to meet deadlines. An accident can result in harm to an employee or client. It can damage morale and image. It can also generate lost work days, and other costs to a facility. The U.S. Bureau of Labor Statistics reports that industries with high rates of employee injuries are foodservice, hospitals, and nursing homes.

What causes accidents? Initially, there is the presence of a risk, or situation that is potentially dangerous. Accidents when because someone is not paying attention. Examples of safety risks appear in Figure 17.6. As you can see from these examples, a risk sets the stage for an accident to occur. For example, a sharp knife sitting in a sink full of soapy water is an invitation for an employee to reach his hand in and get cut. Water accumulating on the floor raises the likelihood that someone walking there will slip.

Figure 17.6 Safety Risk Examples

- A pile of boxes obstructs a hallway where many employees need to walk or in aisle of storeroom or freezer.
- A ladder has a broken rung.
- A slicer has a frayed power cord.
- A puddle of water is accumulating on the floor.
- A pot has a loose handle.
- The hot water temperature is set too high.
- A loose tile sits awkwardly on the floor.
- A sharp knife is sitting in a sink full of soapy water.
- Knives in the kitchen have become dull, requiring an employee to use more pressure when using them.

- A cart used for transporting coffee has a loose wheel.
- The safety guard for a slicer or mixer is missing.
- An urn of hot coffee is balanced precariously on several trays on the counter.
- The safety valve on a steam-jacketed kettle is clogged.
- Broken mugs appear on the floor in the dishroom.
- Hallways or stairways are poorly lit.
- Heavy boxes are placed on higher shelving.

Glossary

Risk
The likelihood of a potential dangerous situation

Risk Management
Managing the possibility of dangerous situations to employees, clients, or the organization

Safety and Safety Inspections

Risks are situations a Certified Dietary Manager can pinpoint and correct through routine inspection. The most important thing to do is simply to notice the risk and take action. A tool for accomplishing this is a safety inspection checklist. Figure 17.7 shows an example of a safety inspection checklist. Others are available in other foodservice management textbooks, food safety textbooks, and even from insurance companies and fire departments. (Copies of these forms are available through the online *Supplemental Textbook Material— Foodservice*, in an editable format that you can customize to your facility.)

A self-audit such as this one helps organize everything when examining the operation for risk. A **structured inspection process** is one that has an established plan, time, forms and evaluation, and is essential to help monitor safety needs on a routine basis.

Who should perform a safety inspection? The task of conducting a safety audit may be rotated among small teams or work groups. Ideally, a Certified Dietary Manager delegates responsibility to groups of employees while retaining final responsibility and accountability. Involving all employees in safety audits builds awareness and commitment.

Frequency of a safety inspection may vary from one facility to the next but should follow an established schedule. Some perform weekly inspections and others do it bi-weekly. Regardless of the frequency, build a state of daily watchfulness for risk among all employees.

There may be a facility-wide safety team that visits each area of the workplace. This is a valuable resource and a new set of eyes reviewing the environment. If the facility is being inspected by a team, welcome the opportunity and learn all you can. Likewise, if someone in your department is invited to join a safety team, realize that this can be an excellent learning experience.

Any identified significant risks should be corrected on the spot or the piece of equipment taken out of service. When a safety inspection has been completed, carefully review the results. Some Certified Dietary Managers use a column on the inspection form itself to note corrections made with a date and time.

Some of the ongoing risk prevention activities in a food production dining services department involve equipment maintenance. When a steam release valve is clogged or an electrical cord is frayed, the Certified Dietary Manager needs to identify this and take quick action to place any dangerous equipment or location "off limits" and arrange for repairs. For detailed ideas about risks common in a foodservice operation and possible interventions, refer to Figure 17.8. Note that this is a great list of rules for any type of facility.

Employee Practices

Beyond risks, employee practices have a great influence on safety. Even in a safe environment an employee can make an error that results in injury. In fact, a majority of food production accidents occur when an employee simply is not paying attention or thinking about his or her action.

Here are some examples:

- A cook is feeling rushed to get the hot entrée out to the dining room. She grabs a pan without using a pot holder.

Figure 17.7 Safety Inspection Self-Audit

The following checklist covers both physical factors in the properly and work practices of personnel. During your inspection be as aware of unsafe acts as you are of unsafe conditions.

AREA	Y	N	COMMENTS
Receiving Area:			
Are floors in safe condition? Are they free from broken and defective floor tiles/boards? Are they covered with nonskid material?			
Are employees instructed in correct handling methods for various containers that are received?			
Are garbage cans washed daily in hot water?			
Are garbage cans always covered?			
Are garbage cans leak-proof and adequate in number and size?			
If garbage disposal area is adjacent to a part of the general receiving area, is there a program that keeps floors and/or dock areas clear of refuse?			
Is there a proper rack for holding garbage containers? Are garbage containers on dollies or other wheel units to elminate lifting by employees?			
Are adequate tools available for opening crates, barrels, cartons, etc. (hammer, cutter, cardboard carbon opener, and pliers)?			
Storage Area:			
Are shelves adequate to the bear weight of items stored? Are employees instructed to store heavy items on lower shelves and lighter materials above?			
Is a safe ladder provided for reaching high storage?			
Are cartons or other flammable materials stored at least two feet from light bulbs?			
Are there screen guards on the light bulbs?			
Is a fire extinguisher located at the door?			
Are employees carefully instructed in the use of detergents to prevent irritation or dermatitis, etc.?			
Do you have a program for disposal of broken glass or china?			
Where controls are in a passageway, are they recessed or guarded to prevent breakage or accidental starting?			
Are dish racks in safe condition (if wooden, free from broken slats and smoothly finished to elminate spintering: if metal, free of sharp corners that could cause cuts)? Are these racks kept off the floor to prevent tripping?			

Continued...

Figure 17.7 Safety Inspection Self-Audit

AREA	Y	N	COMMENTS
Serving Area			
Are steam tables cleared daily and maintained regularly? (Are gas or electric units checked regularly by a competent service person?)			
Are safety valves on equipment operative?			
Are serving counters and tables free of broken parts and wooden or metal slivers and burns?			
Do you have regular inspections of:			
• Glassware?			
• China?			
• Silverware?			
• Plastic Equipment?			
If anything breaks near the foodservice area, do you remove all food from service adjacent to the breakage?			
Are tray rails adequate to prevent trays from slipping or falling off at the end or corners?			
Are floors and/or ramps in good condition (covered with nonskid material, free from broken tile and defective floor tiles/boards)?			
Are these areas mopped at least daily and waxed with nonskid wax when necessary?			
Is there effective traffic flow so that clients do not collide while carrying trays or obtaining foods?			
Dining Areas:			
Are floors free from broken tile and defective floor boards?			
Are floors covered with nonskid wax?			
Are pictures securely fastened to walls?			
Are drapes, blinds, or curtains securely fastened?			
Are chairs free from splinters, metal burns, broken or loose parts?			
Are floors monitored for cleaning up spillage and other materials?			
Is special attention given to the floor adjacent to water, ice cream, or milk stations?			
Are vending machines properly grounded?			
If clients clear their own trays prior to returning to dishwasing area, are the floors kept clean of garbage, dropped silverware, and/or broken glass and china?			
If trays with soiled dishes are placed on conveyor units, are the edges guarded to keep clients from catching fingers or clothing?			
If dishes are removed from dining areas on portable racks or bus trucks, are these units in safe operating condition (for example, are all castors working, all shelves firm)?			

Figure 17.7 Safety Inspection Self-Audit

AREA	Y	N	COMMENTS
Soiled Dish Processing Area:			
Are floors reasonably free of excessive water and spillage?			
Are floor tiles/boards properly maintained and in safe condition (free from broken slats and worn areas that cause tripping)?			
Are all electrical units properly grounded?			
Are switches located to permit rapid shutdown in the event of emergency?			
Can employees easily reach switches?			
Pots and Pans Area:			
Are duckboards or floor tiles/boards in safe condition (free from broken slats and worn areas which could cause tripping)?			
Are employees properly instructed in use of correct amounts of detergent and/or other cleaning agents?			
Are adequate rubber gloves provided?			
Is there an adequate drainboard or other drying area so that employees do not have to pile pots and pans on the floor before and after washing them?			
Do drain plugs permit draining without employees placing hands in hot water?			
Walk-in Refrigerators and Freezers:			
Are floors in the units in good condition and covered with slip-proof material? Are they mopped at least once a week (and whenever spills occur)?			
If floor tiles/boards are used, are they in safe condition (free of broken slats and worn boards which could cause tripping)?			
Are portable and stationary storage racks in safe condition (free from broken or bent shelves and set on solid legs)?			
Are blower fans properly guarded?			
Is there a bypass device on the door to permit exit if an employee is locked in (or, is there an alarm bell)?			
Is adequate aisle space provided?			
Are employees properly instructed in placement of hands for movement of portable items to avoid hand injuries?			
Are heavy items stored on lower shelves and lighter items on higher shelves?			
Are shelves adequately spaced to prevent pinched hands?			
Is the refrigerant in the refrigerator nontoxic? (Check your refrigerator service manual.)			

Continued...

Figure 17.7 Safety Inspection Self-Audit

AREA	Y	N	COMMENTS
Food Preparation Area:			
Is electrical equipment properly grounded?			
Is electrical equipment inspected regularly by an electrician?			
Are electrical switches located so that they can be reached easily in the event of an emergency?			
Are the switches located so that employees do not have to lean on or against metal equipment when reaching for them?			
Are the floors regularly and adequately maintained (mopped at least daily and waxed with nonskid wax when necessary; are defective floor tiles/boards replaced when necessary)?			
Are employees instructed to immediately pick up or clean up all dropped items?			
Are employees properly instructed in the operation of all machines?			
Are employees forbidden to use equipment unless specifically trained in its use?			
Are machines properly grounded?			
Lighting and Exits:			
Is lighting adequate in the:			
• Receiving area?			
• Storage area?			
• Pots and pans area?			
• Walk-in refrigerators and freezers?			
• Food preparation area?			
• Cooking area?			
• Serving area?			
• Serving area?			
• Dining areas?			
• Soiled dish processing area?			
Do doors open into passagewasy where they could cause an accident? (List any such locations.)			
Are fire exists clearly market and passages kept clear of equipment and materials? (List any violations.)			

Figure 17.7 Safety Inspection Self-Audit

AREA	Y	N	COMMENTS
Stairways and Ramps:			
Are they adequately lighted?			
Are the angles of ramps set to provide maximum safety?			
If stairs are metal, wood composition, or marble, have abrasive materials been used to provide protection against slips and falls?			
Are pieces broken out of the casing or front edge of the steps?			
Are clean and securely fastened handrails available?			
If stairs are wide, has a center rail been provided?			
Ventilation			
Is ventilation adequate in the:			
• Receiving area?			
• Storage area?			
• Pots and pans area?			
• Walk-in refrigerators and freezers?			
• Food preparation area?			
• Cooking area?			
• Serving area?			
• Serving area?			
• Dining areas?			
• Soiled dish processing area?			
Other Safety Concerns:			
Do employees wear good shoes to protect their feet against injury from articles that are dropped or pushed against their feet?			
Is employee clothing free of parts that could get caught in mixers, cutters, grinders, or other equipment? Jewelry should be restricted to a single-band ring.			
Are fire extinguishers guarded so they will not be knocked from the wall?			
If doors are provided with a lock, is there an emergency bell or a bypass device that will permit exit from the room should the door be accidentally locked while an employee is in the room?			
Is there a pusher or tamper provided for use with the grinders?			
Are mixers in safe operating condition?			
Do mixers and other dangerous pieces of equipment have protective guards (e.g., blade guard and are they used)?			
Are the mixer beaters properly maintained to avoid injury from broken metal parts and foreign particles in food?			

- A cafeteria server uses a wet rag to wipe the counter, and then to handle a pan for the steam table.
- A pantry employee microwaves a covered tray of food, and then carelessly removes the cover with steam venting towards his hand.
- A cook decides to grab another box of cake mix from the top shelf of the storeroom. He stacks a couple of boxes and climbs up.
- A trayline employee had punched in late and begins running to the trayline.
- A supervisor rushes through the door to the cafeteria without checking to see if the doorway is clear.
- An employee in the dishroom tries to carry too many soiled dishes at a time.

Each of these—and many more—constitutes a situation in which human action is likely to cause an accident. An accident can affect the careless employee, co-workers, or clients, so each employee has a responsibility to everyone in the vicinity to work safely. Common accidents in food production and dining services operations include slips and falls, cuts, burns, and muscle strains. To manage the human factor, a Certified Dietary Manager can take the following actions:

Build awareness. While the Manager is aware of the risk of accidents in the operation, not everyone walking through the doors will automatically have the same awareness. In orientation for new employees and in ongoing training sessions, explain to employees that the food production operation does indeed have hazards, and that each person plays a role in ensuring safety. Make sure that part-time employees also receive this training.

Define expectations. Let every employee know that safety is a priority and ask employees to make safety their priority, too. When possible, share the facility's safety statistics with the work team on an ongoing basis. If they are not optimal, ask the team for a commitment to improve them. Build a goal with objectives and action plans to focus on workplace safety.

Build safety into procedures. As employees are trained to accomplish certain tasks and procedures are written, incorporate specific safety requirements. Explain what tools are required for safe work performance, such as a ladder for reaching high places, a dry pot holder for handling hot pots and pans, a blade guard for the slicer, and so forth. Include actions the employee must take during this procedure to provide protection. For example, a procedure for cleaning electrical equipment includes the basic step of unplugging the equipment first.

Make inspection everyone's job. Whether or not each employee is involved in formal safety inspections, tell employees what hazards to watch for. Ask them to identify and help correct (or report) safety risks.

Ask for caution. Remind employees to be alert, to focus on what they are doing, and to exercise care. Do not allow horseplay or other situations that could cause a safety hazard. Ask employees not to distract each other when they are involved in dangerous tasks. Ask staff to watch out for each other, and alert others when they see a dangerous or careless action in progress.

Include safety when purchasing equipment. Consider the ease of cleaning and maintaining equipment when preparing to purchase new items. Access to electrical supplies, space under the fire hoods, required cleaning procedures, and placement of knobs and doors all impact the ongoing cost of the equipment and the practical use on a daily basis.

Figure 17.8 **Food and Employee Safety Checklist—School Foodservice Department**

PERSONAL SAFETY

- Hands washed frequently and correctly (A handwashing sign is posted).
- Fingernails well trimmed and clean. No nail polish/ artificial nails. Inappropriate jewelry or watches not worn during production and service.
- Hand sinks used for washing hands only. Pot sinks are not used for washing hands.
- Gloves worn when handling ready-to-eat foods without utensils.
- Gloves are changed when task is interrupted and possible contamination can occur. (Example: While making sandwiches, more meat is needed. Employee touches box containing meat and then goes back to making sandwiches).
- Employees trained on lifting heavy objects.
- Employees are in clean and proper uniform, including proper shoes.
- Effective hair restraints are used properly.
- Employee sick reporting log posted.

EQUIPMENT-FOOD SAFETY

- Floors are clean and dry to prevent falls.
- Thermometers calibrated weekly and documented.
- Temperatures of received items documented properly on receiving log.
- Refrigeration equipment maintained at 41°F or below.
- NSF approved cutting boards in good condition and stored vertically for proper draining and quick drying.
- Knives are sharp and stored properly to prevent unnecessary cuts.
- All towels in use are stored in properly concentrated sanitizing solutions. Solution is changed as it becomes dirty.
- Equipment is clean and in good repair: Hot holding equipment, coolers/freezers, can openers (including blade), drawers and racks, exhaust hood and filters.
- Gas equipment is working properly and gas lines are checked regularly for proper operation.
- Can openers are clean and in good working order to prevent employee cuts.
- Steam equipment is in good working order and operated correctly to prevent employee injury.
- Proper handling of hot pans (pot holders) is available to prevent burns.
- Kitchen garbage containers are clean and not overflowing.
- There is good lighting in the department work areas.
- If used: Dishmachine is working properly, temperatures are within range and documented. minimum temperatures for heat sanitizing compartments is 180°F (165°F for stationary racks).
- If used: three-compartment sink is properly set up for warewashing; sanitizing sink is free of suds and temperature is a minimum of 171°F and documented.
- There are proper fire extinguishers available and all staff knows how to use them.

FOOD SAFETY

- FIFO (First In, First Out) method of inventory management.
- Documentation of 'keep' or 'discard' on every food item before meal starts.
- Initial and batch temperatures documents.
- Holding temperatures documented every two hours for 'keep' items.
- Documentation of cooling temperatures on all left-over 'keep' items, (At least two temperatures are taken).
- Food reheated to 165°F or above and documented on production sheet.
- Documentation is complete on production guide for items prepped, items sold, and items left. Numbers match and if not, reasoning is documented.
- All foods are properly wrapped/contained, labeled and dated. **No expired foods**.
- Food is stored a minimum of 6" off floor.
- Unwashed produce stored below ready-to-eat items (Example: Raw broccoli below lunch meat)
- No outside food stored in coolers or freezers.

(Continued...)

Figure 17.8 **Food and Employee Safety Checklist—School Foodservice Department** *(Continued...)*

CHEMICAL SAFETY

- Chemicals clearly identified.
- Chemicals are stored away from food and food-related supplies.

- Safety Sheets are available for all chemicals in the event of an unplanned exposure.
- Sanitizing solutions prepared in correct concentrations and documented.

Source: adapted from the MN School District 196 Food Safety Checklist, used with permission.

Provide specific safety training. At least one in-service session per year should focus on employee safety. Even tenured employees should undergo periodic review sessions to keep safe practices paramount in their minds. The more specific the training, the more effective it will be. In other words, name situations that employees need to notice. Name practices in each work area that need to be avoided. Name actions an employee can take to ensure safety.

Involve Worker's Compensation Insurance. They may offer to do an audit of the kitchen. Recommendations might include:

- Wear non-skid shoes or hand mitts.
- Use fire resistant aprons when using the deep fryer.
- Provide gloves and goggles in the chemical room.
- Use an approved step ladder.

Offer ongoing reinforcement. As you walk through food production areas from day to day, observe what employees are doing. If you see an unsafe practice tell the employee on the spot. If you see a safe practice praise the employee. Safety, like sanitation, is a way of life. If the Certified Dietary Manager makes that an expectation, the employee will remember its importance.

Fire Safety

The potential for fire exists in all food production and dining services operations. Possible causes of fire include: unemptied grease traps, grease build-up on exhaust vents, equipment malfunction, faulty or frayed electrical cords, improper storage of flammable items, ignition of trash because of cigarettes being improperly discarded, or food left unattended during preparation. Employees must be familiar with possible sources and kinds of fire, the locations of fire suppression equipment, and the actions to take in the event of a fire. As with all safety issues, a self-audit is a strong preventative tool. A sample fire safety audit appears in Figure 17.9. (Copies of this form are available in the *Supplemental Textbook Material—Foodservice*).

When responding to a fire, the first few minutes or even seconds are the most important. A fire requires three conditions: fuel, oxygen, and a heat source. The goal in extinguishing a fire is to remove one or more of the required elements. Fires are classified according to the material combusting, as shown in Figure 17.10. Extinguishing a Class A fire may require removing the heat or the fuel source while Class B and Class C fires generally require the removal of oxygen. Fire extinguishers have an identification system that indicates which type of fire they will extinguish.

Putting It Into Practice

4. A foodservice employee notices that every time he comes near the food mixer, he gets an electrical shock. What is the first step you should take for his safety?

Figure 17.9 Fire Safety Audit

DESCRIPTION	Y	N	CORRECTIVE ACTIONS
Hoods and vents are cleaned and free of grease.			
Power cords are not frayed or damaged.			
Broiler, salamander broiler, grill, fryer, and range top are clean and free of grease build up.			
Smoking is limited to designated areas.			
Cigarette butts are being disposed of properly.			
Combustible materials such as paper supplies, are properly stored—away from heat sources.			
Staff are following safe work practices, e.g., hot pads are kept away from heat sources.			
Preventative maintenance on electrical equipment is up-to-date.			
Fire extinguishers are charged and operable.			
Smoke detectors are functioning properly.			
Supplies are stored in a manner that will not interfere with the sprinkler systems.			
Annual training is conducted and documented.			

Figure 17.10 Fire Extinguishers

CLASS	TYPE OF FIRE	RECOMMENDED EXTINGUISHER	COMMENTS
Class A	Normal combustible materials	Foam, soda acid, pump tank (plain water), gas cartridge, multipurpose dry chemical	
Class B	Grease and oil	Foam, carbon dioxide, multipurpose dry chemical, ordinary dry chemical	Never use plain water or a water exstinguisher. This spreads the fire.
Class C	Electrical	Carbon dioxide, multipurpose dry chemical, ordinary dry chemical	Never use plain water or a water extinguisher. This can cause electrical shock.

The best all-purpose fire extinguisher for a food production operation is the multipurpose dry chemical type. Extinguishers should be inspected regularly to ensure that they are still properly charged.

Employees should receive annual training about fire safety. Training should include the emergency response procedures. Topics to address include:

- Fire prevention plan and responsibilities.
- Location, purpose, and use of devices in the department, such as heat detectors, smoke detectors, fire alarm box and fire extinguishers.
- How to respond to a fire.
- Sounding the alarm.

- How to use a fire extinguisher.
- How to protect yourself if clothing catches fire.
- Evacuation plan and exit routes.
- Procedures for protecting/evacuating clients in case of an emergency.

During training, employees should walk through the facility and locate signaling devices, and they should also walk the evacuation routes (not just view them on a map). It is also a good idea for employees to practice using a fire extinguisher in a controlled environment. In some facilities, a fire safety officer or team will conduct fire safety training.

A common failing in fire response is waiting to see whether the fire will become serious before calling for help. In fact, some employees may hesitate, trying to extinguish a fire on their own. It is always safer to call for help, even if it may not be needed. A Certified Dietary Manager should specifically direct employees to sound the alarm, even if the fire seems small. Training aids that can help employees remember some basic response techniques, are described in Figure 17.11.

Figure 17.11 Training Aids for Fire Response

RACE	PASS	STOP, DROP, AND ROLL
Steps for responding to a fire: 1. **Remove** everyone from danger 2. Turn on the **Alarm** 3. **Confine** the fire 4. **Extinguish** fire, if it can be done safely	Steps for using a fire extinguisher: 1. **Pull** the pin 2. **Aim** at the base of the fire 3. **Squeeze** trigger and keep extinguisher in an upright position 4. **Sweep** across the base of the fire	**Stop, Drop, and Roll** if your clothes catch on fire.

Heat Exhaustion

Another safety concern in a food production environment is heat stress. Any time employees find themselves in a hot, humid environment, everyone should be alert to symptoms of heat stress. Timely intervention can prevent serious problems. When a person becomes overheated, symptoms such as profuse sweating, muscle cramps, and skin rash may occur. These are early signs of heat exhaustion, a medical condition in which the body cannot cool itself quickly enough.

If left untreated, this condition can progress to symptoms of pale/clammy skin, weak and/or rapid pulse, low blood pressure, headache, intense thirst, weakness, dizziness, nausea and vomiting. Intervention is important to prevent heat exhaustion from leading to heat stroke. In heat stroke, a person may develop a high fever (>102°F), experience seizures, or become unconscious. This is a medical emergency. Interventions are described in Figure 17.12.

A Certified Dietary Manager needs to be aware of heat-related risks and prevent problems by using air conditioning and fans, encouraging employees to wear lightweight, loose-fitting clothing that conforms with the dress code, encouraging employees to take breaks if they are working in heat, and most importantly—encouraging employees to drink plenty of fluids when working in heat, even if they don't feel particularly thirsty. (Note: The FDA Food Code requires that employee beverages must be in a closed container.)

Putting It Into Practice

5. You are observing a new employee as she disassembles and cleans the slicer. She puts on safety gloves, disassembles the slicer, takes the portable pieces to the dishmachine and runs them through. What safety step has she overlooked?

Figure 17.12 Interventions for Heat Exhaustion

FIRST AID	DO NOT...	CALL 911 IF
• Have the person lie down in a cool place. Elevate the person's feet about 12 inches. • Apply cool, wet cloths (or cool water directly) to the person's skin and use a fan to lower body temperature. Place cold compresses on the person's neck, groin, and armpits. • If alert, give the person beverages to sip (such as Gatorade), or make a salted drink by adding a teaspoon of salt per quart of water. Give a half cup every 15 minutes. Cool water will do if salt beverages are not available. • For muscle cramps, give beverages as above and massage affected muscles gently, but firmly, until they relax.	• **DO NOT...** underestimate the seriousness of heat illness. • **DO NOT...** give the person medications that are used to treat fever (such as aspirin or acetaminophen). They will not help; and they may be harmful. • **DO NOT...** give the person salt tablets. • **DO NOT...** give the person liquids that contain caffeine. • **DO NOT...** use alcohol rubs on the person's skin. • **DO NOT...** give the person anything by mouth (not even salted drinks). If the person is vomiting or unconscious.	Call immediately for emergency medical assistance (911) if: • The person loses consciousness or experiences a change in alertness (e.g., confusion or seizures). • The person has a fever over 102˚F. • Other symptoms of heat stroke are present (like rapid pulse or rapid breathing). • The person's condition does not improve, or worsens despite treatment.

Source: U.S. National Library of Medicine

Government Regulations—OSHA

The Occupational Safety and Health Act of 1970 was passed to "assure safe and healthful working conditions" for today's employees. It mandates that employers provide a safe work environment for employees. In 1971, the Occupational Safety & Health Administration (OSHA) was established to enforce this regulation. In some cases, OSHA enforcement is handled by state agencies.

OSHA is involved in all aspects of employee safety on the job. It provides standards to ensure a safe work environment. OSHA requires the maintenance of safety records, the filing of safety reports, and strict adherence to good safety practices. Employers are required to maintain records of employee accidents and to report serious accidents and fatalities to OSHA.

OSHA periodically inspects businesses to monitor the level of compliance. If a business is found to be in violation of a health and safety regulation OSHA may issue a citation, fine the employer, or in some cases, order the employer to close the business until compliance is attained.

OSHA also provides training information for employers, employees, compliance tools, and references on its Web site at www.osha.gov. Specifically, OSHA standards relate to safe equipment, electrical safety, machine usage, fire safety, accident prevention, and sound ergonomic practices. Guidelines listed in the Safety Inspection and Fire Safety Audits provided in this chapter reflect many of the OSHA standards.

To comply with OSHA standards, a Certified Dietary Manager needs to review standards, monitor and correct hazards, report and document injuries, and provide ongoing training for employees. Employers are required to display a poster prepared by the Department of Labor summarizing the major provisions of the Occupational Safety and Health Act and telling employees how to file a complaint. The poster must be posted in a conspicuous place where employees and applicants for employment can see it.

Accident Investigation and Reporting

If an accident or injury occurs in the operation, it is the manager's responsibility to report the situation—and it is the law. It is likely the facility has an accident or incident reporting form that must completed. See Figure 17.13 for an OSHA sample reporting form. OSHA advises completing a reporting form within seven days of an incident and keeping it on file for five years after the incident.

The form is a tool to help gather all relevant information to support systematic information review. The manager and other reviewers need to look for causes and identify ways to prevent this type of accident from recurring. The employer (the facility) must maintain record-keeping for OSHA. It is important to realize that the form contains confidential employee information. Always handle the form in a confidential manner, sharing it only with those in the facility who need to review it in order to help manage safety concerns.

Putting It Into Practice

6. Your new employee just smashed her finger, resulting in an injury. What is the first action you should take?

Figure 17.13 Safe Food Handling: Personnel

OSHA's Form 301
Injury and Illness Incident Report

Attention: This form contains information relating to employee health and must be used in a manner that protects the confidentiality of employees to the extent possible while the information is being used for occupational safety and health purposes.

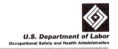
U.S. Department of Labor
Occupational Safety and Health Administration

Form approved OMB no. 1218-0176

This *Injury and Illness Incident Report* is one of the first forms you must fill out when a recordable work-related injury or illness has occurred. Together with the *Log of Work-Related Injuries and Illnesses* and the accompanying *Summary*, these forms help the employer and OSHA develop a picture of the extent and severity of work-related incidents.

Within 7 calendar days after you receive information that a recordable work-related injury or illness has occurred, you must fill out this form or an equivalent. Some state workers' compensation, insurance, or other reports may be acceptable substitutes. To be considered an equivalent form, any substitute must contain all the information asked for on this form.

According to Public Law 91-596 and 29 CFR 1904, OSHA's recordkeeping rule, you must keep this form on file for 5 years following the year to which it pertains.

If you need additional copies of this form, you may photocopy and use as many as you need.

Completed by _____

Title _____

Phone (____) ____-____   Date ___/___/___

Information about the employee

1) Full name _____

2) Street _____
   City _____ State _____ ZIP _____

3) Date of birth ___/___/___

4) Date hired ___/___/___

5) ☐ Male
   ☐ Female

Information about the physician or other health care professional

6) Name of physician or other health care professional _____

7) If treatment was given away from the worksite, where was it given?
   Facility _____
   Street _____
   City _____ State _____ ZIP _____

8) Was employee treated in an emergency room?
   ☐ Yes
   ☐ No

9) Was employee hospitalized overnight as an in-patient?
   ☐ Yes
   ☐ No

Information about the case

10) Case number from the *Log* _____ *(Transfer the case number from the Log after you record the case.)*

11) Date of injury or illness ___/___/___

12) Time employee began work _____ AM / PM

13) Time of event _____ AM / PM   ☐ Check if time cannot be determined

14) **What was the employee doing just before the incident occurred?** Describe the activity, as well as the tools, equipment, or material the employee was using. Be specific. *Examples:* "climbing a ladder while carrying roofing materials"; "spraying chlorine from hand sprayer"; "daily computer key-entry."

15) **What happened?** Tell us how the injury occurred. *Examples:* "When ladder slipped on wet floor, worker fell 20 feet"; "Worker was sprayed with chlorine when gasket broke during replacement"; "Worker developed soreness in wrist over time."

16) **What was the injury or illness?** Tell us the part of the body that was affected and how it was affected; be more specific than "hurt," "pain," or "sore." *Examples:* "strained back"; "chemical burn, hand"; "carpal tunnel syndrome."

17) **What object or substance directly harmed the employee?** *Examples:* "concrete floor"; "chlorine"; "radial arm saw." *If this question does not apply to the incident, leave it blank.*

18) **If the employee died, when did death occur?** Date of death ___/___/___

Public reporting burden for this collection of information is estimated to average 22 minutes per response, including time for reviewing instructions, searching existing data sources, gathering and maintaining the data needed, and completing and reviewing the collection of information. Persons are not required to respond to the collection of information unless it displays a current valid OMB control number. If you have any comments about this estimate or any other aspects of this data collection, including suggestions for reducing this burden, contact: US Department of Labor, OSHA Office of Statistical Analysis, Room N-3644, 200 Constitution Avenue, NW, Washington, DC 20210. Do not send the completed forms to this office.

OSHA defines a **work-related injury** or illness as one that results in days away from work, restricted work activity or job transfer, medical treatment (beyond first aid)—or in the most extreme case—loss of consciousness or death. In addition, a needlestick, hearing loss, or tuberculosis infection may require reporting under certain circumstances.

As a critical personnel policy, all employees need to report any accident or injury to a supervisor. If an accident occurs, the steps are to first take care of the employee, obtaining first aid or medical help as needed. Second, complete the accident reporting form. During this process include questions about how the accident occurred and how the accident could have been prevented. If the employee is in condition to discuss this, ask the employee to make suggestions. Finally, follow internal procedures for handling the emergency and completing the form.

As accidents are tabulated and analyzed in the facility (such as by a safety committee or safety officer), review the accident statistics and trends. Target areas that need improvement and use the steps outlined above to improve the safety record. Accident review should become an integral part of quality assurance activities.

Ergonomics in Foodservice

Another area of increasing concern today is the ergonomics of foodservice work. **Ergonomics** is the science of fitting the work environment to the employee. A key objective of ergonomic analysis and intervention is to prevent injury related to repetitive motions and related work factors.

Repetitive motion injuries are common in many industries including food production and dining services. Unlike an accident or sudden event, a repetitive motion injury occurs gradually, over time. It comes from the motions an employee makes, over and over.

Examples of repetitive motion include:

- Using a scoop over and over to portion applesauce into bowls.
- Bending down to lift boxes and placing them on a shelf over and over again.
- Reaching for a plate cover and turning to place it on a tray moving along the trayline over and over.
- Racking plates for the dishmachine again and again.

Examples of injuries that can result from repetitive motions include:

- Carpal tunnel syndrome. This is an inflammation of tendons in the wrist, causing numbness or tingling.
- Tendonitis. This is inflammation of a tendon, anywhere in the body. A tendon is connective tissue that attaches muscles to bones.

More broadly, experts are also looking at other factors that cause injury to muscles, nerves, tendons, ligaments, and joints. In addition to repetitive motion, factors such as awkward posture, force, and vibration can bring on injury. A broader term for injury related to work environment and tasks is **musculoskeletal disorders (MSDs)**. These are disorders affecting any part of the systems of skeleton, muscles, and tendons.

Today, safety experts in all industries focus a great deal on how the work environment can be designed to help prevent these injuries. First, ask employees to report and investigate symptoms that may indicate development of an MSD. These include:

- Painful joints
- Pain in wrists, shoulders, forearms, knees
- Pain, tingling or numbness in hands or feet
- Fingers or toes turning white
- Shooting or stabbing pains in arms or legs
- Back or neck pain
- Swelling or inflammation
- Stiffness
- Burning sensation

In addition, review any information that becomes available in the workplace that can help pinpoint MSDs that are occurring. Look carefully at workstations, at the posture of employees, and at movements. Look for opportunities to improve the work environment to minimize injury. Train employees how to use good body mechanics. Figure 17.14 lists ergonomic hazards in foodservice, along with solutions.

Figure 17.15 lists examples of training points and interventions in the food production and dining services workplace for preventing MSDs.

Some ergonomically sound techniques for food production and dining services employees are illustrated in Figure 17.16. Most of the recommendations are easy to implement but sometimes hard to remember.

Safety Data Sheets

Every department is required to maintain a notebook of **Safety Data Sheet (SDS)** for each "hazardous" chemical or product used within the food production or dining services areas. Until recently, manufacturers and vendors provided printed material that included information such as health risks, handling instructions, first aid and safe disposal of the products. While some manufactures still provide a SDS printed sheet, most have gone to an online availability of the information to be downloaded and printed by the department for access by employees in the event of an accident or spill.

Putting it Into Action

Training, policies and procedure, audits and inspections are all important pieces of the safe workplace. Ensuring access to appropriate and well maintained equipment helps protect staff from injuries. However, the most important component of safety on the job is the employee. The role of the manager is to develop a culture of safety, and when observing unsafe practices or equipment misuse address the issue. The entire department staff and clients benefit when you hold employees accountable for their compliance to safety regulations.

Glossary

Safety Data Sheet (SDS)
A printed information sheet for each "hazardous" chemical or product used within the department

Figure 17.14 Ergonomic Hazards and Solutions

Dietary employees must perform many lifting, reaching, and repetitive tasks as part of their job duties. Employee activities in this area, if occuring with sufficient duration, magnitude, and/or frequency, may create a musculoskeletal disorder (MSD).

Potential Hazard: Reaching/Lifting:

Are floors in safe condition? Are they free from broken and defective floor tiles/boards? Are they covered with nonskid material?

Possible Solutions

Assess worksites for ergonomic stressors and identify and address ways to decrease them such as:

- Provide height-adjustable workspaces appropriate for the task being performed, so that workers can keep elbows close to the body. For example, lower countertops, or use height adjustable countertops or stands, or provide work stands for employees.
- Redesign or reposition tasks to allow elbows to remain close to the body (e.g., turn boxes over on side to allow easier access).
- Avoid awkward postures (e.g., reposition work in front of worker so that he does not have to reach above or behind to get supplies).
- Use mechanical aids to reduce the need to lift. Use a spring device to automatically lift a load (e.g., use automatic plate and cup riser dispensers).
- Lighten a load that needs to be lifted or get help when lifting.
- Train workers to use proper lifting techniques.

Potential Hazard: Repetitive Motions

Rapid hand and wrist movements from frequent cutting, chopping, or scooping may lead to hand disorder,s such as tendonitis or carpal tunnel syndrome. Example: A kitchen worker scoops ingredients with a flexed wrist.

Possible Solutions

Assess worksites for ergonomic stressors and identify and address ways to decrease the,m such as:

- Rotate workers through repetitive tasks.
- Use mechanical aids for chopping, dicing, or mixing foods (e.g., food processors, mixers).
- Select and use properly designed tools. For example, kitchen scoops or kitchen knives that allow the wrist to remain straight.
- Maintain a neutral (handshake) wrist position.
- Restructure jobs to reduce repeated motions, forceful hand exertions, and prolonged bending.

Source: http://www.osha.gov/SLTC/etools/hospital/dietary/dietary.html

Figure 17.15 Musculoskeltal Disorders (MSDs): Training Points

- Use proper lifting techniques.

- Lighten the load; do not try to lift too much at once.

- Provide mechanical aids for lifting as warranted.

- Avoid reaching or working above shoulder height.

- Seek to avoid motions that require bending the wrists. Instead, try to keep wrists comfortably straight as much as possible.

- Teach safe postures: As often as possible, elbows should be at 90° angles, shoulders should be relaxed and low; and arms should be close to the body.

- Be sure standing workers are working at comfortable counter heights that do not require them to bend excessively.

- Avoid repeated twisting and arrange the work area to support this.

- For workers involved in prolonged repetitive movements, provide frequent breaks from the task.

- Rotate workers through jobs to reduce the repetition of movements on any one worker.

- As possible, minimize the amount of force or pressure a worker must use to accomplish a task.

- Look for utensils with ergonomically designed grips, especially for utensils that are used repeatedly. These are thicker than ordinary handles and may minimize strain.

- Ask a qualified expert, such as an occupational health nurse, to train employees to stretch safely to avoid injury.

- Talk with workers and ask them what steps they believe could make their jobs more comfortable.

Figure 17.16 **Ergonomically Sound Techniques**

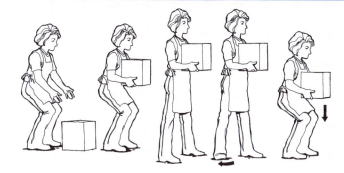

Lifting

1. Get close to the load. Bend at the hips and knees. Firmly grasp the load.

2. Keep head and shoulders erect. Lift, using legs for power.

3. Maintain a wide base.

4. To transfer the load, turn with your feet. Do not twist at the wrist.

5. Lower the load by bending at the hips and knees.

Straight Wrists

Avoid the situations illustrated below. Instead, keep wrists as straight as possible.

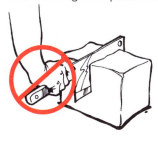

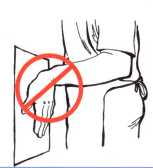

Holding a Can

Avoid picking up a large can with one hand.

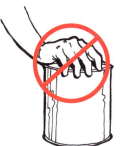

Instead, pick up a large can with two hands on the sides.

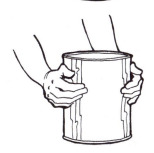

Source: The Grossbauer Group. Used with permission.

Safe Food Handling: Purchasing, Receiving and Storage

Overview and Objectives

Ensuring food safety depends on selecting a safe food vendor, obtaining food from approved sources, and carefully controlling the receiving, storage, and distribution practices. After completing this chapter, you should be able to:

✓ Identify appropriate grades and inspections for food

✓ Procure food and water from approved sources

✓ Verify the quality and quantity of food supplies and equipment received

✓ Check supplier invoices against facility purchasing order

✓ Recognize the hazards associated with types of food packaging

✓ Recognize the signs of contamination upon receipt and in storage

✓ Process rejections for unacceptable products

✓ Label, date and monitor food to ensure rotation

✓ Prevent environmental contamination of food

✓ Establish and maintain security procedures

Purchasing

For a food production operation purchasing is the first step in the flow of food. Food and water must be purchased from **approved sources**. An approved source is one that is inspected based on federal, state, or local laws and has appropriate HACCP procedures in place. CMS guideline F371 specifies that food be procured "from sources approved or considered satisfactory by Federal, State of local authorities". See the *Supplemental Textbook Material—Foodservice* for the most recent version of CMS F371. Vendor specifications should include:

- Quality standards such as grading and HACCP verification
- Wholesomeness indicators such as inspection.

In addition, delivery times and intervals may also be included in the vendor specifications. The manager needs to exercise careful planning when purchasing food. Purchasing excessive quantities of food can result in spoilage, increased costs, and an increased likelihood of foodborne illness. Perishable products—such as fresh produce, fresh seafood, fresh meats, eggs, and dairy products—should be purchased in a quantity that can be used within a short time period.

Glossary

Approved Source
A source that is inspected based on federal, state, or local laws and has appropriate HACCP procedures in place

Non-perishable foods such as canned and frozen foods can be purchased in quantities that allow for longer storage times, if desirable.

Inspection

All food shipped in interstate commerce (from one state to another) must meet the requirements of one or more federal laws. The U.S. Department of Agriculture (USDA) has established uniform standards for state and federally inspected meats, poultry, and eggs. **Inspection** is a mandatory process that addresses wholesomeness and safety of fresh meats, dairy products, and produce. Some products that are not shipped across state lines may have to be inspected by state programs with their own standards—some higher than those of federal programs. Food production operations may only purchase meat, poultry and eggs that have been inspected by the USDA or by a state department of health or agriculture. Inspected food is considered to be safe for consumption. However, inspection does not imply any quality standard.

Seafood and fish must be purchased from approved suppliers. This is especially important for molluscan shellfish such as oysters, scallops, mollusks, and clams because they may be consumed raw or undercooked. To ensure safety when received, these foods must be accompanied by a certification that documents where and when they were harvested (**Shellfish Identification Tags**). This certification must be kept for 90 days to allow time for evidence of a Hepatitis A virus infection. The Public Health Service maintains lists of Certified Shellfish Shippers. Suppliers should be selected from this list or from state-approved lists.

Grading

Grades are classifications of foods by a descriptive term or number to ensure uniform quality and give an indication of desirability. **Grading** is a voluntary process. Most grades are assigned by government agencies and follow strict guidelines. Grades refer to attributes such as visual appearance, color, size, marbling, and uniformity.

Canned vegetables and fruits are usually graded and each vendor has its own terminology. Beef, veal, pork, and lamb are graded by the USDA. For beef, the USDA grades are: prime, choice, select, standard, commercial, utility, cutter, and canner. The last three grades are not used in food production operations. Examples of inspection stamps and grade shields appear in Figure 18.1.

Figure 18.1 USDA Inspection Stamps and Grade Shields

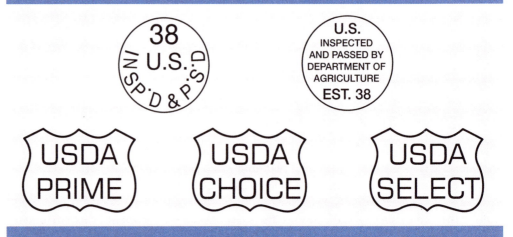

Putting It Into Practice

1. On which foods should you look for an inspection stamp when receiving a food order?

Vendor Selection

Selecting a vendor is an important part of the purchasing process. The Certified Dietary Manager should consider the extent to which the potential vendor will be able to meet the quality, service, and cost expectations of the food production operation. The relationship between the manager and the vendor should be based on mutual understanding, cooperation and trust.

Selection of a vendor is a business decision. Although a personal history with a sales representative is a valuable asset, the final decision should be based on the needs of the organization. Visits to the vendor's distribution center and inspections of delivery vehicles are advisable in the process of selecting a vendor. (Note that food prepared in the home cannot be served in quantity foodservice operations.)

Determine if the facility has a purchasing agreement and if you are required to purchase exclusively with a vendor. Many managers spend time weekly meeting with a number of sales representatives from multiple vendors. While access to a local market or vendor can be helpful for the occasional missing item, professional organizations purchase the majority of their inventory from a limited number of prime vendors.

In today's marketplace, most healthcare and school operations participate in a **Group Purchasing Organization (GPO)**. The GPO functions as a contract buying program that negotiates favorable pricing for items most frequently used by their members. Not all items, nor all brands, purchased are covered by the GPO pricing program. Even items not on the GPO contracted price are usually less expensive through the prime vendor than through the local or back-up vendors. If the facility does have a GPO program available, it is generally to the manager's benefit to access the purchasing agreement. Another advantage of the GPO is they typically pre-approve the vendors for safety, sanitation and delivery services.

Some of the considerations leading to selection of a safe food vendor include:

- Is the vendor inspected by an independent source to ensure food safety?
- Can the supplier provide you with written proof of government inspection for meats?
- Does the vendor have a Hazard Analysis Critical Control Point (HACCP) system in place?
- Are the vendor's delivery vehicles clean and well maintained?
- Are the delivery trucks for refrigerated foods adequately refrigerated?
- If purchasing frozen foods: do delivery trucks have freezer sections?
- Can the vendor provide business references?
- Can the vendor meet the delivery needs (daily, weekly, monthly) of the facility to ensure a safe flow of food?
- Does the vendor have a reputation for providing quality products?
- Will the vendor allow staff to inspect products upon receipt?
- Is the vendor cooperative if you refuse products because of food safety concerns?
- Where is the vendor located relative to the foodservice operation?

Once a reputable vendor is found, it is important to monitor quality continuously to ensure that the vendor has a long-term commitment to providing safe, quality food.

Glossary

Group Purchasing Organization (GPO)
A contract buying program that negotiates favorable pricing for its members

Receiving

Receiving is an important phase in the flow of food through a food production operation. Food items should be carefully inspected before being placed into storage. The person receiving must be knowledgeable of food safety, quality standards, and purchasing specifications. It is essential that food is inspected immediately upon delivery. Product not meeting the facility's quality and safety standards should be refused and returned to the vendor.

If possible, schedule deliveries at times convenient for the receiver to inspect food carefully or change the scheduled work time of receiving staff to be available at the time of planned deliveries. Even government inspected foods must be examined since federal inspection programs do not inspect food at every step in the flow of food from producer to vendor to foodservice operation. Storage areas should be prepared to accept new deliveries; staff should also be available to compare the invoice to the order and store the food immediately.

Of special concern today is fish, such as large tuna or farm-raised (aquaculture) fish that might be consumed raw or undercooked, as in sushi. If you purchase frozen fish for this purpose, it must contain a label indicating that is was properly frozen. (These fish may contain a parasitic worm that can infect your clients.)

Purchased juice products, including pureed fruits and vegetables that are served to highly susceptible populations, such as the sick and the elderly, must contain a label stating that the products have been pasteurized.

Potentially hazardous foods must be received at a temperature of 41°F or below.

A frozen food must be received in a frozen state and at 0°F or below in most cases. Carefully inspect refrigerated and frozen foods for any sign of temperature abuse during transportation and delivery. For instance, large ice crystals are evidence that frozen food was thawed and refrozen—and should be rejected at delivery. A receiving checklist (Figure 18.2) can help employees check and the document condition of foods (a downloadable version of the checklist is available in the online *Supplemental Textbook Material—Foodservice*).

When receiving food:
- Reject food in damaged packaging.
- Check for inspection stamps, date codes, labels/tags for fish or juice.
- Check the temperature of frozen and refrigerated foods, including milk.
- Verify freshness by color, odor, touch, and package condition.
- Look for signs of pest infestation and/or spoilage.

Figure 18.3 shows how to check temperature of foods, and Figure 18.4 shows quality and safety indicators to check for many common foods.

Figure 18.2 Receiving Checklist

Received by: _____   Date: _____   Page #: _____ of ____

Item	Item Matches P.O.	Actual Temp.[1]	Packaging Intact?		Use-By Date Valid?		Accepted	Rejected[2]	Stored[3]
			Y	N	Y	N			

1   Receive refrigerated food at 41°F or below. Receive frozen food at 0°F. Ice cream may be received at 6°F - 10°F.
2   If rejected, write comments on the back of this form.
3   Check to confirm that the item was stored.

Figure 18.3 Verifying Food Temperature During Receiving

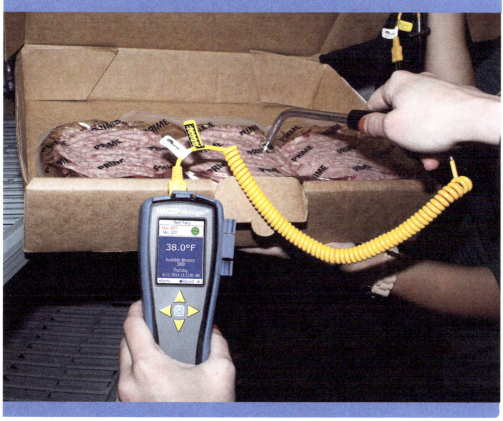

Courtesy: Cooper-Atkins

Figure 18.4 Quality Indicators for Receiving Safe Food

FOOD ITEM	ACCEPT	REJECT
Fresh Beef	• Light pink to bright red color (aged beef may be darker) • Firm and elastic	• Dark brown or greenish color, sour or rancid smell
Fresh Poultry	• Slightly yellow appearance • Firm flesh • Not sticky to touch • Received at or below 41°F	• Dark appearance under wings • Sticky to touch
Marine Foods	• Gills of fresh fish are pink • No iridescence (shimmering) • Eyes clear, not sunken	• Excessive fish or ammonia smell
Milk and Dairy Products	• Intact packging • Clean containers • Butter with firm texture • Cheese free of mold • Received at or below 41°F	• Damaged or leaking containers • Expired dates
Egg and Egg Products	• Clean eggs, uncracked shells • Received at or below 45°F	• Cracked or dirty eggs
Fresh Produce	• Bright color, no mold or wilt	• Signs of insect damange or plant disease • Bruises or soft produce
Canned Foods	• No dents • All foods labeled	• Dented or rusted cans
Dry Goods	• Intact packaging	• Ripped or torn packaging
Frozen Fish	• Labeled that it was properly frozen	• If label is missing • If large ice crystals are present
Molluscan Fish	• Contains a shellfish ID tag	• If tag is missing
Juice or Pureed Fruits/ Vegetables	• Is labeled "pasteurized"	• If not pasteurized

Food Packaging

Technologies for packaging food to promote safety are constantly evolving. Some of the technologies used are discussed below.

Modified Atmosphere Packaging (MAP). Most spoilage microorganisms are **aerobic,** meaning they need oxygen to grow. In modified atmosphere packaging, oxygen is commonly replaced with a mixture of ozone, carbon dioxide or nitrogen. This type of packaging can extend freshness by maintaining a reduced-oxygen environment. Many food products are now packaged this way including vegetables, salad greens, fresh pasta, meat, fruit, cheese, seafood, and pre-prepared foods such as sandwiches and bakery products.

Although the packaging can extend shelf life, it will not always prevent microbial growth. For example, an **anaerobic** pathogen such as Clostridium botulinum may thrive in this low-oxygen environment. Another concern with MAP foods is that they may not "look" or "smell" spoiled when, in fact, they may have become unsafe for consumption. It is up to the manufacturer to protect the client from illness by providing storage instructions and date markings on how to store and handle the product safely. It is up to the operator to make sure that these products are received and stored properly. Thus when receiving and storing MAP foods, you should:

- Read the label. Note that recommended handling practices vary from product to product.
- Check for a **time/temperature indicator (TTI) strip**. This strip changes color if the product is outdated or has been temperature abused.
- Check for an expiration date or use-by date on the package. Do not use packages past recommended dates.
- Check for air bubbles; vacuum packaged foods should be free of air bubbles.
- Maintain MAP packaging under refrigeration.
- Keep MAP packaging sealed until ready to use them. Once a MAP package has been opened, the advantages of a low-oxygen environment disappear. Pathogens can now grow more rapidly.

Modified Atmosphere Packaging (MAP) techniques are very safe and provide advantages. However, a Certified Dietary Manager must nevertheless recognize and control hazards, as with any food product.

Ultra High Temperature Processing (UHT). UHT products are treated by flash sterilization and then packed into sterilized, airtight containers. Milk that is processed using the UHT (shelf-stable milk) can be stored at room temperature for the time period indicated on the label. The most common UHT products are dairy products but the use is expanding to fruit juices, wine, soups, and stews. After opening, the product must be refrigerated and used within the time listed on the product label. For instance, a milk-based soup that was processed with UHT has the following directions on the label: "After opening, keep refrigerated and use within 7-10 days."

Storage

Proper storage is an important aspect of food protection. Storage is more complex than simply having adequate space. Storage involves the variables of light, temperature (see Figure 18.5), ventilation, and air circulation. Food must be stored 6" above the floor, on clean, slatted racks or shelves, and in a manner that prevents environmental or cross-contamination. Slatted shelving allows for proper air circulation around food and should

Putting It Into Practice

2. While checking in an order you notice that one jar of mayonnaise in the case has a bulging lid. What should you do?

not be covered with foil or other material. Food must also be stored away from walls and ceilings. Food not intended for further preparation before serving must be stored in a way that prevents contamination from food requiring preparation.

Figure 18.5 Storage Temperatures

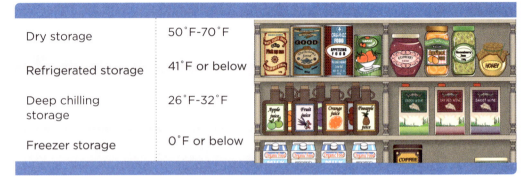

Dry storage	50°F–70°F
Refrigerated storage	41°F or below
Deep chilling storage	26°F–32°F
Freezer storage	0°F or below

For instance, raw foods—such as meat—should never be stored above ready-to-eat foods—such as fresh fruit, salads, or desserts. The raw food may splash or drip onto the ready-to-eat food and result in cross-contamination. Food may not be stored in locker rooms, toilet areas, dressing rooms, in garbage rooms, mechanical rooms, under sewer lines that are not adequately shielded, under open stairwells, under a water leak, or near any other potential source of contamination. Chemicals must never be stored near food.

Every food has a shelf life, which is the amount of time the product can be expected to remain reasonably safe if properly stored. Foodservice staff must monitor the dates on foods to ensure foods are used before expiration. New deliveries should be stored behind previous deliveries to ensure that the oldest product is used first. This method of stock rotation is called **First In, First Out (FIFO)**.

Certain foods may be difficult to identify after they are removed from their original packaging. Foods such as salt and sugar look the same, but if they are mixed up for clients on special diets it can be disastrous. Some oils or granulated foods may look like cleaning compounds. Packaged food labels contain nutrition information as well as valuable ingredient information that may be needed for consulting with clients with allergies. For those reasons, containers holding food or food ingredients that are removed from original packaging for use in the foodservice operation should be labeled with the common name of the food and the date the package was opened.

When storing raw meats, fish and pork should be kept separate from poultry because of the possible higher bacterial count in the poultry. As mentioned, meats should be stored below ready-to-eat foods to avoid drippage during thawing.

Food storage areas must be equipped with thermometers accurate to ±3°F. The temperature of storage areas should be monitored not less than once a day and the actual temperatures documented on a temperature log (Figure 18.6) (A downloadable version of the temperature log is available in the online *Supplemental Textbook Material— Foodservice*).

Figure 18.6 Storage Temperature Log

Storage Area: _____ Page #: _____ of _____

| Date | Storage Temp. | | Comments/Corrective Actions |
	AM	PM	

Dry storage: 50°F-70°F | Refrigerated Storage: 41°F or below | Deep chilling storage: 26°F-32°F | Freezer Storage: 0°F or below

Dry storage area temperatures should be maintained between 50°F-70°F. For short-term holding of perishable foods, maintain refrigerators between 34°F-41°F. Sometimes a food is not quite as cold as the temperature around it. Maintaining refrigeration temperatures below 38°F will help ensure that actual food temperatures remain out of the hazard zone. The Food Code suggests placing a thermometer in the warmest part of the refrigerator. New technology allows employees to measure a simulated product temperature for better accuracy.

Ideally, meats, poultry and fish should be stored in a deep chilling unit. Very low temperatures may damage food and affect quality for some items such as produce and dairy products. Often separate coolers are used for produce and dairy with slightly higher thermostat settings. A summary of suggested practices for storing food appears in Appendix C and in the online *Supplemental Textbook Material—Foodservice*, a printable copy of the food storage guidelines.

> NOTE: Detailed information on food safety and foodborne illness is covered through the food handler certification programs. Check with state and local regulations for specific requirements regarding food handler certification or food handler cards.

Figure 18.7 provides a summary of guidelines for purchasing, receiving, and storing food.

Putting It Into Practice

3. You are storing the following items in a cooler: a case of lettuce, a case of cottage cheese, a case of chicken breasts you want to thaw, and a bowl of tuna salad prepared for tomorrow's lunch. Where would you place these items in your cooler and why?

Figure 18.7 Guidelines for Purchasing, Receiving and Storing Food

ITEM	PURCHASE	RECEIVE	STORE	SHELF LIFE
Meat	• USDA or state inspected	• Receive frozen at 0°F • Receive refrigerated at 41°F or below	• Store frozen at 0°F or below • Store refrigerated at 41°F or below, separate from poultry	• Fresh beef: 6-12 months in freezer; 3-6 days in refrigerator • Ground beef: 3-4 months in freezer; 1-2 days in refrigerator
Poultry	• USDA or state inspected	• Receive frozen at 0°F • Receive refrigerated at 41°F or below	• Store frozen at 0°F or below • Store refrigerated at 41°F or below	• 6 months in freezer; 1-2 days in refrigerator
Fish and Shellfish	• From an approved supplier • Shellfish must have shellfish identification tag	• Receive frozen at 0°F • Receive refrigerated at 41°F or below	• Store frozen at 0°F or below • Store refrigerated at 41°F or below, separate from poultry	• All: 2-4 months in freezer • 1-2 days in refrigerator
Milk and Dairy Products	• Pasteurized milk and milk products	• Receive frozen (ice cream) at 6°F to 10°F • Receive refrigerated at 41°F	• Store frozen at 0°F or below • Store refrigerated at 41°F or below • Unopened UHT package may be stored at room temperature	• Milk: Use by expiration date on carton • Ice cream: 6 months in freezer

Product Recalls

Periodically, manufacturers identify quality issues that affect the safety or integrity of their product in the marketplace. Issuing a product recall is a major process for the manufacturer and distributor to coordinate. If a product has been designated for recall, typically the distributor contacts all customers who have purchased the specific lot numbers of the item and advises the customer on the appropriate steps for disposal. Normally, the vendor does not want to "pick up" the product from a facility. Many of the major vendors also list complete details of product recalls on their website.

Summary

Ensuring the safety of the food served to clientele starts with the vendor and their acquisition of food from approved growers. The purchase, delivery, and storage within the department is designed to maintain the quality and safety of the food until the time of preparation. In the next chapter, food safety shifts to the actual preparation and presentation of meals for the clients.

Safe Food Handling: Food Preparation

Overview and Objectives

Did you ever consider how many processes food goes through before we actually consume it? Safe purchasing, receiving and storage procedures are just the beginning of processes needed to keep our food safe. In this chapter, we will evaluate foodborne diseases and their causes, explain all phases in the flow of food, and review HACCP guidelines. After completing this chapter, you should be able to:

✓ Identify potentially hazardous foods and foodborne pathogens and their control

✓ Recognize the causes, symptoms, and types of foodborne illnesses including biological, chemical and physical types

✓ Monitor time and temperature to limit growth of or destroy microorganisms

✓ Prevent cross-contamination of food

✓ Identify appropriate techniques for temperature retention

✓ Ensure the safe cooling of food

✓ Establish critical limits

✓ Establish the corrective action to be taken when critical limits are exceeded

✓ Establish procedures to identify and monitor critical control points (CCP)

✓ Establish effective recordkeeping systems that document HACCP

✓ Anticipate emergency preparedness procedures necessary to assure a safe food supply

✓ Develop a crisis management plan to address an outbreak of foodborne illness

Foodborne Illness: Causes & Preparation

Foodborne illness is a major public issue. In 2011, the Food Safety Modernization Act was implemented to expand and improve the security and safety of our nation's food supply. This was historic legislation designed to build a new system of food safety oversight. Why do we need this important legislation? According to the Center for Disease Control (CDC), "each year, foodborne illness strikes 48 million Americans, hospitalizing a hundred thousand and killing over three thousand."

In addition, many people experience foodborne illness and do not report it, brushing off symptoms as "the flu". A **foodborne illness** is a disease that is transmitted by food. The most frequent cause is harmful microorganisms—or poisons produced by harmful

Glossary

Foodborne Illness
A disease that is transmitted by food

microorganisms. Symptoms vary according to the cause of the illness and the person who is afflicted. However, common symptoms may include vomiting, diarrhea, fever, and headache. In some cases, death is a very real risk.

Some individuals are more susceptible to foodborne illness than others. Their symptoms may be more severe, and their risk of death may be higher. Preschool age children, the elderly, pregnant women, and persons with weakened immune systems are considered to be high-risk groups, also called **highly susceptible populations (HSP)**. Serving these groups requires special awareness of their increased vulnerability—and sometimes special precautions in ingredient selection and meal preparation.

Often, when there is one case of foodborne illness, there are more cases related to the same food item. A **foodborne illness outbreak** occurs when two or more persons become ill after ingesting the same food and a laboratory analysis confirms that food was the source of the illness. If foodborne illness is caused by a chemical, this is also defined as an outbreak, even if there is only one case.

The annual cost of foodborne illness is estimated to be $152 billion. According to the CDC, more than 250 different types of diseases are caused by contaminated food or beverages. New strains of harmful foodborne microorganisms are constantly evolving.

Food Hazards

Food can become unsafe in a number of ways. There are many **hazards** in the environment that affect the safety and quality of food served. Hazards are present in air, water, foods, on work surfaces, and on the hands and bodies of dining services employees. Food-related hazards fall into three major categories: biological, chemical, and physical, as shown in Figure 19.1. The presence of substances in food that could cause harm is called **contamination**.

Figure 19.1 Food Hazards

BIOLOGICAL	CHEMICAL	PHYSICAL
• Bacteria	• Pesticides	• Dirt
• Parasites	• Toxic Metals	• Hair
• Viruses	• Cleaning Chemicals	• Broken Glass
• Fungi		• Metal Shavings
• Natural Toxins		
• Prions		

Biological Hazards

Biological hazards include bacteria, viruses, parasites, and fungi. Viruses and bacteria are most commonly cited in foodborne illness outbreaks but all present a threat to the safety of the food supply. Bacteria are plentiful in the environment and in our bodies. While some serve useful purposes, others cause serious foodborne illnesses. Microorganisms that cause foodborne illness are called **pathogens**.

Pathogens may already be in the food supply or may be introduced at any time from the point of harvest to the processor, manufacturer, distributor or at the food production operation. Improper operating procedures and food preparation practices allow pathogens to survive and grow. In turn, these events increase the risk of foodborne illness (see Figure 19.2).

Glossary

Highly Susceptible Populations
Persons who are more likely to experience foodborne disease because they are immunocompromised, preschool age children, pregnant women or older adults

Foodborne Illness Outbreak
Occurs when two or more cases of a similar illness result from eating a common food

Hazards
Biological, chemical, or physical property that may cause an unacceptable consumer health risk that must be controlled

Contamination
The presence of biological, physical, or chemical substances in food that could cause harm

Biological Hazards
A living organism such as bacteria, viruses, parasites or fungi that can cause harm to humans

Pathogens
Microorganisms that cause foodborne illness

Figure 19.2 Causes of Foodborne Illness

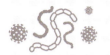

| Pathogens are naturally present in the food supply. | Contamination or mishandling occurs during processing, transport, storage, preparation, and/or service. | Pathogens may grow. New pathogens may be introduced. Other biological, chemical, and physical contaminants may also enter food. | Food is consumed and foodborne illness results. |

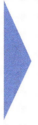

Bacteria

There are many types of bacteria, with differences in their growth habits and requirements. **Anaerobic** bacteria grow in an environment with little or no oxygen. These bacteria might contaminate canned foods or modified atmosphere packaged products. They may also grow in the center of large quantities of food. **Aerobic** bacteria require oxygen to grow.

Many bacteria associated with foodborne illness can grow either with or without oxygen and are called **facultative**. When growth conditions are unfavorable some bacteria form spores, exist in a dormant state, and then begin growing again when conditions are ripe. Spores are difficult to kill and can function as a foodborne illness timebomb. Sound food protection practices can keep them under control.

Types of Illness

Exactly how pathogens cause illnesses varies. Some microorganisms enter the body in an active state and continue to grow. The type of illness that results is called a **foodborne infection**, because the person who eats the food is literally infected with the pathogens. For example, Salmonella bacteria enter the body in a live state and grow in the body, causing fever, nausea, diarrhea, and other symptoms. This illness is called salmonellosis.

Other microorganisms produce a poison or toxin that may not be destroyed in cooking. The bacteria may not be alive anymore, but their toxins nevertheless cause illness. This type of illness is called **foodborne intoxication**. For example, Clostridium botulinum bacteria produce a toxin. The illness that results from eating an affected food is called botulism.

Finally, some microorganisms enter the body in a live and growing state—and produce toxins in the body. The resulting illness is a **toxin-mediated infection**. Shiga toxin-producing E. coli bacteria (STEC), for example, operate this way causing an illness that involves severe diarrhea and vomiting.

Types of Pathogens

Due to environmental and growth conditions, most pathogens favor certain foods. For example, Listeria bacteria are often associated with unpasteurized cheese and processed meats, Salmonella with eggs, Shiga toxin-producing E. coli with ground beef, and Norwalk virus with shellfish.

The Certified Dietary Manager should be able to recognize symptoms that could signal foodborne illness and warrant medical evaluation. However it is important to note that

Glossary

Facultative
Can grow with or without the presence of oxygen

Foodborne Infection
When pathogens enter the body in an active state and continue to grow (e.g., Salmonella)

Foodborne Intoxication
An illness that occurs from the toxin or poison left from bacteria that are no longer alive (e.g., Clostridium botulinum)

Toxin-Mediated Infection
When live bacteria enter the body and produce a dangerous toxin (e.g., E. coli bacteria)

control mechanisms for foodborne illness are fairly universal. A comprehensive set of food protection practices can prevent illness from a wide range of pathogens. The CDC lists the top five pathogens causing illness, hospitalization, and death: Norovirus (a virus, formerly called Norwalk virus), Salmonella (bacteria), Clostridium Perfringens (bacteria), Campylobacter (bacteria), and Staphylococcus aureus (bacteria). These top five pathogens are highlighted on the following pages (Figure 19.3).

Conditions for Bacterial Growth and Toxin Formation

To protect clients from foodborne illness, first consider the conditions that allow bacteria to grow or toxins to develop. The conditions are similar to what humans need: air, food, moisture, and warmth. Bacteria require food for themselves. Often, they favor food high in protein, such as meat. But sometimes, they settle for vegetables, fruits, and other plant foods. In addition to food, bacteria grow most rapidly in an environment that also provides them with moisture, warmth, neutral or slightly acid pH, oxygen at a level favored by the bacteria and time. Moisture is measured as available water (a_w) in a food. Examples of food with a high a_w content include meat, cheese, and produce. Meats, fresh fruits, and fresh vegetables, for example, have an a_w of close to 1.0, while crackers have an a_w of 0.1.

The term pH describes level of acidity or alkalinity. Optimal conditions for microorganisms are typically neutral or slightly acidic. Generally, as foods become more acidic, they are less likely to support bacterial growth. Meats, fish, and vegetables tend to be slightly acidic and support bacterial growth. Foods that are very acidic, with a pH below about 4.2, do not favor bacterial growth. Based on a_w and level of acidity, you can see why traditional methods of food preservation use techniques like dehydrating food products (to *reduce* a_w) and pickling or adding vinegar (to reduce pH to extremes where bacteria cannot thrive).

Time and temperature are critically interrelated in controlling bacterial growth and formation of toxins. When all other conditions are suitable for microorganisms, a key question is: How much time does the microorganism have in which to flourish? For example, in one environment bacterial growth may be controlled if temperature and time are managed. However, if the temperature is the same, but the bacteria have twice as much time to grow, there may be a hundred times more bacteria present. The more time a microorganism has under favorable conditions, the more it will multiply or produce toxins. This is one reason that holding time, cooling (for hot foods), reheating time (for leftovers), storage time, and other time-related factors are important for ensuring safe food. Conditions that help bacteria grow can be summarized by the acronym, **FOTTWA**, shown in Figure 19.4.

Glossary

FOTTWA
Acronym for the conditions needed for bacterial growth: Food, Oxygen, Temperature, Time, Water, Acidity

PHF/TCS
Abbreviation for Potentially Hazardous Food (Time/Temperature Control for Safety) designation of foods that require control of time and temperature for safety

Putting It Into Practice

1. What type of contamination is most likely to occur from unwashed hands?

Figure 19.3 Common Foodborne Pathogens

TYPE	SOURCE	SYMPTOMS AND COMPLICATIONS	PREVENTION
Bacillus cereus Bacteria	Milk, cereals, rice, and starchy foodstuffs	Diarrhea, fever, chills, and dehydration. Onset is usually within 12-50 hours.	Keep food out of the hazard zone. Keep dry products away from moisture.
Campylobacter jejuni Bacteria	Raw meat, poultry and shellfish, contaminated water and unpasteurized milk	Muscle pain, headache and fever followed by diarrhea, abdominal pain and nausea. Onset is usually 2-5 days.	Thoroughly cook meat and poultry. Use pasteurized milk and products. Control time/temperature. Use clean utensils. Use chlorinated drinking water.
Clostridium botulinum Bacteria	Grows in anaerobic environment—canned and reduced oxygen packaged foods or soups and sauces that have been improperly cooled. Also found in honey. Produces a toxin.	Double vision and difficulties in speaking, swallowing and breathing. May result in nerve damage and life-threatening illness. Illness is called botulism. Onset is usually 12-48 hours.	Dispose of canned foods that are leaking or bulging, or are dented or damaged. Inspect vacuum-packaged foods for tears and time/temperature abuse.
Clostridium perfringens Bacteria	Naturally present in the soil. Any raw food may contain the spore or bacteria. Called the "cafeteria germ" because many outbreaks result from large quantities of food being held at room temperature or cooked too slowly.	Abdominal pain and diarrhea. Onset is usually 8-22 hours.	Thoroughly cook foods containing meat or poultry. Maintain food at safe temperatures. Cool foods quickly by dividing into small, shallow containers. Use ice as an ingredient, use an ice bath, or use a blast chiller. Reheat refrigerated foods adequately.
Listeria monocytogenes Bacteria	Commonly found in the intestines of animals and humans, in milk, soil, and leafy vegetables. Also found in unpasteurized dairy products and processed meals.	In adults: sudden onset of fever, chills, headache, backache, abdominal pain, and diarrhea. In newborns: may cause respiratory distress, refusal to drink, and vomiting. Can cause miscarriage or stillbirth in pregnant women. Onset 3-70 days.	Avoid unpasteurized milk and dairy products. Cook ground meats thoroughly. Maintain food temperature out of the hazard zone. Bacteria may grow at refrigerated temperatures, so follow use-by and sell-by dates on processed foods.
Salmonella enteritidis Bacteria	Often found in meat and poultry products. Can survive in frozen food and grow with or without oxygen. Common cause is poor personal hygiene or cross-contamination.	Nausea, vomiting, cramps, and fever. Onset is within 12-36 hours. Can be fatal to high-risk groups, such as the elderly.	Avoid serving raw eggs or undercooked poultry. Never pool eggs. Use pasteurized egg products. Sanitize work surfaces and utensils. Cook food thoroughly.
Shiga toxin-producing *Escherichia coli* **(STEC)** Bacteria	Ground beef has been implicated in several severe outbreaks. Beef was often contaminated during processing and then mishandled during preparation. Also found in raw seed sprouts, lettuce, unpasteurized milk.	Produces a toxin which causes hemorrhagic colitis. Symptoms include abdominal cramps, watery diarrhea, nausea, vomiting, and low-grade fever. Acute kidney failure is a possible complication. Onset is usually 3-8 days.	Cook ground beef to 155°F for 15 seconds or more. Reheat properly. Use good sanitation and hygiene practices. Store and hold foods properly.

(Continued...)

Figure 19.3 **Common Foodborne Pathogens** *(Continued...)*

TYPE	SOURCE	SYMPTOMS AND COMPLICATIONS	PREVENTION
Shigella Bacteria	An infected foodservice employee (carrier) or contaminated water supply are frequently cited sources. Prepared salads, gravies, and milk have been implicated.	Symptoms include diarrhea, fever, chills, and dehydration. Onset is usually within 12-50 hours.	Ensure a safe source of water. Restrict foodservice employees with infectious disease from the foodservice operation. Ensure good personal hygiene.
Staphylococcus aureus Bacteria	Illness is caused by a toxin. Improperly sanitized equipment and poor handwashing practices are culprits. Ham, cold meats, custards, cream-filled desserts are implicated foods.	Nausea, vomiting, and abdominal cramps. Can be fatal to elderly, infants, and other high-risk populations. Onset 1-6 hours.	Keep food out of the hazard zone by storing and cooking properly. Ensure good personal hygiene. Do not allow employees with infected cuts to handle food.
Yersinia enterocolitica Bacteria	Found in meats, oysters, fish, and raw milk. Poor sanitation and food preparation practices contribute to outbreaks.	Fever, headache, nausea, abdominal pain, and diarrhea. Onset 24-48 hours.	Heat food thoroughly to destroy the bacteria. Practice effective handwashing.
Giardia Bacteria	Found in contaminated water, infected food handlers, possibly fresh produce.	Diarrhea, abdominal cramps, bloating, weight loss, or malabsorption. Typical onset is 1-2 weeks after contact; may last 6 weeks or much longer. Person may have no symptoms.	Practice proper handwashing and good personal hygiene. Use approved water sources.
Anisakis Parasite	Roundworm found in fish, transmitted through ingestion of raw or partially cooked marine foods.	Can be painful and is often misdiagnosed as appendicitis, Crohn's disease or gastric ulcer. Can require surgery to remove the parasite.	Cook marine foods thoroughly to destroy the parasite.
Trichinella spiralis Parasite	Roundworm found in pork and wild game. Illness caused by consuming pork that was not thoroughly cooked.	Muscle pain and fever.	Thoroughly cook pork to destroy parasites.
Hepatitis A Parasite	Virus is transmitted from one person to another through food. Water, shellfish and salads are frequently implicated foods.	Fever, abdominal pain, loss of appetite and jaundice. Typical incubation time is 10-15 days, but can be up to 50 days.	Practice proper handwashing and good personal hygiene. Restrict infected persons from foodservice operation.
Norovirus Virus	Contaminated shellfish or foods washed in contaminated water. Employees infected with the virus.	Nausea, vomiting, diarrhea and abdominal pain.	Avoid serving raw shellfish. Observe good personal hygiene and cooking practices.
Vibrio vulnificus Bacteria	Contaminated shellfish, especially from warm seawater.	Fever, skin lesions, collapse, cystic shock.	Avoid serving raw shellfish.

Figure 19.4 Conditions for Bacterial Growth: FOTTWA

Food	Food must contain appropriate nutrients for growth. Bacteria generally required protein and carbohydrates.
Oxygen	Some bacteria require oxygen (aerobic). Some bacteria cannot tolerate oxygen (anaerobic). Others grow with or without oxygen (facultative).
Temperature	Temperature is probably the most critical factor in the growth of bacteria. The hazard zone of 41°F-135°F is the range in which microorganisms grow and produce toxins most rapidly.
Time	A single bacterial cell can multiply into 1 million cells in 5 hours under ideal conditions. A general rule is that food in the hazard zone for 4 or more hours may be unsafe.
Water	Moisture is measured based on water activity (available water or a_w). Pathogens generally grow in foods with an a_w value greater than 0.85.
Acidity	Many pathogens tend to prefer conditions that are near a pH of 4.3-7.5, which is neutral or slightly acid.

Foods that require control of time and temperature, in order to prevent growth of pathogens or formation of toxins are called potentially hazardous foods (time/temperature control for safety), or PHF/TCS. Examples include: meat, poultry, eggs, fish, seafood, cut melons, raw seed sprouts, garlic/oil mixtures, baked potatoes, cooked plant foods such as beans or rice, and some fresh vegetables (e.g., lettuce, tomatoes). These foods typically contain the nutrients, available water, and acidity levels that bacteria require for growth. Many plant foods are **PHF/TCS**. In fact, foodborne illness outbreaks over recent years have been traced to plant foods such as chopped parsley, lettuce, spinach, fresh berries, green onions, tomatoes, fruit juices, and other products.

> Shell eggs that have been treated to destroy possible Salmonella bacteria are ommited from the list of PHF/TCS. These are often called pasteurized shell eggs.

The 2013 FDA Food Code definition of PHF/TCS emphasizes the fact that PHF/TCS requires control of both time and temperature to control hazards. The old definition targeted foods that might support "rapid and progressive growth" of pathogens. Today, however, "rapid" is not as meaningful. Pathogens do not need to grow rapidly to create illness. Prolonged, progressive growth, such as that of Listeria bacteria in lunch meats or hot dogs held under refrigeration for extended periods of time, is enough to cause illness.

Hazard Zone

An awareness of FOTTWA is the first step towards understanding how to prevent growth of harmful bacteria. Many food protection practices involve controlling temperatures. The temperature range in which most bacteria grow rapidly is called the **hazard zone**. The hazard zone is the range from 41°F -135°F, as shown in Figure 19.5. This temperature

Glossary

Hazard or Danger Zone

The temperature range in which most bacteria grow rapidly (41°F - 135°F range is also commonly known as the danger zone. The terms hazard zone and danger zone can be used interchangeably. (Individual states and local authorities may use slightly different temperatures or time guidelines based on their criteria. For purposes of this textbook, the FDA Food Code is the basis for the standards cited.)

The Certified Dietary Manager can minimize bacterial growth during preparation and service by controlling the time food spends in a temperature range favorable to bacterial growth. In general, temperature control means keeping cold food cold and hot food hot, while minimizing the time a food spends in the hazard zone. In fact, a potentially hazardous food that is allowed to remain in the hazard zone for a <u>cumulative time of four hours</u> or more during all phases of receiving, storage, preparation and service is *considered unsafe to eat.*

Figure 19.5 Hazard Zones

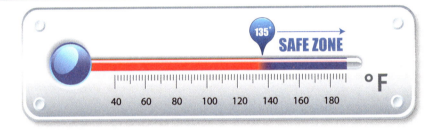

The safe temperature zone for hot foods is 135°F or higher

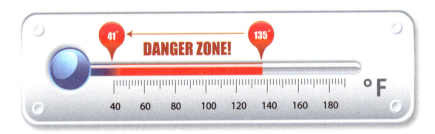

The hazard zone is the temperature range between 41°F and 135°F, where pathogens grow most rapidly.

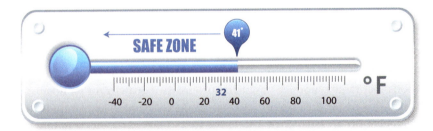

The safe temperature zone for cold food is 41°F or below.

Putting It Into Practice

2. In the following recipe, which foods would be considered potentially hazardous?
   - 1 lb. boneless chicken breast 1/2" pieces
   - 3 cups fat-free chicken broth
   - 2 cups diced potatoes with onion
   - 2/3 cups frozen mixed vegetables
   - 3 Tbsp. flour
   - Salt, pepper, sage, thyme to taste

Virus

A **virus** is the smallest and simplest form of life known. Viruses can be transmitted from a dining service employee to a client on the food but do not grow or multiply in food. Viruses need a living host such as humans, animals, or fish in which to grow. Fish and shellfish can also be sources of foodborne viruses. Preventing viral foodborne illness requires health screening of employees, removing employees from the work schedule who may have viral illness, sound personal hygiene habits, and careful selection of marine foods.

Parasite

A **parasite** is a small or microscopic organism that lives within another organism called a host. The parasite can be transmitted from animals to humans if food is not cooked thoroughly. For example, Trichinella is a parasite found in pork (rarely seen in commercially grown pork in the United States and Europe) and wild game. It's actually a roundworm that causes an infection (trichinosis) in the person who consumes it. Cooking pork to the proper temperature and holding that temperature for a recommended minimum time destroys the parasite.

Fungi

Molds and yeasts are types of **fungi**. Some play a role in food processing. For example, yeasts are used in the production of bread and molds are used in the processing of cheese. However, molds and yeasts can also be a threat to food safety. Molds grow well on most types of food and appear as brightly colored, fuzzy growth. Certain molds produce a toxin which can result in a foodborne illness. Toxins produced by fungi, called mycotoxins, may be found in dry and/or acidic foods. Guidelines for handling food that has mold appear in Figure 19.6.

Figure 19.6 Guidelines for Handling Foods Containing Mold

Some foods that develop mold must be discarded. Other foods can be used, but first cut out the mold and at least an inch of food under and around it.

DISCARD	CUT AND USE
• Cucumbers	• Bell Peppers
• Tomatoes	• Broccoli, Cauliflower
• Spinach, Lettuce, Leafy Greens	• Cabbage
• Bananas, Peaches, Melons	• Garlic, Onions
• Berries	• Potatoes
• Breads, Cakes, Rolls, Flour	• Turnips
• Soft Cheeses like Brie or Mozzarella	• Zucchini, Winter Squash
• Lunch Meat and Cheese (slices)	• Apples, Pears
• Yogurt, Tub Spreads, Cream Cheese	• Hard Cheeses like Cheddar or Swiss
• Canned Foods	
• Peanut Butter	
• Juices	
• Cooked Leftovers	

Glossary

Fungi
Molds or yeast that can cause an illness or produce a toxin that causes the illness

Prions

Prions are biological agents in a very unique category. They are small, protein-like particles responsible for illnesses such as bovine spongiform encephalopathy (BSE), commonly know as "mad cow disease". Unlike other pathogens, they are not affected by conditions for pathogen growth (FOTTWA). They are not destroyed by heat, as many pathogens are. They cause infection only when one animal (or person) consumes food made from an animal infected with the prion. For example, the mad cow outbreak in Great Britain in the 1980s was traced to feeding cows with meat and bone products that came from infected sheep. Human infection is extremely rare but government officials are taking many precautions to protect the U.S. food supply from potentially infected meat. Chronic Wasting Disease (CWD) in deer and elk is also caused by a prion. CWD is present in 12 U.S. states and deer and elk meat from these locations should not be consumed.

Yeasts

Yeasts are not a significant cause of foodborne illness but can contaminate food and cause it to spoil. Yeasts prefer sweet, liquid foods and are well known for fermenting cider and fruit juices. An indication of yeast spoilage is a fermenting, alcoholic smell, and discoloration.

Natural Toxins

Toxins can occur naturally in foods such as fish, shellfish, mushrooms, and certain plants. A foodborne illness called ciguatera (pronounced "sig-wah-terrra") is caused by consuming fish that has, in turn, ingested toxins present in algae. Shellfish can also be toxic due to algae they consume. An example of shellfish-related illness is paralytic shellfish poisoning. Scombroid poisoning is the result of eating certain varieties of fish that release a toxin called histamine when they begin to spoil. Mushroom poisoning can result from eating certain varieties of mushrooms. Generally these toxins are not destroyed by cooking. So the best protection is prevention: purchase seafood and mushrooms only from approved sources. See the online *Supplemental Textbook Material—Foodservice* for more information.

Chemical Hazards

Chemical hazards include pesticides that are sprayed on food, preservatives used to maintain food, toxic metals in cooking equipment and utensils, and chemical cleaning materials used in the foodservice operation.

Preservatives and Food Additives

Some chemicals are added to food to help preserve the quality. Sulfites are one example that is used for fresh fruits and vegetables, shrimp, lobster, and wine. Sulfites may cause an allergic reaction in some people so sulfiting agents added to a product in processing plant must be declared on labeling. Do not use a sulfiting agent on raw produce.

Other chemicals added to enhance food quality that may cause allergic reactions are nitrites/nitrates in meats and MSG (monosodium glutamate) used in Asian or Latin American foods.

Allergens

Food allergies are a separate, but classified as chemical, type of food-related illness warranting the attention of Certified Dietary Managers. The FDA Food Code has added an emphasis on food allergies: "Food allergy is an increasing food safety and public health issue affecting approximately 4% of the U.S. population or twelve million Americans." The 2013 FDA Food Code lists the following topics that managers need to know regarding food allergies:

- The eight major food allergens
- Food allergen ingredient identities and labeling
- How to avoid cross-contamination during food preparation and service.

A food allergy is an adverse reaction to food that involves the immune system. An allergic reaction depends upon the allergen, a specific protein in the food that triggers an immune system response. For example, the protein in peanuts or eggs may function as an allergen for sensitive individuals. Figure 19.7 shows the foods associated with the most common food allergies. The best control measure to use in the foodservice department is to prevent cross-contamination between allergenic and non-allergenic ingredients. For a full discussion on food allergies, see Chapter 4 in the *Nutrition Fundamentals and Medical Nutrition Therapy* textbook.

Figure 19.7 **The Most Common Food Allergens**

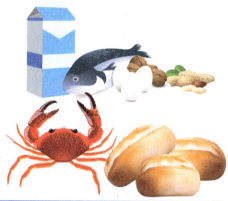

- Milk
- Eggs
- Fish
- Shellfish (e.g., crab, lobster, shrimp)
- Tree Nuts (e.g., almonds, pecans, walnuts)
- Wheat
- Peanuts
- Soybeans
- A food ingredient derived from one of these: peanut oil, baked goods containing eggs, sauces containing wheat flours, etc.

Pesticides

Chemicals used to keep produce grown in the United States free from plant diseases and insect infestations are regulated by the government and should not cause foodborne illness when applied at recommended levels. But some foods originate from international sources with less government regulation and monitoring. Wash all fresh fruits and vegetables to remove chemical residues before serving.

Toxic Metals

Metals that can cause foodborne illness include cadmium, antimony, lead, zinc, and copper. Antimony, zinc, and copper may cause contamination after prolonged contact with acid foods. Carefully select foodservice equipment to control this hazard.

Cleaning Supplies

Cleaning products may also cause contamination when improperly used or stored. Cleaning supplies and other toxic materials must be stored separately from the food preparation and service areas. Never use a food container to store chemicals, and never use chemical containers to store food. Containers used for cleaning—such as buckets and pails—should be clearly marked and dedicated for use in cleaning only.

Putting It Into Practice

3. A Certified Dietary Manager notices a client wheezing after eating a stir-fry dish that was fried with peanut oil. What should the manager do first? Why might this have happened?

Physical Hazards

Physical hazards are foreign materials that enter food accidentally. Examples are glass fragments, pieces of bone, metal shavings, staples from produce crates, and other objects that fall into food and cause serious physical harm or injury. Methods or techniques to prevent contamination of food from physical hazards include: visually inspecting food during preparation, maintaining equipment in good repair, keeping food covered to prevent fragments from falling into it, and discarding food that has been exposed to broken dishware.

Foodborne Illness Prevention

Foodborne illness is a real and present danger. This places a great responsibility on every Certified Dietary Manager and food production and dining services staff member to protect clients. It is essential to take steps to protect food and control hazards. The steps follow the movement of food throughout your operation—from purchasing ingredients to receiving and storing, to preparing and serving food, to managing leftovers.

United States government research indicates that the five top causes of foodborne illness outbreak are:

- Improper holding temperatures
- Contaminated equipment
- Poor personal hygiene
- Inadequate cooking
- Food from unsafe sources

A Certified Dietary Manager must ensure safe practices in all phases of foodservice management. How do we know what is a safe practice? The Food and Drug Administration (FDA) has developed a set of food protection standards, called the FDA Food Code, which provides the basis for this chapter.

Anyone managing a food production operation must be aware of the constant hazards that can result in foodborne illness. In the U.S. today, foodborne illness is a serious public health concern. In some cases, failure to observe food safety practices can result in illness, hospitalization, or even the death of a client. While the responsibility is grave, we fortunately have a wealth of knowledge about the factors that can cause foodborne illness and the means to control them. This is the charge of every Certified Dietary Manager.

The movement of food through the various stages of purchasing, receiving, storage, preparation, transport, holding, service, cooling, and reheating is called the **flow of food**. Each step in this flow presents hazards and challenges for food protection. In this section, we will focus on the latter segment of this flow, beginning with food preparation.

Preparing Safe Food

Temperature is a critical variable and must be monitored at each step in the flow of food. To ensure safe handling, keep temperature logs in all storage, preparation, and service areas. Involve all staff members in monitoring temperatures and be sure all staff is trained in the proper procedures for recording food temperatures.

Time is also an important control technique for food protection. Label all food items with the latest time for use when moving it from storage to preparation areas. Once food has been removed from a monitored, temperature-controlled environment, serve or dispose of it within four hours. For instance, if meals are served through room service and the lunch entrée was prepared at 10:00 a.m. for a room service request, it must be served or refrigerated properly before 2:00 p.m.

Dispose of food if it is in unmarked containers or if the expiration date has passed. Communicate food labeling and monitoring practices to all members of the food production and dining services team.

Cross-Contamination

During all phases of food preparation and service, food production and dining services professionals must take steps to prevent cross-contamination. **Cross-contamination** is the transfer of pathogens from any item to food. The source of contamination may be a non-food item, such as a work surface, another food item, or the hands of a foodservice employee. Figure 19.8 identifies examples of how cross-contamination can occur. To prevent cross-contamination:

- Follow proper procedures for cleaning and sanitizing equipment and utensils.
- Observe handwashing practices and standards for glove use.
- As much as possible, isolate raw foods from ready-to-eat or prepared foods in all phases of the flow of food.

Figure 19.8 Examples of How Cross Contamination May Occur

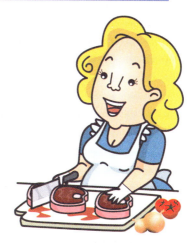

- A foodservice staff member prepares tuna salad while wearing gloves and then puts a pan of macaroni and cheese into the warmer without changing gloves and washing hands.
- A cook dices beef for stew on a cutting board and then chops onions on the same board without cleaning and sanitizing the surface between jobs.
- A cook uses the same spatula to put raw burgers on the grill and to remove cooked burgers from the grill.
- A foodservice staff member allows raw egg mixture to splash over prepared foods near the steam table.
- An employee picks up trash from the floor and then enters the walk-in refrigerator without first washing hands.

Raw fruits and vegetables must be thoroughly washed in water to remove soil and other contaminants. They should be washed before being cut, combined with other ingredients, cooked, served, or offered for service in a ready-to-eat form.

Pathogens like Salmonella or chemicals such as pesticides may be present on the outside surface of fruits and vegetables. The 2013 FDA Food Code says, "All fresh produce, except commercially washed, pre-cut, or bagged produce, must be thoroughly washed under running, potable water before eating, cutting, or cooking." This is required even if you plan to peel the produce prior to eating. If using pre-washed, bagged produce in an opened bag, it must be considered a potentially hazardous food.

Ice that is used for displaying fresh produce or cooked shellfish cannot be used further for cooking or service.

Glossary

Cross Contamination
The transfer of pathogens from any item or human to food

Thawing

Foods must be thawed in a manner that avoids placing the food in the hazard zone for an excessive amount of time. Frozen food should never be thawed at room temperature. Following are four options for thawing food safely:

- Thaw gradually under refrigeration that maintains the food temperature at 41°F or less.
- Thaw completely submerged under cold, potable, running water (70°F or less), with water pressure sufficient to continuously agitate any food particles off the surface. With this method, thawing time should be less than two hours, or until food reaches 41°F. This method may not be effective for thawing large pieces of meat.
- Thaw during the cooking process by cooking frozen food in the oven in a continuous process.
- Thaw and cook single-service items completely in the microwave from a frozen state and then cook immediately.

Food that is removed from the freezer to thaw gradually under refrigeration should be date-marked to indicate the date by which the food should be consumed. The food should be consumed seven days or less after the food was removed from the freezer and should be held at 41°F or below.

Slacking

Slacking is the process of moderating the temperature of frozen foods before preparation (such as deep-fat frying). For example, when deep-fat frying chicken nuggets that are at -10°F, maybe bring them up to 25°F first. Regulations about slacking PHF/TCS foods vary from one jurisdiction to another.

The FDA Food Code says that if slacking is used you should:

- Maintain the temperature of the food being slacked at or below 41°F, under refrigeration.
- Maintain the product at any temperature, as long as the product remains frozen.

Cooking

Cooking is a very important step in the flow of food. Failure to cook PHF/TCS food thoroughly can cause foodborne illness. Cooking food thoroughly destroys most (but not all) biological hazards.

For PHF/TCS foods, the FDA Food Code suggests cooking standards that combine time and temperature. An **endpoint temperature** is the temperature a food reaches at the end of cooking.

Endpoint temperature should be measured with a calibrated measuring device such as a thermometer or thermocouple. Measure in the part of the food that is heated last—usually the center or thickest part of the food. See Figure 19.9 for more tips on measuring temperatures.

Glossary

Endpoint Temperature
The temperature a food reaches at the end of cooking

Figure 19.9 Measuring a Food Temperature

Food Item

- Insert thermometer into geometric center or into thickest portion.
- Insert away from the bone, fat or gristle on a food product.
- Insert sideways into small items.

Food Packaging

- Fold bag over the thermometer or probe for bulk milk or liquids.
- Place between frozen packages of food.

General Guidelines

- Wait 5-10 seconds for an accurate reading.
- Sanitize thermometer after each use.
- Submerge until at least two inches deep in milk and other liquids.

In addition, the Food Code specifies that when measuring the temperature of thin foods, use a temperature measuring device (thermometer) with a suitable, small-diameter probe. Typically this is a **thermistor** or **thermocouple thermometer** rather than a **bi-metallic stem thermometer**. A bi-metallic stem thermometer needs to contact food all along its sensitive stem, often about three inches, in order to obtain a valid reading. In contrast, small, thin probes available with thermocouple or thermistor thermometers may capture an accurate reading with less contact surface.

After using a thermometer probe, always clean and sanitize it with an isopropyl alcohol wipe. The Food Code stipulates that a thermometer is like a utensil because it contacts food and therefore requires sanitization.

For any thermometer, calibration is also essential (see Figure 19.10). A thermometer used for measuring food temperatures should be accurate to ±2°F. Note that this is more rigorous than the calibration requirement for a thermometer used to measure ambient temperatures in storage areas.

Reaching a specified temperature alone is not adequate for ensuring destruction of pathogens. Cooks should be instructed to hold the endpoint temperature for a specified length of time, as shown in Figure 19.11. For mixed foods, such as casseroles and soups, find the ingredient with the most stringent time and temperature standard—and apply that standard.

Cooks should monitor and record cooking times and temperatures in a log, as shown in Figure 19.12. A downloadable version of the Endpoint Temperature Log is available in the online *Supplemental Textbook Material—Foodservice*.

Some PHF/TCS foods pose special concerns. Cooking pork and game animals is imperative to destroy possible parasites. Ground meats and seafood have an increased surface area resulting from grinding. This creates more opportunity for pathogens to flourish. Stuffed foods, such as ravioli or stuffed turkey, also provide favorable breeding ground for foodborne pathogens. The FDA time and temperature standards reflect these concerns.

Glossary

Bi-Metallic Stem Thermometer
A stem style thermometer made of two metals

Thermocouple or **Thermistor Thermometer**
A smaller, thin probe that gives an accurate reading with less contact surface

Figure 19.10 Calibrating a Bi-Metallic Thermometer—Slush Method

STEP 1	Fill an insulated container (like a foam cup) full of potable, crushed ice.
STEP 2	Add cold water and stir.
STEP 3	Allow time for the mixture to come to a 32°F temperature (about 4-5 minutes).
STEP 4	Insert a bi-metallic stemmed thermometer into the geothermal center of the cup (away from the bottom and sides).
STEP 5	Hold thermometer until the temperature stabilizes and record the temperature.
STEP 6	Repeat two times to verify the temperature reading.
STEP 7	If the temperature is not 32°F, use pliers on the calibration nut under the top of the thermometer to adjust the temperature to 32°F.

Figure 19.11 Cooking Time and Temperature Guide (Suggested Minimums)

FOOD ITEM	TEMP.	TIME	COMMENTS
All whole cuts of meat such as pork, steaks, roasts, and chops	145°F	15 sec.	Allow the meat to rest for three seconds before consuming.
Poultry, game, stuffed fish, stuffed meat and stuffed pasta	165°F	15 sec.	
Chopped or ground seafood or meat (includes ground beef, ground pork, veal, lamb, and mechanically tenderized meat)	155°F	15 sec.	
Fish, seafood, meats not listed above	145°F	15 sec.	
Eggs on steam table	155°F	15 sec.	Cooked to hold
Egg, single-serving	145°F	15 sec.	Cooked to order
Fruits and vegetables	135°F	No time standard	
Food cooked in microwave	165°F	Hold 2 min. after cooking	

Note: These are standards recommended in the 2013 FDA Food Code and the 2011 Update Bulletin. Please consult your local standards, which may be different. Also review manufacturers' instructions for processed foods.

Figure 19.12 Endpoint Temperature Log

Date: _____ Page #: _____ of _____

ITEM	TIME	TEMP.	COOK'S INITIALS	ENDPOINT ✔*

• Check to indicate that this was the endpoint of cooking.

New to the 2013 Food Code are greater controls for partially cooking a product with the expectation of fully cooking it at a later date or time. Cook-chill and Sous-vide systems are required to maintain a HACCP plan and record keeping system that can be provided to regulatory agencies. The use of par–cooked meats for finishing just prior to service on a room-service or cooked to order line or the practice of par-cooking foods such as large roasts must now establish and follow a written HACCP plan. The plan has to ensure that the stages of cooling, storage, reheating to 165°, cooling, and storage are completed within time and temperature parameters that adequately prevent pathogen survival and growth. They must also be clearly labeled so they are not accidently served to the client in a partially cooked state.

Highly Susceptible Populations

If serving a highly susceptible population, be aware that both eggs and juice receive special attention in the Food Code. Generally avoid using fresh, shell eggs for food preparation. Instead, use pasteurized egg products for quantity cooking. Pasteurized in-shell eggs are fine for both single-service and quantity production. (The use of shell eggs, pasteurized shell eggs and liquid eggs was discussed in Chapter 4.)

With the implementation of juice HACCP regulations in 2002, juices must be treated by the processor to control foodborne illness risks through a HACCP process (e.g., pasteurized). Juices made on site must use a HACCP plan for managing juice-related hazards. Note that juice, as defined in the Food Code, includes liquids, purees, or concentrates.

For highly susceptible populations, the Food Code cites the FDA and CDC health advisories to avoid eating fresh seed sprouts, such as mung bean or alfalfa sprouts. It also stipulates that raw or undercooked meats, such as raw, marinated fish, soft-cooked eggs, or rare meat may not be served. (In foodservice operations serving a general population, this may be permitted as long as the operation provides a consumer advisory about the associated risks.)

Due to the incident and impact of E. coli on young children, a children's menu may not list undercooked hamburger or other ground meat.

Putting It Into Practice

4. A foodservice employee is preparing French toast for a special brunch. He uses a spatula to transfer the egg-wash covered French toast to the griddle. He flips the French toast on the griddle and uses the same spatula to transfer the cooked French toast to the steamtable pan for service. Is this a concern and why or why not?

Microwave Cooking

When preparing food in a microwave:

- Rotate or stir the food item throughout or at the midpoint of cooking to distribute heat evenly.
- Cover to retain surface moisture.
- Cook to a temperature of at least 165°F in all parts of the food item.
- Allow to stand covered for two minutes before serving to obtain temperature equilibrium.

Serving Safe Food

During service, a combination of time and temperature is used to prevent or slow microbial growth. PHF/TCS foods must be held out of the hazard zone as much as possible, as shown in Figure 19.13.

Figure 19.14 illustrates examples of monitoring temperature during preparation and service.

Figure 19.13 Safe Food Handling: Food Preparation

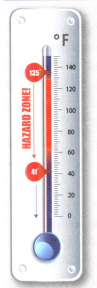

Above 135°F
Hold hot foods above 135°F to prevent growth of microorganisms. Cook food to recommended time/temperature standards to destroy microorganisms.

41°F -135°F
Hazard Zone

Below 41°F
Hold cold food below 41°F to slow bacterial growth and extend shelf life.

Figure 19.14 Monitoring Temperatures During Preparation and Service

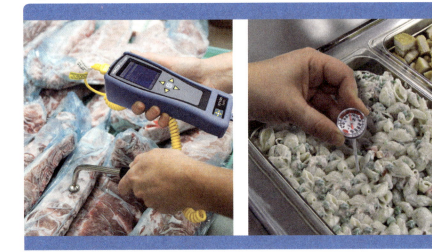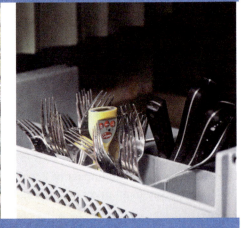

Images courtesy of Cooper-Atkins

A log (Figure 19.15) can help employees monitor and document holding temperatures, which should be measured at least every two hours.

Figure 19.15 Holding Temperature Log

Date: _____ Page #: _____ of _____

ITEM	TIME	TEMP.	COOK'S INITIALS	CORRECTIVE ACTION

Keep food out of the Hazard Zone: Hold cold foods below 41°F. Hold hot foods above 135°F.

Hot Holding

Hot foods must be held at 135°F or above, with the exception of roasts cooked to a time and temperature shown in Figure 19.11. Stir foods during holding to redistribute heat throughout the food product. Keep food containers covered to retain heat and to prevent environmental contaminants from entering the food.

Steam tables and food warmers are examples of equipment that may be used to retain heat and control food temperatures. Steam tables are not meant to cook foods—only to hold them after cooking. Food warmers (also called "hot-box") are usually equipped with an ambient thermometer. Steam tables usually have a temperature control knob but generally do not measure the actual food temperature. When holding hot foods for service, measure the food temperature at least every two hours. If the food temperature falls into an unsafe range, immediately follow procedures for reheating previously cooked food. When re-stocking hot food products, finish one pan before bringing in a refill; do not pour new product on top of older product.

Cold Holding

Cold food must be held below 41°F. Holding food below this temperature slows the growth of bacteria. Special considerations are required for using ice as a coolant. Packaged food may not be stored in direct contact with ice or water if the entry of water is possible due to the nature of the packaging or its positioning in the ice or water. Ice that has been used as a coolant may not be used as a food or food ingredient. Unpackaged food may not be stored in direct contact with undrained ice, with these exceptions:

- Whole, raw fruits or vegetables—such as celery or carrot sticks or whole potatoes— may be immersed in ice or water.
- Raw chicken and raw fish that are received immersed in ice in shipping containers may remain in that condition while in storage awaiting preparation or service.

During holding and service, utensils should be kept in the food. Utensil handles should be kept above the top of the food and the container. Between uses, a utensil can be stored in water that is at least 135°F. During service, food on display must be protected from contamination. During transport, food items must be maintained out of the hazard zone and food must be covered to prevent contamination.

Self-Service Food Bars

Self-service food bars, such as buffets and salad bars, present special food protection risks. Client actions and habits create the potential for contamination. Label all food items in self-service areas to discourage clients from sampling food items. Sneeze guards must be used on service lines, salad bars, and display cases. Self-service food bars should be monitored by dining services employees trained in food protection practices. Clients are required to use a clean plate for each service from a food bar to prevent contamination from soiled dishes and utensils.

Ready-to-Eat Foods

The FDA Food Code has specific guidelines for serving ready-to-eat food that is edible without additional preparation to achieve food safety such as bakery items (breads, rolls, cakes, pies), fruits and vegetables that are served raw, or dried meat products such as jerky or beef sticks. Self-service of these foods must include utensils or effective dispensing methods that protect the food from contamination.

Cooling

Large food masses such as roasts, turkeys, and large containers of rice, refried beans, or soup/stews take longer to cool because of the mass of food. According to the FDA Food Code, PHF/TCS food should be cooled from 135°F to 41°F within a total maximum time of six hours. The first step of this process must get food down to 70°F within the first two hours.

If food starts at room temperature, such as canned tuna, cool it down to 41°F within a maximum total time of four hours. Figure 19.16 identifies methods for speeding the cooling process. Once cooled, food should be covered, dated, and labeled according to date marking standards.

Figure 19.16 Proper Cooling Methods

- Place food in a shallow container (2" deep) to increase surface area and reduce cooling time.
- Divide a large food mass into several smaller masses (e.g., a 20 lb. roast into five 4 lb. pieces).
- Stir the food in a container placed in an ice water bath.
- Use rapid cooling equipment such as a blast chiller.
- Add ice as an ingredient.

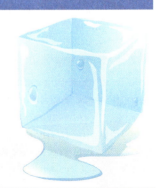

Date Marking

PHF/TCS food prepared in the food production operation and held at or below 41°F should be labeled at the time of preparation with the date by which the food should be consumed. Prepared foods should be used within seven days or less of preparation if held at 41°F or below.

The practice of date marking is detailed in the FDA Food Code. When a date is marked on a food product, it indicates the date by which the product must be used or discarded. A key objective of this practice is to address the time element of bacterial growth. The longer a PHF/TCS food remains in storage, the more opportunity Listeria bacteria have to grow—and they can do so even at or below 41°F.

Date marking applies not only to leftovers. Generally, after opening a package of PHF/TCS food it must be date marked as well. It should be used or discarded it within seven days, counting the day the package was opened as Day 1.

Certain products, such as hard cheeses or cheeses that contain up to 50% moisture (e.g., cheddar, Parmesan, gorgonzola, jack), yogurt, sour cream, buttermilk, and certain shelf-stable processed meat products are exempt from date-marking procedures. Date-marking guidelines also do not apply to deli salads obtained from a food processing plant, because they apply processes to prevent bacterial growth. Instead, refer to the manufacturer's use-by date. Remember that if PHF/TCS food in storage is not maintained at or below 41°F, it should still be discarded.

Reheating

Frozen, ready-to-eat food taken from a commercially prepared, intact package must be heated to at least 135°F for hot holding. Reheating for hot holding should be done as rapidly as possible.

A previously cooked food (a food that was prepared, cooked, and cooled in the food production operation) must be reheated to an internal temperature of 165°F for a minimum of 15 seconds. This process must be completed within two hours.

Reservice of food is also governed by the FDA Food Code. Food that is unused or returned by the client may not be offered to others. If the food is individually packaged, such as crackers, salt, pepper, or sugar packets, it may be reserved if the packaging is in sound condition. No food, including secure packets, may be reserved if it is returned from clients in medical isolation or quarantine.

Summary

Referring to the conditions for growth of pathogens, FOTTWA, it is clear that a Certified Dietary Manager has many opportunities to ensure food safety in the process of food production, continuing through service and management of leftovers. In all, time and temperature are critical factors for making food safe.

HACCP Basics

Hazard Analysis Critical Control Point (HACCP) is an important development in food protection. The HACCP system is a preventative food safety program that greatly reduces the likelihood of foodborne illness. HACCP (pronounced has-sip) was developed years ago to ensure a safe food supply for astronauts. It is now being implemented throughout the food processing and service industries.

HACCP uses a systematic approach to identify, evaluate, and control food safety hazards. It focuses on the flow of food rather than on individual procedures. A Certified Dietary Manager who uses HACCP principles in combination with basic sanitation and a solid employee training program can prevent, eliminate or reduce the occurrence of foodborne illness in his/her facility.

Glossary

HACCP
Hazard Analysis Critical Control Point

Putting It Into Practice

5. You observe a foodservice staff member replenishing chili on the steam table. She carefully records the temperature. Then she adds fresh chili to the batch in the steamtable being careful to thoroughly stir the two batches together. Is this a concern? Why or why not?

HACCP builds on essential food safety practices that should already be in place. These are called standard operating procedures (SOPs). They include the sanitation guidelines outlined in the FDA Food Code and discussed in other chapters of this book—such as practices for:

- Purchasing, receiving and storing food
- Personal hygiene policies
- Procedures for thawing, cooking, holding, and cooling food
- Procedures for cleaning and sanitizing

They are prerequisites for implementing an effective plan. Without them, any HACCP plan may fail.

Although using HACCP is not directly part of the Food Code, the FDA recommends implementing this procedure throughout the food industry. HACCP plans may be required in food production operations processing juice in-house, preparing pureed food, or operating a cook-chill system. Furthermore, school foodservice operations participating in the National School Lunch program are required to have HACCP plans. The local health department may require implementation of a HACCP system.

The success of HACCP is dependent on a number of variables. Certified Dietary Managers learn the principles and concepts and demonstrate their ability to effectively organize a HACCP system by applying their knowledge. In turn, it is essential that the managers educate and train all members of their food production and dining services team on the principles of HACCP and their role in its implementation.

Implementing a HACCP System

A HACCP system revolves around seven principles, summarized in Figure 19.17.

Figure 19.17 Seven Principles of HACCP

1	Analyze hazards.
2	Identify critical control points (CCPs).
3	Establish critical limits for critical control points (CCPs).
4	Establish procedures for monitoring critical control points (CCPs).
5	Establish corrective actions.
6	Establish a record-keeping system.
7	Establish procedures to verify that the system is working.

1. Analyze Hazards

Identify hazards associated with foods in recipes and on menus. These items could be hazardous due to ingredients, the processes involved in preparation, how the product is held or handled during service, or its ultimate use. Hazards may vary from one food production operation to another—even with the production of the same menu item. Differences include:

- Ingredient sources
- Product formulations
- Processing or packaging techniques
- Preparation methods and equipment
- Storage and service plans
- Who will be consuming the food
- Employees' understanding of safe food practices.

Figure 19.18 lists some questions to ask when deciding what hazards are present.

While HACCP is concerned with the safety of all food, particular attention should be given to PHF/TCS foods. These foods can support progressive bacterial growth or development of toxins. It's also important to examine the flow of food through the food production system. As you track each PHF/TCS food, where are the hazards? Where could dangerous microorganisms have an opportunity to grow? Developing a flow chart or diagram of food movement can help identify hazards and control points.

2. Identify Critical Control Points

Points in the flow of food at which a potential hazard can be controlled or eliminated are called **control points**. Control points occur throughout the flow of food, such as during receiving, storage, thawing, cooking, holding, and chilling, and are generally addressed through standard operating procedures. For each control point, ask this question: Could loss of control here lead to an unacceptable health risk? If so, it's called a **critical control point (CCP)**. To determine whether a step is a CCP, refer to the CCP Decision Tree (Figure 19.19). Critical control points vary depending on the food item being prepared and the preparation techniques being used. Often, cooking to recommended time and temperature standard becomes a CCP. However, in a cook-chill operation, blast chilling food to a recommended temperature within a specified time is also a CCP.

Following the CCP Decision Tree, there is generally only one CCP for any food or menu item. However, advice varies: some HACCP examples include only one step in the flow of food and designated as a CCP while in other models there are several. Whether one or several, CCPs are designated for any given recipe is not an issue, either way, you are implementing critical control. However, beware of designating too many steps as CCPs. This can make the system too complex for employees to carry out. Instead, review the standard operating procedures and use them as control points (not CCPs with documentation requirements) as appropriate.

3. Establish Critical Limits for Critical Control Points

There must be a **critical limit** for each CCP identified. A critical limit defines the limits of certain properties that are accepted for a given product at a given stage in the flow of food. It is observable and measurable. For a cooked food, a critical limit might specify minimum internal temperature for the endpoint of cooking, along with the minimum time that temperature must be held. The standards used for critical limits should come from the local food code, the FDA Food Code, or a similar guideline.

Putting It Into Practice

6. How would you cool the following products:
   1. Chicken salad made from canned chicken
   2. Beef stew

Figure 19.18 Analyzing Hazards: Questions to Ask

Q Does the food contain any sensitive ingredients that may present known hazards (e.g., Salmonella, Staphylococcus, aflatoxin)?

Q What are the sources (e.g., geographical region, specific supplier)?

Q Does the process include a controllable processing step that destroys pathogens? If so, which pathogens?

Q Does the microbial population change during the normal time the food is stored prior to consumption?

Q Does the layout of the facility provide an adequate separation of raw materials from ready-to-eat (RTE) foods if this is important to food safety? If not, what hazards should be considered as possible contaminants of the RTE products?

Q Will the equipment provide the time-temperature control that is necessary for safe food?

Q Is the equipment properly sized for the volume of food that will be processed?

Q Can the equipment be sufficiently controlled so that the variation in performance will be within the tolerances required to produce a safe food?

Q Is the equipment reliable or is it prone to frequent breakdowns?

Q Is the equipment designed so that it can be easily cleaned and sanitized?

Q To what degree will normal equipment wear affect the likely occurrence of physical hazard (e.g., metal) in the product?

Q Is the package clearly labeled "Keep Refrigerated" if this is required for safety? Does the package include instructions for the safe handling and preparation of the food by the end user?

Q Is each package and case legibly and accurately coded? Does each package contain the proper label?

Q Can employee health or personal hygiene practices impact the safety of the food being processed?

Q Do the employees understand the process and the factors they must control to assure the preparation of safe foods?

Q Will the employees inform management of a problem which could impact safety of food?

Q What is the likelihood that the food will be improperly stored at the wrong temperature?

Q Would an error in improper storage lead to a microbiologically unsafe food?

Q Will the food be heated by the consumer?

Q Will there likely be leftovers?

Q Is the food intended for the general public?

Q Is the food intended for consumption by a population with increased susceptibility to illness (e.g., infants, the aged, or immunocompromised individuals)?

Source: FDA

Figure 19.19 CCP Decision Tree

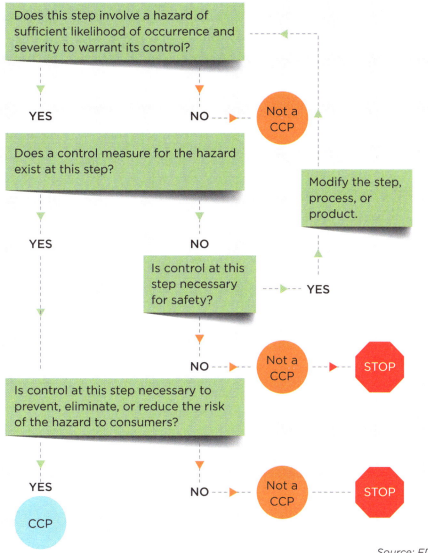

Source: FDA

4. Establish Procedures for Monitoring CCPs

Determine how and by whom CCPs will be monitored. **Monitoring** procedures may be included in standardized recipes. Observe and measure to determine whether critical limits are met. Critical limits may also be included in recipes and food production personnel should be required to measure all CCPs and document them in HACCP logs (such as the Cooking Temperature Log in Chapter 18).

5. Establish Corrective Actions

When monitoring shows that a critical limit has not been met, there must be an established procedure to follow. These procedures, called **corrective actions**, are specific to each food production operation. Corrective actions should be clearly written and understood by food production personnel. For example, when baking meatloaf (a CCP), the critical limit is to reach 155°F for a minimum of 15 seconds. You check the temperature in the deepest part of the meatloaf at the end of cooking and it's only 140°F. A corrective action might be to return the meatloaf to the oven immediately and continue

Glossary

Monitoring
Checking that a processing or handling procedure does not exceed the established critical limit at each critical control point.

Putting It Into Practice

7. You are preparing leftover rice for storage. If the rice was prepared on January 9, what would you put on the label?

cooking to reach 155°F for 15 seconds. Other examples of corrective actions might be: contacting the Certified Dietary Manager for direction, reheating immediately to a specific temperature, or disposing of food that was improperly cooked.

6. Establish a Record-Keeping System

A record-keeping system documents HACCP activities and includes time and temperature monitoring records. Use forms to document the flow of food products, time and temperature, and corrective actions. Maintain daily HACCP logs in a notebook accessible to all members of the food production team. The HACCP log may identify critical limits to check and include a place for employees to document corrective actions taken. Be alert to **dry lab**, the practice of entering time and temperature measurements without actually taking them. Dry lab will undermine the success of any HACCP program.

7. Verify the System Is Working

Calibration of temperature monitoring devices and review of HACCP logs for accuracy and completeness will help to verify the system is fulfilling its mission to improve food safety. Review HACCP logs, records of monitoring CCPs, and corrective actions taken by staff members. Conduct random checks to ensure that CCPs are being monitored appropriately by staff and that temperature monitoring equipment is working properly. Figure 19.20 lists some activities a manager may use in the **verification** process.

Figure 19.20 HACCP Verification Activities

- Establish of appropriate verification schedules
- Review of the HACCP plan for completeness
- Confirmation of the accuracy of the flow diagram
- Review of the HACCP system to determine if the facility is operating according to the HACCP plan
- Review of CCP monitoring records
- Review of records for deviations and corrective actions
- Validation of critical limits to confirm that they are adequate to control significant hazards
- Validation of HACCP plan, including on-site review
- Review of modifications of the HACCP plan
- Sampling and testing to verify CCPs

Source: FDA

HACCP and Planning

When analyzing HACCP records, look for patterns that indicate a need for employee training, equipment repair or replacement. Sometimes HACCP information will indicate a need to change kitchen layout, menus, ingredient selection, preparation methods, processes, or procedures. These records can provide a valuable tool for planning and refining a safe food production system. Consider the flow of food, and update the HACCP plan as changes are made.

Glossary

Corrective Actions
The procedure to follow when monitoring shows that a critical limit has not been met

Dry Lab
Recording temperatures without actually taking them

Verification
The use of equipment to determine that the HACCP system is in place and achieving the desired objectives

Putting It Into Practice

8. In a traditional baked chicken breast recipe, what would the critical control point(s) be?

For example, HACCP logs may indicate that it is difficult to meet cooling recommendations for tuna salad. Upon review of the flow of food for tuna and mayonnaise, you realize that food preparation is starting with ingredients at room temperature. Corrective Action: Change the procedure and pre-chill potentially hazardous ingredients.

In another example, when reviewing the plans to re-design the kitchen, map out the flow of food for key menu items. The current layout presents opportunities for contamination that could be avoided: The trash room occasionally overflows into an area where fresh meats are received and food waste from dining service is being processed very close to the cold food preparation area. Corrective Action: Work with an architect to specify that food receiving and preparation areas must be isolated from sources of contamination.

In another example, observations highlight the hazard associated with cross-contamination. Corrective Action: Use color-coded cutting boards to reinforce safe practices among employees.

The Process Approach to HACCP

In a food production operation, HACCP may take a different form than in a food processing or packaging environment. The FDA explains "The resources available to help you identify and control risk factors common to your operation may be limited." The report advises that a "complete HACCP system" is ideal, but variations are acceptable, as long as the plan is designed to control risks and incorporate "some, if not all" of the HACCP principles. Because each set of procedures for production and service is different, "HACCP has no single correct application," according to the FDA.

In a process approach, assign sets of food flow charts to process-related categories and manage them as groups. See Figure 19.21 for examples. The FDA suggests three types of processes:

- **Process 1:** Food preparation with no cook step, where the flow of food is: receive > store > prepare > hold > serve. Examples: salads, cold sandwiches.
- **Process 2:** Preparation for same-day service, where the flow of food is: receive > store > prepare > cook > hold > serve. Examples: baked chicken, meatloaf.
- **Process 3:** Complex food preparation, where the flow of food is: receive > store > prepare > cook > cool > reheat > hot hold > serve. Examples: casseroles in which meats or other ingredients are cooked and cooled the day before assembly, or leftovers that are reheated and served at another meal.

There can be variations in these processes, but they characterize the foodborne illness risks fairly well; examples of the risks are outlined in the FDA Annex. Process 3 includes at least two trips through the hazard zone, so it carries the greatest risks. It clearly requires carefully managed temperature control, especially in cooling and reheating steps. Date marking and storage are also important.

Target food-flow steps involving the hazard zone and apply controls to manage the hazards in all processes. For Process 1, where there is no cooking to destroy potential pathogens, controls focus more on purchasing specifications, receiving check-in, date marking, and storage time and temperature. For Process 2, cooking (endpoint temperatures) and holding will require your most active managerial control.

Putting It Into Practice

9. What is the best way to train staff on HACCP plans?

Figure 19.21 Process Examples

PROCESS 1: No Cook | Example: Fruit Salad

	Receive	Control measures: known source, receiving temperatures
	Store	Control measures: proper storage temperatures, prevent cross-contamination, store away from chemicals
	Prepare	Control measures: personal hygiene, restrict ill employees, prevent cross-contamination
	CCP: Cold Holding	Critical limit: hold at 41° or below,* Check and record temperatures
	Serve	Control measures: no bare hand contact with ready-to-eat food, personal hygiene, restrict ill employees

PROCESS 2: Same-Day Service | Example: Baked Chicken

	Receive	Control measures: known source, receiving temperatures
	Store	Control measures: proper storage temperatures, prevent cross-contamination, store away from chemicals
	Prepare	Control measures: personal hygiene, restrict ill employees, prevent cross-contamination
	CCP: Cook	Critical limit: internal temperature of 165°F for 15 seconds.* Check and record temperatures
	CCP: Hot Hold	Critical limit: hold at no less than 135°F. Check and record temperatures
	Serve	Control measures: no bare hand contact with ready-to-eat food, personal hygiene, restrict ill employees

PROCESS 3: Complex Food Preparation | Example: Beef and Bean Tamale Pie

	Receive	Control measures: known source, receiving temperatures
	Store	Control measures: proper storage temperatures, prevent cross-contamination, store away from chemicals
	Prepare	Control measures: personal hygiene, restrict ill employees, prevent cross-contamination
	CCP: Cook	Critical limit: Cook to 165°F for at least 15 seconds.* Check and record temperatures
	CCP: Cool	Critical limit: Cool to 70°F within two hours and from 70°F to 41°F or lower within an additional four hours.* Check and record temperatures
	CCP: Reheat	Critical limit: heat to 165°F for at least 15 seconds.* Check and record temperatures
	CCP: Hot Hold	Critical limit: Hold for hot service at 135°F or higher.* Check and record temperatures
	Serve	Control measures: no bare hand contact with ready-to-eat food, personal hygiene, restrict ill employees

Thermometer icon means that taking a temperature is necessary; Clipboard icon means recording data is necessary.

*Accessed May 2015 in 2013 FDA Food Code. Source: USDA. Guidance for School Food Authorities: Developing a School Food Safety Program Based on the Process Approach to HACCP Principles, 2005.

Figure 19.22 Examples of Hazards and Control

MEASURES FOR SAME-DAY SERVICE ITEMS

Process 2: Preparation for Same-Day Service

Example Products:	Baked Meatloaf	Baked Chicken
Biological Hazards	Salmonella spp.	Salmonella spp.
	E. coli O157:H7	Campylobacter
	Clostridium perfringens	Clostridium perfringens
	Bacillus cereus	Bacillus cereus
	Various fecal-oral route pathogens	Various fecal-oral route pathogens
Control Measures	Refrigeration at 41°F or below	Refrigeration at 41°F or below
	Cooking at 155°F for 15 seconds	Cooking at 165°F for 15 seconds
	Holding at 135°F or above OR time control	Holding at 135°F or above OR time control
	Good personal hygiene (no bare hand contact with ready-to-eat (RTE) food, proper hand-washing, exclusion/restriction of ill employees)	Good personal hygiene (no bare hand contact with ready-to-eat (RTE) food, proper hand-washing, exclusion/restriction of ill employees)

Source: Accessed in 2015 from the 2013 FDA Food Code, page 575

Processes may also emerge for menu items. A chicken salad sandwich, for example, may include elements of Process 3 (receive, store, prepare, cook, cool) and Process 1 (store, prepare, hold, serve). Figure 19.22 illustrates examples of hazards and controls for foods prepared for same-day service.

If foods are grouped according to their flow in the operation, mapping out a flow for each individual menu item is not required, says the FDA, adding that "a hazard analysis on individual food items is time and labor intensive and generally unnecessary." Managing the steps in a process as a SOP "achieves the same control of risk factors as preparing a HACCP plan for each individual product," suggests the report.

Summary

HACCP is a proactive method for managing food safety. It allows a Certified Dietary Manager to focus resources where they are needed most, at critical control points (CCPs) in the flow of food. Although not specifically required for most food production and dining services operations today, HACCP is a great idea because it is an effective management tool for control. HACCP builds upon standard operating procedures. It requires documentation and monitoring. In food production, it is not necessary to create a detailed HACCP flow chart for every food in order to implement the HACCP concepts. Instead, a manager can group foods according to the types of preparation processes used.

NOTE: Detailed information on food safety and foodborne illness is covered through the food handler certification programs, for example ServSafe®. Check with state and local requirements for specific requirements regarding food handler certification or food handler cards.

Safe Food Handling: The Physical Plant

Overview and Objectives

The 2013 FDA Food Code uses the term "active managerial control" to describe a dining services facility's responsibility for developing and implementing controls to "prevent, eliminate, or reduce the occurrence of foodborne illness risk factors." This chapter outlines the active managerial control for regulations, employees, physical facilities, equipment maintenance and environmental controls. After completing this chapter, you should be able to:

✓ Identify federal safety laws/regulations for a facility

✓ Conduct routine maintenance inspections of equipment and correct problems identified

✓ Manage a preventive maintenance program and manufacturer guidelines for equipment maintenance

✓ Prepare a safety inspection checklist and inspection report of hazards

✓ Identify appropriate environmental controls for water supply, waste disposal and ventilation

✓ Assure cleaning and sanitation of equipment and utensils

✓ Follow an integrated pest management (IPM) system

✓ Organize equipment workflow for use, placement and access to supplies, hand sinks and lavatory facilities

 Section **A** Manage Regulations and Crisis

Federal Safety Laws and Regulations

Regulatory inspections are part of everyday life in food production and dining services facilities. Regarding sanitation, regulatory inspections will be assessing the control over the foodborne illness risk factors. The FDA lists the elements of an effective food safety management system in the 2013 Annex. It includes principles for protecting food products throughout the flow in a food production facility. The elements also include the following:

1. Certified food protection managers who have shown a proficiency in required information by passing a test that is part of an accredited program

2. Standard operating procedures (SOPs) for performing critical operational steps in a food preparation process

3. Equipment and facility design and maintenance

4. Record keeping

5. Manager and employee training

6. Ongoing quality control and assurance

Food production and dining services operations must comply with many local, state, and federal regulations. Each of the elements above are required for some state and federal regulations. Not all guidelines are always required because each state may interpret federal laws differently.

Regulations

Each of the three branches of the government is involved in protecting the safety of the food supply and public health. See Figure 20.1 for an explanation of each. Congress and the Senate comprise the legislative branch and they pass laws regarding food handling and protection. Agencies like the FDA, within the executive branch of the government, develop regulations to implement the laws. The judicial branch reviews the policies and procedures of regulatory agencies to protect the rights of both private businesses and the public. Laws usually state broad objectives and need to be interpreted. Regulations are more specific and give guidance on how to comply with the law. Several regulations may be necessary to implement one law.

A food production and dining services operation may be required to comply with a number of different laws and regulations regarding safety and sanitation. Laws and regulations addressing food protection are present at the federal, state and local level. It is important for the Certified Dietary Manager to learn about standards and expectations of different regulatory agencies and to develop policies and procedures to achieve compliance. Local laws may be stricter than state laws. In this case, the dining services operator must comply with the most stringent standard. When in doubt, the Certified Dietary Manager should consult a representative of the regulatory agency or their administrator to review the regulations.

Local or Municipal Laws and Regulations

Depending on the size of the community and the number of dining operations it has, the county or municipal government may have a department of health or food protection that enforces local laws.

State Laws and Regulations

All states have a department charged with protecting the safety of food produced, served, and transported in the state. The office may be within the department of public health or the department of agriculture.

Federal Laws and Regulations

Federal laws and regulations exist to protect food safety by requiring inspection, controlling food additives, and regulating the transport of food across state borders.

FDA Food Code

The FDA Food Code is a framework upon which an effective retail food safety program can be built. Today, the FDA's purpose in maintaining an updated model food code is to assist food control jurisdictions at all levels of government by providing them with a scientifically sound technical and legal basis for regulating the retail segment of the food industry. The retail segment includes those establishments or locations in the food distribution chain where the consumer takes possession of the food.

Figure 20.1 Regulatory Agencies and Resources

FOOD AND DRUG ADMINISTRATION (FDA)

The FDA, an agency of the Department of Health and Human Services Public Health Service, is responsible for ensuring the safety and wholesomeness of all foods sold in interstate commerce except for meat, poultry and eggs, all of which are under USDA jurisdiction. FDA develops standards for the composition, quality, nutrition, and safety of foods. It collects and interprets data on nutrition, food additives, and environmental factors, such as pesticides, that affect foods. FDA also sets standards for certain foods and enforces federal regulations for labeling, food and color additives, food sanitation, and safety of foods. FDA monitors recalls of unsafe or contaminated foods and can seize illegally marketed foods.

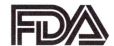

DEPARTMENT OF AGRICULTURE (USDA)

Through inspection and grading, the USDA enforces standards for wholesomeness and quality of meat, poultry, and eggs produced in the United States. USDA food safety activities include inspecting poultry, eggs, domestic and imported meat, and inspecting livestock and production plants. The USDA is also responsible for making quality (grading) inspections for grain, fruits, vegetables, meat, poultry, and dairy products (including cheeses). The USDA's education programs target family nutritional needs, food safety, and expanding scientific knowledge.

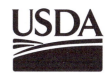

CENTERS FOR DISEASE CONTROL AND PREVENTION (CDC)

An agency of the Department of Health and Human Services, CDC becomes involved as a protector of food safety—including responding to emergencies when foodborne illnesses arise. It directs and enforces quarantines while administrating national programs for prevention and control of vector-borne diseases (diseases transmitted by a host organism) and other preventable conditions. It maintains statistics on foodborne illnesses.

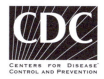

NATIONAL MARINE FISHERIES SERVICE (NMFS)

A part of the Department of Commerce, NMFS is responsible for seafood quality and identification, fisheries management, habitat conservation, and aquaculture production. NMFS has a voluntary inspection program for fish products. Its guidelines closely match regulations for which FDA has enforcement authority.

DEPARTMENT OF HEALTH & HUMAN SERVICES, CENTERS FOR MEDICARE & MEDICAID (CMS)

Provides guidance to surveyors for regulatory tags that include F tag 371 §483.35(i)—Sanitary Conditions, and the requirement at 42 CFR 483.65(b) (2) regarding preventing the spread of infection. Even if you are surveyed by CMS, you will also have to follow your local and state sanitation regulations.

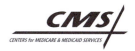

LOCAL GOVERNMENTS

State and local government agencies cooperate with the federal government to ensure the quality and safety of food produced within their jurisdictions. FDA and other federal agencies help state and local governments develop uniform food safety standards and regulations and assist them with research and information. States inspect restaurants, retail food establishments, dairies, grain mills, and other food establishments within their borders. In many instances, they can embargo illegal food products, which gives them authority over fish, including shellfish, taken from their waters. FDA provides guidelines to the states for this regulation. Many states have their own fish inspection programs. The FDA also provides guidelines for state and local governments for regulation of dairy products and restaurant foods.

The Food Code is neither federal law nor federal regulation and it does not replace local regulations. Rather, it represents FDA's best advice for a uniform system of regulation to ensure that retail food is safe and properly protected and presented. Although not federal requirements (until adopted by federal bodies for use within federal jurisdictions), Food Code provisions are designed to be consistent with federal food laws and regulations, and are written for ease of legal adoption at all levels of government.

The most current FDA Food Code recommendations may or may not apply in the particular jurisdiction, so it is important to become familiar with all sanitation regulations that apply to the facility.

Inspections

One way agencies and governments assess compliance with regulations is through the inspection process. The FDA recommends that food production and dining service operations be inspected once every six months. An inspection often begins with an inspector or sanitarian identifying him or herself and presenting the appropriate identification. *If an inspector does not present identification, be sure to ask for it.* In most cases inspections are unannounced. In some areas of the country, inspections only occur in response to complaints. In other areas, routine inspections can be expected by every food operation. Some operations may be inspected by several different agencies.

Inspection Process

When interacting with inspectors or surveyors, remember to show professional courtesy. The manager or senior supervisor on duty should accompany the inspector during the visit to answer questions that the inspector may have. It is appropriate to ask the inspector questions if you do not understand a regulation or violation. The key to success with inspections is to view them as a resource and not a hindrance. Inspectors are well trained in the area of food protection and are a source of valuable information.

Areas that an inspector will probably address include such areas as:

- Food purchasing practices, including use of approved sources and potable water.
- Food storage practices, including the cleanliness and temperature of food storage areas, indication that proper stock rotation methods (FIFO) are being used, labeling and dating practices for food products, protection of food in storage from cross-contamination, and proper storage of chemicals away from food preparation areas, in clearly marked containers.
- Food preparation and service practices, including the thawing, cooking, holding, transporting, serving, cooling, and reheating of food. The inspector may want to review temperature logs, measure temperatures, review date-marking procedures, and observe staff work habits.
- Personal hygiene of employees, including the cleanliness of staff, use of disposable gloves and utensils to avoid hand contact with food, presence of any staff with reportable symptoms or illnesses, and accessibility and use of handwashing sinks and supplies. The inspector may interview staff about work habits and practices. See *Management in the News in the online Supplemental Textbook Material— Foodservice.*
- Cleaning and sanitization practices, including manual and mechanical warewashing practices, proper dilution of chemical sanitizers, and proper water temperature. The inspector will tour the premises and inspect equipment to determine overall cleanliness. The inspector may request a copy of cleaning schedules.

- The inspector will likely evaluate the facilities, including safe water supply, proper sewage disposal and backflow prevention with air gap or approved device, absence of pest infestation, and pest control methods and techniques employed.

While the FDA Food Code provides a sample risk-based inspection form and guidelines, the form and criteria used locally may vary. Have food temperature logs and staff training records available for the inspector. Some facilities are required to have a manager certified in dining services sanitation on the premises at all times. Be sure that the proper records and evidence of certification are available and current.

An inspector who discovers minor infractions will establish a deadline for correction. Correct violations immediately—if possible, even before the inspector leaves the premises. The inspector may note that the correction has been made and remove the violation from his/her evaluation prior to leaving the facility. Take notes during inspection. The notes will help make any necessary improvements and are a resource to prepare for future inspections. A health inspector can serve as a resource, too. If there is anything you don't understand—ask.

If a serious problem or imminent health hazard is noticed, the inspector may order the facility to close immediately. A food production and dining services operation that fails to correct problems by established deadlines risks fines and loss of the permit to operate.

HACCP-Based Inspections

Some local health departments have changed their inspection process to one based on HACCP principles. Instead of traditional inspections that focus on the observed food operation, a HACCP-based inspection focuses on the flow of food. This style of inspection is more likely in a production kitchen or a location with satellite service of prepared food sent to a remote dining service (i.e. a pre-plated cook-chill service). The inspector will review HACCP logs during the visit allowing the inspector to inspect food safety practices over a long period of time rather than just on the day of the inspection.

Inspection Preparation

An inspector will usually leave a written report that notes areas for improvement and any violations. Study the written report to identify why violations occurred and to develop an action plan to avoid having the same violation occur a second time. To improve compliance during inspections, follow these guidelines:

- Plan and Prepare: Obtain a copy of applicable regulations and review them in advance. For questions about the regulations, contact the regulatory agency that enforces them. Develop policies and work practices that comply with the guidelines.

- Use Self-Inspection: Conduct routine self-inspections to identify issues before they become a problem. Ask an inspector for blank inspection reports or create self-inspection forms specifically for the dining services operation. Several examples of self-inspection forms are included in this textbook. Correct problems that are discovered during self-inspections.

- Network: Through professional organizations, discuss regulations and compliance issues with peers. Identify common strategies and resources.

- Train and Educate Staff: Train all staff members in safe food preparation practices and regulations applicable to their own jobs.

Putting It Into Practice

1. List some steps to prepare your staff for a sanitation inspection.

Emergency or Disaster Preparedness

A disaster is a sudden change, often an unstable condition, that requires decisive action to be taken. Often an emergency endangers the health of a client or employee, or it threatens the safety and security of the dining services operation. A disaster can occur in any type of dining services operation. Some examples of crisis situations are:

- Fire
- Flood
- Tornado or hurricane
- Utility (water or gas) loss
- Delivery driver strike
- Food tampering by client or employee
- Sudden illness of an employee or client
- Workplace violence
- Bomb threat
- Robbery or theft
- Vandalism
- Act of terrorism
- Foodborne illness outbreak

Emergency Plan

Imagine being the Certified Dietary Manager of a dining services operation that has been flooded and is without utilities. What if the dining services operation were at a hospital, nursing home or other facility where the expectation is to continue providing meals? How can this work? How could you be sure that the food being served is safe? To handle such a situation properly, it is necessary to plan in advance. Anticipate the type of crisis situations that your operation might face and develop a plan of action. Examples of advance planning and preparation for crisis situations are:

- A nursing home maintains a supply of bottled water and a one-week supply of disposable dishes for use in the event the water supply becomes contaminated or water service is lost.
- A correctional facility maintains an emergency menu and food supply for use in case power is lost or weather prohibits delivery of food.
- A fire evacuation plan is established for a fine dining restaurant and employees are trained in the use of fire extinguishers.
- Employees at a hotel are trained in procedures to follow if they receive a bomb threat, such as what to listen for and what to ask the caller.
- A hospital has an agreement with a regional food supplier to provide a refrigerated truck.
- A fast food restaurant has an established procedure to follow if they receive a complaint about foodborne illness.
- Emergency phone numbers for police, fire, and medical personnel are posted by each telephone in a college dining hall.
- Employees of a correctional facility are trained in non-violent intervention techniques.
- A resort maintains a crisis management manual with procedures to follow in the event of most emergency situations.

Putting It Into Practice

2. What principles of purchasing must you keep in mind even if you are in a crisis?

A Certified Dietary Manager should always have a written plan about how to feed clients in an emergency. Food preparation in situations where power is lost or food deliveries are impossible may require a pre-planned menu that includes foods that do not require cooking, such as peanut butter sandwiches, fresh or canned fruit, and similar items. In creating a plan, consider what supplies are likely to be on hand, how to handle a severe staffing shortage if employees cannot get to work, and whether the operation will feed extra people. In some healthcare facilities, an emergency staffing plan may include drawing on employees from other non-client care departments. Staff need to be aware of the emergency plan so they will be ready to activate it at any time.

> A hurricane preparedness plan is a standard when working at a large hospital in Jackson, Mississippi. There was no plan for the three days without water when the city pipes froze one winter. Although the basic problem was not the same, the fact that a plan had been thought out and contacts established within the community allowed the staff to act on parts of the plan instead of reacting to the crisis.

Foodborne Illness Outbreak

A dining services operation may at some time receive a complaint about foodborne illness. Every dining services operation should have a plan in place to deal with such complaints. Questions that should be asked of the complainant include:

- What is your name, address and phone number?
- When did you eat at the dining services operation (day and time)?
- What were you served?
- When did you become ill?
- Have you sought treatment? Where?
- Was anyone else with you when you ate at the dining services operation?
- If yes, are they ill and what did they have to eat?

Do not accept responsibility for the illness or agree to pay for medical care. Encourage the complainant to seek medical care if they indicate a need, but do not state that the facility will pay for medical care. (That is a decision to be made by the Administrator and the facility's Risk Manager/Lawyer.) If the suspect food is still in service, immediately take it out of service and save it. In many hospitals and larger senior living communities there is an employee health or infection control nurse to contact as a first step. He/she will know if other employees have reported similar illnesses. Alert the senior leadership team of the reported complaint, the possibility of others being affected and the need for any immediate action. Senior leadership may decide to contact the liability insurance carrier and to interview staff involved in the preparation of the suspect food.

After receiving the complaint, contact the local department of health. Reporting the complaint to local public health officials should be done quickly to prevent possible illness from spreading further. A laboratory analysis of the suspect food can help to confirm the presence of foodborne pathogens—or establish the safety of the item. Some facilities even have a procedure to save a plate of food from each meal served.

The local health department will investigate the complaint of foodborne illness. A team of investigators will likely interview the victim, visit the dining services operation to interview management and personnel, take samples of suspected food items, and evaluate the food protection practices of the dining services operation. HACCP logs can provide a record of food handling practices in the facility.

Since dining services staff may be carriers of an illness, the team may request that cultures be taken from all staff to detect the presence of a communicable disease. Bacterial sampling of work surfaces and equipment may also be done to determine if they are contaminated. During an investigation, it is very important for management and personnel to cooperate fully.

Managing the Crisis Communications

In the event of a crisis situation, there should be one designated person responsible for contact with members of the media. All other staff should decline answering questions and refer members of the press to the designated spokesperson. Before answering any questions, the spokesperson should determine the facts surrounding the emergency or crisis situation. In many cases, the spokesperson should consult with legal counsel before answering questions if possible. During an emergency, spokespersons are also encouraged to follow these do's and don'ts:

- Do provide factual information.
- Don't speculate, guess or provide false information.
- Do develop a prepared statement of exactly what information you want to release and then follow your statement.
- Don't feel obligated to answer all of the questions you are asked.
- Do communicate in a clear and concise manner.
- Don't use jargon or shocking descriptions.
- Do ask technical experts to provide explanations of complex situations if necessary.
- Don't allow pointed questions to alarm you.
- Do inform the media that public health and safety is your priority and that you are cooperating with regulatory agencies.
- Don't appear uncooperative or intimidated.

Food Security

In today's world, food security is a growing concern. The FDA recommends that Certified Dietary Managers consider the possibility of food tampering, or other criminal or terrorist actions that may result in unsafe food. Terrorist activity could occur at any point in the flow of food—on the farm, in a food processing facility, in a warehouse, or in a dining services operation. A manager needs to be alert to this possibility and can definitely take proactive steps to help prevent or limit this kind of crisis in a dining services department. FDA advice for dining services operations includes the following:

- Train staff to report any unusual or suspicious behavior.
- Promote security awareness among employees. Ask them to notice and report signs of tampering.
- Supervise and observe dining services activities.
- Screen employees before hiring.
- Provide work assignments and schedules, and insist that each employee wear an ID badge.
- Restrict access. Do not allow employees in work areas when they are off-duty and do not allow others into food storage and food production areas.
- Prevent staff from bringing personal items into non-public food preparation or storage areas.
- Monitor activity in self-service areas, such as salad bars.
- Limit access to and secure storage areas for chemicals used in the operation (e.g., no public access; secure with lock and key).
- Monitor inventory and report unusual changes: disappearance of products, or unauthorized appearance of products.

- Establish a chain of communications. Train staff to inform a designated manager of any concerns.
- Have a crisis response plan and keep all emergency contact numbers for the community readily accessible. Include the FDA emergency number on your contact list: 301-443-1240. Also include the phone number for your state complaint coordinator.

A number of government agencies at all levels, from federal through local, participate in ensuring food safety. A Certified Dietary Manager should be familiar with regulations that apply to the dining services department and work diligently to comply with them on a routine basis. While the FDA Food Code provides a model for sanitation regulations, each health jurisdiction sets its own standards. Routine inspections are a means through which government agencies help to ensure the safety of dining services clients, and additionally, the equipment used to prepare food. The equipment used to prepare food and the physical facilities of the dining services operation have a tremendous impact on the safety of food served. In the next section, we will consider what characteristics enable dining services equipment and facilities to support safe food.

Section B — Manage Physical Facilities

Design and construction of a commercial kitchen and dining services is a specialty niche in the builder's world. The regulations related to wiring, placement of outlets, equipment spacing, air-flow and hood space make kitchen design both interesting and difficult. Equipment specifications and local regulations may make adding desired equipment very expensive or even impossible. Work with internal engineering staff to identify opportunities and placement for new equipment.

Equipment representatives may be able to assist in the selection of a new stove but a commercial kitchen designer is recommended for major projects or remodels. They can help design a space that is efficient, uses the most appropriate equipment for the type of service being provided, and help navigate the approval process with local authorities. Never "just add" a major piece of equipment to a kitchen or dining room without first verifying that it meets safety and mechanical regulations for the location.

The following comments are based on commonly used guidelines and recommendations. Local regulations and specifications may differ.

Construction Materials and Considerations

Floors, Walls, and Ceilings

The materials for floors, walls, and ceilings are selected on the basis of ease in cleaning, resistance, and durability. Utility service lines should not be unnecessarily exposed and should not obstruct or prevent cleaning. Walls and ceilings are often light in color to distribute light and to make any soil more noticeable.

Floors

The floor in food preparation and utility areas should be easy to maintain, wear-resistant, slip-resistant, and non-porous. Common materials for floors are quarry tile, terrazzo, and sealed concrete. Other materials may be used in dining rooms. For instance, tightly woven carpeting would be acceptable in a dining room but not in a food preparation or storage area.

Vinyl tile is not recommended, even for dining rooms, because it is difficult to maintain and wears out quickly. Ceramic tile is a common floor finish for public restrooms and other high traffic areas. Floor mats, if used, should be easy to remove and to clean.

Floor Drains

Floors that are flushed with water for cleaning or are subject to frequent liquid spills should have adequate drains to allow the liquids to drain off by themselves.

Walls

The best wall finish in food preparation areas is structural glazed tile or ceramic tile. Both withstand heat, grease, and frequent cleaning. Structural glazed tile is also resistant to impact from movable carts and equipment, which is important to prevent chips. Surfaces that are chipped or cracked allow microorganisms to attach themselves.

Floor and Wall Junctures

Coving is required at the juncture of floors and walls. Coving at a floor-wall joint facilitates cleaning by preventing accumulation of bits of food that attract insects and rodents.

Ceilings

A wide variety of construction materials is available for ceilings, including: acoustical tile, painted drywall, painted plaster, and exposed concrete. Acoustical tile is a common choice because it is economical and has sound-absorbing qualities. Special non-absorbent acoustical tiles have been developed. Tiles are easier to replace when needed.

Heating, Ventilation, Air Conditioning Systems

Heating, Ventilation, and Air Conditioning (HVAC) systems should help maintain appropriate temperatures and air flow. The elements of an HVAC system—including hoods, vents and filters—should be inspected and cleaned on a regular basis to ensure efficient operation and to prevent the risk of a fire from grease build-up. Hoods can be commercially cleaned to eliminate grease build-up, which is a fire hazard. All preparation and work areas where odors, fumes, or vapors accumulate should be vented to the outside. Heating, ventilating, and air conditioning systems should be designed and installed so that make-up air intake and exhaust vents do not cause contamination of food, food contact surfaces, equipment or utensils. Vents and hoods should be maintained in a clean condition and air filters, if used, should be changed regularly.

Lighting

Lighting should be: adequate so that dirt and soil are visible, easy to clean, and bright enough to prevent accidents from poor lighting. Lighting is measured in foot-candles. Work areas require 50 foot-candles of light. Storage areas and walk-in coolers require at least 10 foot-candles. In food preparation and warewashing areas, lighting must be shielded and shatter-resistant.

Special Area Considerations

Dry Storage Areas

Storage areas should be well ventilated, dry, and constructed of easy-to-clean surfaces. Concrete or tile floors, cement block walls with epoxy paint, and acoustic ceilings are common for all storage areas except those that are refrigerated. Three- or four-level metal shelving is commonly used in storage areas. Slatted or louvered shelves are recommended for storage areas because they permit proper air flow. Storage areas should be maintained at 50°F - 70°F.

Warewashing Areas

Warewashing areas should be designed so that they are easy to sanitize and can withstand wet conditions. Common construction materials include slip-resistant quarry tile floors, ceramic or structural glazed tile walls, and moisture-resistant acoustic ceilings.

Preparation Areas

A major consideration in preparation areas is work surfaces. A common material used in the construction of work surfaces is stainless steel. Stainless steel is non-corrosive, non-absorbent, and non-toxic—making it a very suitable material for use in dining services operations. All food contact surfaces must be accessible for cleaning and sanitizing.

Toilet and Handwashing Facilities

Toilets should be conveniently located but separate from food preparation areas. The number of toilets and sinks required will vary by the size of the dining services operation and is usually determined by state and local regulations. Separate restrooms for employees and clients are recommended. The doors to toilet areas must be tight-fitting and self-closing.

Dining Services Equipment

Equipment Standards

Many utensils and products intended for household use are not appropriate for use in dining services operations. A Certified Dietary Manager should purchase only equipment that is intended for use in the dining services industry. In general, dining services equipment should be designed to be easily cleaned, maintained, and serviced—either in the assembled or disassembled state.

Metal pieces such as slicer blades and mixer pieces should be made of heavy gauge metal and checked frequently for nicks or broken areas.

One way to identify properly designed and constructed equipment is to look for the NSF International mark. (See Figure 20.2) The NSF International mark of approval is a recognized standard of acceptance for many pieces of equipment. This seal assures the manager that the equipment meets certain construction standards for sanitation and safety.

Another important standard is the Underwriter's Laboratories (UL) mark, which indicates compliance of the equipment with electrical safety standards. (See Figure 20.2) UL has developed nearly 20 safety standards for the commercial dining services industry. Only equipment meeting these standards can display the blue UL sanitation certification mark. The following are examples of characteristics to look for when purchasing dining services equipment:

- Easy disassembly for cleaning
- Durable, corrosion resistant and non-absorbent
- Materials that do not impart any significant color, odor, or taste to food
- Smooth surfaces free of pits, crevices, ledges, bolts and rivet heads
- Coating materials that are resistant to cracking and chipping
- Rounded edges and internal corners with finished, smooth surfaces.

Putting It Into Practice

3. The dining services assistant comments that the cooler temperature seems warm but the cooler temperature log indicates that the cooler hasn't varied more than three degrees throughout the day. What is the first action you should take?

Refrigeration Equipment

Refrigeration equipment is important to food protection. To ensure maximum performance of refrigeration units, follow these steps:

- Check to see that gaskets and hinges fit tightly and that there is no air leaking.
- Clean or replace the air filter.
- Clean the condenser.

Figure 20.2 Equipment Standards Marks

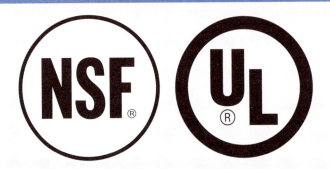

Some dining services operations connect thermostats on refrigerators to security or other monitoring equipment. Maintenance or management personnel can be notified immediately if the equipment fails—rather than discovering food spoilage several hours after the fact. Thermal barriers made of flexible, overlapping, PVC strips can be mounted on the doors of walk-in refrigerators and freezers to help maintain temperatures even when the door is opened. There should be room inside or on the door for a temperature log that is filled out three times a day. Take the actual food temperature if there has been a disruption in service or if it appears the thermometer is off.

Equipment Installation

Equipment that is fixed because it is not easily mobile should be installed so that it is spaced to allow access for cleaning along the sides, behind and above the equipment. Equipment that is not easily movable should be sealed to the floor or elevated on legs that provide at least 6" (15 cm) clearance between the floor and the equipment. Equipment mounted on concrete bases or on small steel legs can interfere with proper cleaning. Easier access for cleaning can also be provided by mounting equipment on wheels so it can be moved or by using wall-mounted equipment.

Cutting Boards

Surfaces such as cutting blocks that are subject to scratching and scoring should be resurfaced if they can no longer be cleaned and sanitized effectively or they should be discarded if they cannot be resurfaced. Wooden cutting boards may be prohibited in some areas; if used, they must be made of hard maple. Cutting boards made of food-grade seamless hard rubber or acrylic are recommended.

Color-coded cutting boards are available: red for meat, yellow for poultry, white for dairy, green for fruits and vegetables, beige for cooked poultry, and blue for seafood. Even a two-board combination (such as red for raw foods and beige for cooked foods) will reduce the risk of cross-contamination.

Thermometers

Monitoring proper storage, cooking, holding, cooling and reheating temperatures is vital to food protection. The most common thermometer used in dining services is the bi-metallic stem type. Bi-metallic stem thermometers are made of two metal strips which are joined together. The expansion and contraction of these strips move a pointer on a dial face. Bi-metallic thermometers need to be calibrated on a regular basis to ensure accuracy. Technology offers some alternatives to bi-metallic thermometers. As more dining services operations implement HACCP food safety programs, other types of dining services thermometers are becoming more common.

Thermocouple and Thermistor

The probes of these electronic thermometers can measure the temperature of food and provide a digital display. Some have additional electronic features, such as the ability to store temperature readings. Most have interchangeable probes, which allows matching the probe to the food or equipment. A thermometer with a small, thin probe allows for greater accuracy in checking temperatures of thin foods, such as ground beef patties, fish filets, or strips of meat for stir-fry. In fact, the Food Code stipulates using one of these for thin foods. (See Figures 20.3 and 20.4.)

An important consideration with any type of temperature-measuring device is cross-contamination. A thermometer used to measure the temperature of a raw food and then used to monitor a prepared food can contaminate the prepared food with bacteria. Probes should be sanitized with an approved sanitizer after each use. Dining services storage areas should be equipped with thermometers to measure the ambient temperature. Grill and oven thermometers may be used to verify the calibration of cooking equipment.

Figure 20.3 Monitoring Temperature of a Thin Food, Like Salmon Steak

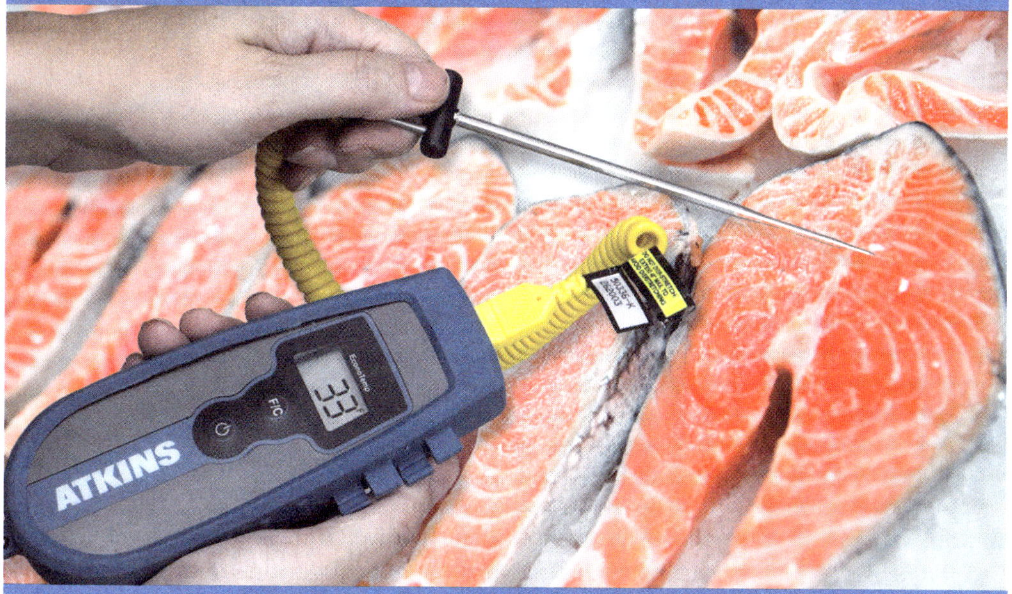

Image courtesy of Cooper Atkins

Figure 20.4 Verifying Temp. of Salad with Bi-Metallic Stem Thermometer

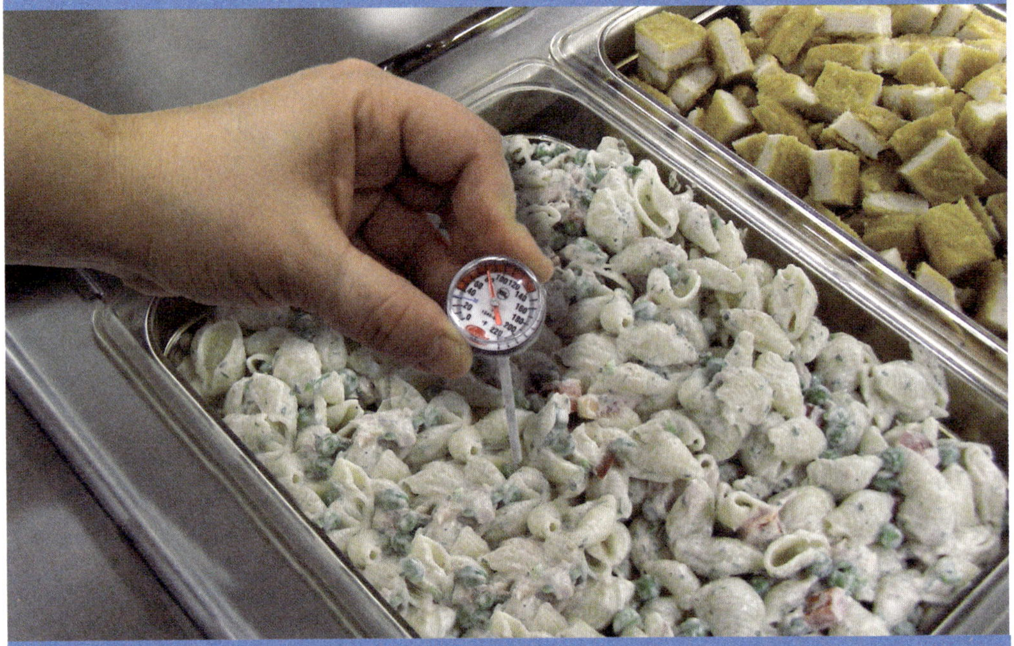

Image courtesy of Cooper Atkins

Clean-In-Place Equipment (CIP)

Clean-in-place equipment must be self-draining and designed so that cleaning and sanitizing solutions circulate throughout a fixed system and contact all food-contact surfaces. Clean-in-place equipment that cannot be disassembled for cleaning should have access points to allow inspection of interior food contact surfaces. CIP equipment and pieces that can be disassembled need the same steps for cleaning and sanitizing: wash, rinse, sanitize, air dry.

Equipment Calibration

Storage equipment is essential for maintaining proper food temperatures. Cooking and holding equipment—such as ovens, grills, steam tables and food warmers—should be calibrated on a regular basis. Equipment that is not calibrated may not cook food thoroughly or hold food at a safe temperature.

Putting It Into Practice

4. You are observing a new employee as she disassembles and cleans the slicer. She puts on safety gloves, disassembles the slicer, takes the portable pieces to the dishmachine and runs them through. She carefully washes the blade of the slicer and then reassembles the slicer. What step(s) has she overlooked?

Mechanical Warewashing Equipment

Dishwashers must be equipped with a temperature measuring device that indicates the temperature of water in each tank and the temperature of water during the sanitizing final rinse. Warewashing machines should be equipped with internal baffles, curtains, or other means to minimize internal cross-contamination between the solution in the wash and rinse tanks. In mechanical dishwashing, adequate dwell time is also a consideration. Dwell time is the time that dishes spend in contact with heat during sanitization.

Manual Warewashing Equipment

A sink with at least three compartments must be provided for manually washing, rinsing, and sanitizing equipment and utensils. A temperature-measuring device must be provided for frequently measuring the washing and sanitizing temperature of the water. Dishmachine temperatures should be monitored and recorded. Test strips may be used to monitor concentration of chemical sanitizing agents. Newer machines should be equipped to dispense detergents and sanitizers automatically. It should also have a visual signal or audible alarm to indicate a failure to dispense these chemicals.

Cleanability

Cleaning and maintenance are important considerations when designing a dining services facility and when purchasing equipment. A well-designed dining services operation utilizes materials that are durable, non-porous and easy to clean. Regulations for dining services operations have changed considerably over the last several years, so it is important to consult new standards before making any construction, remodeling, or major purchasing decision. The sanitary design of a dining services facility is often governed by a variety of laws, including public health, building, and zoning. The primary consideration for the sanitary design of dining services facilities is cleanability. **Cleanability** is the extent to which an item is accessible for cleaning and inspection and ease with which soil can be removed by normal cleaning methods.

Some examples of how food safety can be part of a facility design are:

- Equipment is easily dissembled.
- Finishes are durable and easy to clean.
- Equipment is attached to the wall, eliminating legs, which makes it easier to clean under the equipment.
- Equipment racks have a minimum number of legs.
- Garbage disposals are placed in work areas to facilitate waste disposal.
- Shelves under tables are designed to be portable, so they can be cleaned easily.

Developing a Cleaning Program

Maintaining a clean environment for food preparation is an important part of food safety. The presence of bacteria and the likelihood of foodborne illness increase if a dining services operation fails to use appropriate cleaning and sanitizing techniques. Equipment, food contact surfaces, and utensils must be clean to sight and touch. The food contact surfaces of equipment should be free of any encrusted grease deposits and other soil accumulations. The plumbing under the dishmachine should be clear of rust and lime build-up. Non-food contact surfaces should be kept free of dust, dirt, food residue and debris. A philosophy of clean-as-you-go should be instilled in all dining services staff. A cleaning program will most likely be effective if the Certified Dietary Manager incorporates a system of self-inspection and training.

Maintaining a clean dining services operation requires that Certified Dietary Managers use their skills in planning, organizing, staffing, training, and directing. The manager must first determine what the cleaning needs of the operation are and when these functions need to be carried out. The manager should then determine who will be responsible for carrying out the cleaning. Some cleaning may be done by contract personnel, but most will be completed by dining services employees. The manager should provide adequate staffing so that employees will be able to carry out the planned cleaning activities. The manager should train employees in proper cleaning techniques and safe use of chemicals. Finally, the manager should evaluate the cleaning program on an ongoing basis to ensure its effectiveness and to correct any identified problems.

A written schedule, such as that in Figure 20.5, can be developed to outline the cleaning program and the position responsible for the task on a daily basis. When compared to the posted work schedule, identifying the individual employee from day to day is easily done.

A self-inspection checklist (Figure 20.6) can be used to evaluate the effectiveness of the cleaning program. Depending upon the condition of the department, the self-inspection may be a daily or weekly task for the manager.

Detailed instructions on proper cleaning techniques should be incorporated into employee training programs, both during the orientation phase and as part of the ongoing in-service education program. An example of this appears in Figure 20.7.

Cleaning Products

Detergents are powerful dirt-removing cleaning agents. Types of cleaning products are described in Figure 20.8. A cleaning supply vendor can assist in selecting the right chemical for the right job. Or, the local or state regulatory agency may be able to provide a list of approved chemical products. Factors in selecting a detergent include:

- Dissolvability: how well the detergent disperses with water.
- Wetting ability: how well it saturates the surface of the object to be cleaned.
- Emulsification ability: how well the detergent suspends the fats in water and keeps them suspended.
- Free rinsing ability: how well the detergent keeps soil from returning to the cleaned object.
- Deflocculation ability: how well the detergent puts lumps of food-soil in suspension in water.
- Non-toxicity: the extent to which the detergent is free of toxins and other elements harmful to humans.
- Corrosiveness: how great a corroding effect the detergent has on the surface of the item to be cleaned.

Wiping Cloths

Cloths used for wiping up food spills should be used for no other purpose and be stored in a sanitizing solution. Dry or moist cloths that are used with raw animal foods must be kept separate from cloths used for other purposes and kept in a separate sanitizing solution. Sponges should not be used on any food-contact surface.

Clean vs. Sanitary

Clean does not mean sanitary. **Clean** means free of visible dirt or debris. Cleaning is accomplished by physical and/or chemical means and is a two-step process:

1. Wash with an approved detergent
2. Rinse with clear water

Sanitary means free of harmful levels of microorganisms. It is almost impossible to sanitize equipment and facilities unless they are first clean. Clean dining services equipment may appear safe to use, but if it is not sanitized, then a hidden threat to food safety exists. Equipment and utensils must be sanitized after cleaning. The FDA Food Code defines a thermometer probe as a utensil, too, so it must also be sanitized.

Glossary

Clean
Free of visible dirt

Sanitary
Free of harmful levels of microorganisms

Figure 20.5 Sample Daily Cleaning Schedule

Area: _____ Week of: _____

Item	Person Responsible	Initial When Completed						
		Sun	Mon	Tue	Wed	Thur	Fri	Sat
Grill	Cafe Employee 1							
Fryer	Cafe Employee 1							
Reach-in Refrigerator	Cafe Employee 1							
Food Warmer	Cafe Employee 2							
Steam Table	Cafe Employee 2							
Salad Bar	Cafe Employee 3							
Serving Line	Cafe Employee 3							
Soda Dispenser	Cashier							
Dining Room Table	Cashier							
Floor	Utility Aide							
Garbage Cans	Utility Aide							

Figure 20.6 Sample Cleaning Self-Inspection Checklist

AREA	CLEAN		ACTION TAKEN
	Yes	No	
KITCHEN			
Floors			
Walls			
Ceilings			
Baseboards			
Hoods and Vents			
Light Fixtures			
Counters			
Filters			
Fans			
Garbage Cans			
DINING ROOM			
Floors			
Walls			
Ceilings			
Baseboards			
Light Fixtures			
DRY STORAGE AREA			
Floors			
Walls			
Ceilings			
Baseboards			
Light Fixtures			

Figure 20.7 Sample Cleaning Procedures for Floors

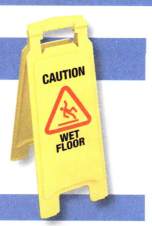

HOW TO CLEAN FLOORS

Equipment Needed:
- Broom
- Dustpan
- Two Mops
- Two Mop Buckets

Supplies Needed:
- Heavy-Duty Detergent

WHAT TO DO		HOW TO DO IT
STEP 1	Sweep	• Sweep the floor with a broom, making sure to get under equipment. • Minimize dust by using short, controlled strokes. • Use dustpan to pick up debris.
STEP 2	Set up mop buckets	• Fill each bucket 3/4 full with hot tap water. • Put the appropriate amount of cleanser in one of the buckets.
STEP 3	Apply cleaner to floor	• Dip first mop into cleanser solution and wring out. • Mop small section of floor using a figure-eight motion. • Allow detergent to loosen soil for a few minutes.
STEP 4	Rinse floor	• Dip the second mop into the rinse water, wring out, and use the mop to pick up the dirt and cleaning solution. • Change detergent solutions and rinse water often.

SAFETY CONSIDERATIONS

- Check product label and refer to MSDS for precautions and emergency procedures in the event of an accident
- Follow manufacturer's directions on detergent label to ensure the proper dilution.
- Use "wet floor" signs to prevent accidental slips and falls.

Sanitizing

Sanitizing is the process of making equipment and work surfaces sanitary. There are two major methods of sanitizing: heat sanitization and chemical sanitization.

- Heat sanitization: The procedure is to expose an object to sufficiently high heat for a sufficient period of time to sanitize it. According to the FDA Food Code, cleaned food contact surfaces can be sanitized by immersion in water that is 171°F or above for at least 30 seconds.

Figure 20.8 Types of Cleaning Products

Alkaline Detergents	The most commonly used detergents. General-purpose alkalines are only mildly alkaline and are usually applied to walls, celings, and floors. Heavy-duty types are highly alkaline for use in dishwashing machines.
Abrasive Cleaners	Effective in scouring off rust, grease, and heavy soil but can scratch certain surfaces such as stainless steel. Use caution with abrasive cleaners, as scratches in food contact surfaces can harbor bacterial growth.
Acid Cleaners	Acid cleaners have more specialized uses, such as deliming dishmachines and removing water spots. Use acid cleaners with caution to avoid skin irritation.
Degreasers	Degreasers are highly alkaline and can remove grease build-up from floors, ovens, and vents. Degreasers are also known as solvent cleaners.

Note: To avoid producing a poisonous gas, never mix chemicals together.

- Chemical sanitization: **Sanitizers** are chemicals that destroy harmful pathogens. The dilution or strength of a sanitizing solution is measured in parts per million (ppm). Dispensing equipment for sanitizers should be calibrated on a regular basis and the strength of a sanitizing solution should be checked with a chemical test strip on a daily basis. Chemical test strips are often available from the chemical supply vendor. Keep in mind that the effectiveness of a sanitizer may be affected by the temperature, hardness, and/or pH of the water in which it is mixed. Also, some chemical solutions lose their strength over time. Chemical sanitizers are summarized in Figure 20.9.

Figure 20.9 Chemical Sanitizers

Product	Dilution in Parts Per Million (ppm)	Water Temperature	Immersion Time
Iodine	12.5 - 2.5	75°F - 120°F	30 seconds
Chlorine	50 - 100	100°F - 115°F	30 seconds
Quaternary Ammonium Compounds	180 - 200	75°F minimum	30 seconds

General guidelines only; follow manufacturer's directions or local regulations.

Glossary

Sanitizers
Chemicals that destroy microorganisms

Putting It Into Practice

5. What cleaner would you recommend to your staff to remove the grease buildup from the back of a range?

Dishwashing

Manual Cleaning and Sanitizing

Manual cleaning and sanitizing is generally done with a three-compartment sink. (Some municipalities are now requiring a four-compartment sink. The additional compartment is designated for pre-scraping.) If using a three-compartment sink, remember to pre-scrape utensils and cooking equipment before placing them in the first sink compartment. The steps in manual cleaning and sanitizing using a three-compartment sink are:

1. Pre-clean to remove loose food soil.

2. Wash in the first sink using an approved detergent with a water temperature of 110°F-120°F.

3. Rinse in the second sink, using clear water.

4. Sanitize in the third sink using an approved sanitizer at the appropriate concentration and temperature. See Appendix E.

5. Allow dishes to air dry and store in a clean, dry, protected area.

Remember to change the water as necessary to maintain the temperatures and to clean the sink after each use. Use cleaned and sanitized drain boards to stack the equipment and utensils during air drying.

Mechanical Cleaning and Sanitizing

While there are various sizes and types of dishwashers (see Figure 20.10), the following steps will apply to most operations. These six steps are necessary in any mechanical warewashing operation. Each step is equally important in obtaining clean and sanitary dishware.

Figure 20.10 Mechanical Dishmachine Temperatures

Type of Machine	Wash Solution Temp.	Sanitizing Rinse Temp.
Stationary rack, single temperature machine	165°F	165°F
Stationary rack, dual temperature machine	150°F	180°F
Single tank, conveyor, dual temperature machine	160°F	180°F
Multi-task, conveyor, multi-temperature machine	150°F	180°F

NOTES:

• The temperature of sanitizing rinse should not exceed 194°F.

• The actual temperature attained within a hot water sanitizing machine (at utensil surface) should be at least 160°F when measured by a thermometer or temperature test strip.

The steps are:

1. Separate: Separate any items that will require special attention, such as items that are heavily soiled or have burned-on residue.

2. Pre-scrape or pre-flush: Excess food soil and pieces of paper straws or napkins will clog the dishmachine, scrap trays, pump and wash arms—and reduce their effectiveness. Excess food soil in the wash tank also uses up more detergent and requires more frequent changes of water in the wash tank.

3. Rack dishes: Proper racking of dishes is essential for getting good results. All of the racks should be filled with similar items. A rack should contain cups only, or plates only, or bowls only, etc. Avoid mixing loads. The dishmachine works by spraying water at the dishes, and if the water cannot reach all of the dish surfaces, the dishes cannot get clean.

4. Wash: Washing dishes requires a properly operating dishmachine and the proper detergent usage. Be sure to use the right detergent, make sure that the machine is set up properly, and see that it is free of paper, straws, and excess food.

5. Perform sanitizing rinse: Rinsing is done automatically and requires only the proper water flow, proper water temperature, and the proper rinse aid. Visually inspect the machine to ensure that the rinse jets are not clogged. Verify that rinse temperature is reaching the appropriate point, that the rinse injector is supplied with the proper rinse aid and that dwell time is adequate.

6. Air Drying: Air drying the dishes requires nothing but time. Wait until the dishes are completely dry before putting them in a clean, dry storage area. Avoid stacking utensils within one another until they are completely dry.

Dish and Utensil Storage

After cleaning and sanitizing, all dishes and utensils must be stored dry, in clean, dust-free areas above the floor, and protected from dust, splashes, spills and other forms of contamination.

Section C   Conduct Equipment Inspection & Maintenance

Preventative Maintenance

Preventative maintenance of equipment and facilities is required as an ongoing process in order to keep food production and dining services facilities in good repair and condition. Preventative maintenance goes beyond the daily cleaning tasks. Some preventative maintenance responsibilities will undoubtedly be carried out by dining services staff, while others may be performed by the facility maintenance staff or through a contract with a commercial equipment maintenance company. It is important to determine what duties dining services and maintenance will perform.

Preventative maintenance includes weekly, bi-monthly, monthly, quarterly, and semi-annual cleaning responsibilities. Figure 20.11 shows a partial preventative maintenance cleaning schedule. When assigning these cleaning duties, it is important to include the who, what, when, and how that are part of any cleaning schedule. How to decide who should do which cleaning duties? Obviously, no one wants to be assigned to clean the grease traps each time. Determining who does what cleaning can be a great topic for a department meeting. Get input from staff as to how cleaning duties should be divided up. One facility uses a job jar and each week and employees pull a job from the jar.

It is the Certified Dietary Manager's responsibility is to make sure that cleaning is done properly and according to schedule.

A checklist should be used to ensure that equipment and facilities are properly maintained, as shown in Figure 20.12. Whatever the schedule, make sure that proper tools, equipment, and cleaning materials are available when needed. The manager is also responsible for making sure that employees are thoroughly trained in the procedure and cleaning materials for each task. For example, one facility noticed a significant increase in the cost of sanitizers. Upon investigation, one of the staff believed that if some sanitizer was good, double the amount would be better. Training needs to include why the concentration of sanitizer is important.

Preventative Maintenance Records

There are different types of preventative maintenance records. Two are temperature logs and equipment repair records.

Temperature Logs

Temperature logs should be established for equipment where maintaining temperature is critical. These logs can be set up on a monthly basis and maintained by an assigned staff person. Temperature logs are essential to help determine the time when the equipment stopped working. Since time and temperature are important in maintaining food safety, temperature logs are part of preventative maintenance. Temperature logs can be useful during inspections if they are maintained and completed appropriately. Figure 20.13 shows a sample of a dishmachine temperature log. Similar logs can be set up for coolers and freezers. A sample of this form is available in the online *Supplemental Textbook Material—Foodservice*.

Figure 20.11 Preventative Maintenance Cleaning Schedule for Facilities and Equipment

What to Clean	When to Clean	How to Clean	Person Responsible	Initial When Complete
Drain Covers	Monthly	Remove and wash thoroughly with detergent or degreaser if necessary		
Walls	Monthly	Wash with detergent or degreaser if necessary		
Ceiling Vents	Monthly	Wash with detergent or degreaser if necessary		
Hood Filters	Monthly	Wash filters, replace if necessary		
Grease Traps	Every two months	Clean with degreaser		
Fans	Monthly	Wipe down blades and fan cover		
Ice Machine	Quarterly	Remove ice, clean interior surfaces with detergent, flush ice-making unit		
Cooler/ Refrigerator	Bi-monthly or more often as needed	Wipe down racks, clean floors, and fan with detergent		
Freezer	Bi-annually	Empty, defrost, wash racks, floors, fans with detergent		
Steamer	Weekly	Use approved de-liming agent		
Dishwashing Machine	Weekly	Use approved de-liming agent		
Dish Racks	Weekly	Scrub with detergent		
Food Carts	Weekly	Scrub with detergent or use steam cleaner		
Garbage Cans	Weekly	Scrub with detergent or use steam cleaner		
HVAC	Every six months	Steam clean		

Figure 20.12 Equipment Cleaning Checklist

EQUIPMENT	CLEAN?		OPERATIONAL?		ACTION TAKEN
	Yes	No	Yes	No	
Oven					
Range Top					
Broiler					
Tilting Skillet					
Fans					
Hood Filters					
Food Carts					
Steamer					
Trunnion Kettles					
Steam Jacketed Kettle					
Dish Racks					
Cooler/Freezer					
HVAC					
Fryer					
Steam Table					
Food Warmer					
Walls					
Ceiling					
Grease Trap					

Figure 20.13 Dishmachine Temperature Log

Month: _____ Year: _____

Instructions: Record temperatures for dishmachine at each meal. Keep this form on the clipboard throughout the month. Report any problems to your supervisor.

DATE	BREAKFAST			LUNCH			DINNER		
	Wash	Rinse	Hold	Wash	Rinse	Hold	Wash	Rinse	Hold
1									
2									
3									
4									
5									
6									
7									
8									
9									

Equipment Repair Records

Certified Dietary Managers should maintain a record of repairs for each piece of major equipment. An equipment repair record that contains the number of repairs and the cost of each is essential when writing a justification for new equipment. The equipment repair record should be established as soon as a new piece of equipment is received. In today's electronic age, there is unlimited data space for computerized equipment repair records, including setting up reminders for periodic maintenance. See Figure 20.14 for a sample equipment repair record form.

Equipment Replacement Decisions

As a Certified Dietary Manager, you will be expected to recommend for purchase or purchase new equipment. The equipment maintenance record will assist in deciding when to purchase, what to purchase, and why. The steps in replacing or purchasing new equipment include:

1. Conducting cost analysis
2. When cost analysis/justification for replacement was written
3. Developing equipment specifications
4. Installation and staff training

These steps will be explored in greater detail in Chapter 22: Manage the Capital Budget.

Water, Plumbing & Waste Management

Working with maintenance or a local plumbing firm during construction times or after emergency situations, such as a flood or tornado, is extremely important. It is the manager's responsibility to make sure that maintenance staff know the local, state, and federal sanitation regulations. One example is the FDA Food Code requirement that a

Figure 20.14 Equipment Repair Record

Name of Equipment:		Brand:		Purchase Date:	Purchase Price:
Model #:		Serial #:			
Name of Manufacturer or Vendor:				Representative's Phone #:	
Warranty Information *(includes recommended preventative maintenance):*				Representative's Email:	

	Date of Repair	COST OF REPAIR	
		Material	Labor
Repair Log *(attach copy of repair bill and name of person doing repair):*			

drinking water system be flushed and disinfected before being placed in service after construction or an emergency situation.

Water can be a vehicle for transmitting harmful microorganisms. Part of the food protection process involves selecting appropriate sources of water, and managing how clean and waste water are handled in the operation through the plumbing system. In addition, food safety requires proper management of refuse.

Sources of Water

Water served in a dining services operation—as well as water used in food preparation, warewashing, and even handwashing—must be **potable**, or safe to drink. An approved source may be the local public water system. Alternately, it may be a non-public water system that meets national primary drinking water regulations, as well as state or local regulations. Water from a non-public source must be sampled and tested at least annually, and the report must be kept on file in the dining services operation. Water must be received through an approved water main or water transport vehicle. Bottled drinking water that meets appropriate standards is also permissible.

Ice is also a form of water and should be made from potable water. It is important to maintain ice machines in good repair and follow basic sanitation practices in serving ice to clients. Figure 20.15 summarizes some key practices to help ensure safe ice.

Glossary

Potable Water
Water that is safe to drink

Figure 20.15 Ice Management Practices

- Close or cover the ice bin when not in use.

- Wash hands following established procedures before scooping or dispensing ice. Realize that hands can transfer microorganisms directly to ice, and freezing temperatures do not destroy all pathogens.

- Use a scoop or designated utensil to transfer ice (do not use glass). Touch only the handle of the scoop.

- Store the scoop in or near the ice bin in a protected manner, or in a sanitizing solution (per your local health regulations), with handle up.

- Clean and sanitize ice scoops regularly.

- Do not store any food products or beverages in or directly above the ice bin.

- Report any concerns about equipment malfunction to a designated supervisor.

- Assure that cleaning compounds are stored and used in such a way that they cannot spill or spray into ice.

- Protect ice supplies from broken china or glasses. If glass breaks or a chemical spills in the vicinity of an ice bin, empty, clean, and sanitize the bin.

- Routinely clean and sanitize the ice collection.

- Follow the manufacturer's instructions for maintenance, which may include de-liming machines and replacing filters.

Source: Food Protection Correction, Dietary Manager Magazine, October 2005.

Plumbing

Plumbing systems also cover handwashing sinks. The FDA Food Code requires that handwashing sinks provide water at a temperature of at least 100°F. Handwashing sinks must be maintained so that they are accessible at all times to employees. Employees may ONLY use chemical hand sanitizers as a substitute for handwashing when food exposure is limited and handwashing sinks are not convenient, such as in an approved temporary food operation like a mobile unit. An amendment to the FDA Food Code requires that toilets and urinals NOT be used for the disposal of mop water.

The plumbing system performs two very important functions. It brings potable water to the operation and it removes waste materials to a sewer or disposal plant. A major consideration for food protection is to avoid any connection between the two functions. Fixtures and equipment that are used for food preparation, cleaning, or sanitizing cannot have a **cross-connection**—a dangerous link between an outlet of a drinkable water system and unsafe water. An unapproved link may allow contaminants to flow into potable water, making it unsafe. A cross-connection is a structural design issue.

If contaminated water does flow into potable water, this process is called **backflow**. For example, if a faucet is located below the flood rim of a sink, when the sink gets too full, dirty water may flow back into the faucet. Sometimes, rather than just flowing back into potable water, contaminated water is actually sucked into the clean water supply. This type of backflow is called **back-siphonage**. Back-siphonage occurs after a loss in pressure in the water supply and water is siphoned back into the drinkable water supply.

Glossary

Cross-Connection
A dangerous link between an outlet of drinkable water with unsafe water

Backflow
When contaminated water flows back into potable water

Back-Siphonage
When water is siphoned back into potable water supply after loss in water pressure

To prevent backflow, plumbing lines should provide for an **air gap**. An air gap is an unobstructed air space between an outlet of drinkable water and the flood rim of a fixture or equipment. For example, space between the flood rim in a sink and the outlet of a faucet is an air gap. If an air gap is not present, then an approved mechanical device to prevent backflow should be installed.

Plumbing should be kept in good repair. Be alert to leaks or drainage issues that might contaminate food or food preparation areas. Get to know the local codes, as plumbing regulations vary. Always use the services of a licensed, qualified plumber for installing or repairing plumbing systems.

Waste Management

Proper management of waste and garbage will help to maintain a clean, sanitary dining services operation and to prevent pest infestations. As quickly as possible, garbage should be removed from food preparation and serving areas. Trash holding areas should be located as far as possible from food.

Garbage cans should be sturdy and easy to clean. They should be equipped with tight-fitting lids and covered when not in use. Garbage cans should be cleaned on a routine basis, and garbage cans with cracks or leaks should be replaced immediately. Indoor trash areas should be cleaned on a regular basis and garbage should be picked up at regular intervals to prevent excess odors and reduce food sources for pests.

If the facility has a recycling program be aware of the local, state, and federal sanitation requirements. For instance, the FDA Food Code requires that recyclables be kept covered if the containers contain food residue or after a recycling container is filled.

Chemical Safety

The use of chemicals is an essential component of a dining services operation. Chemicals are used in cleaning and sanitizing and sometimes in office operations. Chemicals that are stored or used incorrectly pose hazards to food because they can contaminate food and make it unsafe. Chemical safety is an important part of a comprehensive food protection program. In addition, the federal government imposes regulations on chemical use for dining services operations. A related issue is the safe practice for chemically preventing and eradicating pests.

Chemical safety is addressed by **OSHA**, a government agency responsible for protecting the safety of employees, including those in dining services operations. OSHA has issued a regulation requiring employers to inform employees about the possible dangers of chemicals they use to do their jobs and to train them to use chemicals in a safe manner.

The regulation is called the **Hazard Communication Standard**, or Right to Know Law. The purpose of the Hazard Communication Standard is to ensure that all employers receive the information they need to inform employees about chemicals they work with and to train their employees to properly use hazardous substances. It helps in the design and implementation of employee protection programs. It also provides necessary hazard information to employees so that they can participate in and support protective measures.

Safety Data Sheet

By law, a document called a **Safety Data Sheet (SDS)** must be made available by every chemical manufacturer (see Figure 20.16). An SDS should be available for every chemical used in your operation and placed in a location that is readily accessible to all employees.

Glossary

Air Gap
An unobstructed air space between an outlet of drinkable water and the flood rim of a fixture or equipment

OSHA
Occupation Safety and Hazard Administration responsible for enforcing chemical safety standards

Hazard Communication Standard
Law that requires informing employees about chemicals they work with and to design an institute employee protection program

SDS
Safety data sheet required for every chemical that addresses the safe use of the chemical

Putting It Into Practice

7. Where would you expect to find an air gap in your kitchen?

Figure 20.16 Sample Safety Data Sheet

Safety Data Sheet May be used to comply with OSHA's Hazard Communication Standard, 29 CFR 1910 1200. Standard must be consulted for specific requirements.	**U.S. Department of Labor** Occupational Safety and Health Administration (Non-Mandatory Form) Form Approved OMB No. 1218-0072
IDENTITY *(as used on label and list)*	**Note:** Blank spaces are not permitted. If any item is not applicable or no information is available, the space must be marked to indicate that.

SECTION I

Manufacturer's Name:	Emergency Telephone Number:
Address *(Number, Street, City, State, and Zip Code):*	Telephone Number for Information:
	Date Prepared:
	Signature of Preparer *(optional):*

SECTION II—Hazardous Ingredients/Identity Information

Hazardous Components [Specific Chemical Identity, Common Name(s)]	OSHA PEL	ACGIH TLV	Other Limits Recommended	% (Optional)

The SDS addresses safe use of a chemical, as well as hazards, safety precautions, proper disposal practices, and how to deal with accidents. In some cases, the SDS may suggest the use of personal protective equipment, such as rubber gloves or goggles.

Safety Data Sheets are not easy to read, so employees will require orientation in how to use them. Be sure that employees understand:

1) What to use each chemical for

2) How to mix each chemical

3) What protective equipment is required

4) Where to find the MSDS for a chemical

5) How to read it

6) What to do in case of an accident or spill.

Suggested training content is summarized in Figure 20.17.

Putting It Into Practice

8. One of your staff accidently spilled delimer on her arm. What is the first action you should take?

Figure 20.17 Hazard Communication Training Program Content

- Location of Safety Data Sheets (SDS) in the operation
- Inventory list of hazardous chemicals used in the operation
- How to read product labels to learn potential hazards and directions for safe use
- Proper handling, application, storage, and disposal of chemicals
- Use and location of personal protective equipment
- Emergency procedures in the event of a spill or exposure

To comply with the Hazard Communication Standard:

- Review the Hazard Communication Standard.
- Develop an inventory of chemicals used in the dining services operation.
- Request a Safety Data Sheet (These are also available online for easy access and printing) for each chemical used in the operation, and make it available to all employees.
- Make sure that all chemicals are in labeled containers.
- Include safe chemical use in the new employee orientation and as part of annual training for all employees.

Chemical Storage

For food safety, it's also important to store chemicals away from food. Chemicals should be stored in their original containers and be clearly labeled. If transferring is necessary, transfer them only to durable, clearly labeled containers. Containers used to hold and dispense chemicals should be clearly marked and should never be re-used for food storage. Likewise, discarded food containers should never be used for chemical storage because someone may mistake the contents for food.

Medicines

Storage of medicines are also regulated by the FDA Food Code. The Food Code requires that "only those medicines that are necessary for the health of employees" are allowed in the dining services department. They must be labeled with a manufacture's label and located to prevent contamination of food, equipment, utensils, linens, and single-service articles. Refrigerated medicines must be stored in a covered, leakproof container that is identified as a container for the storage of medicines. They must also be located so they are inaccessible to children.

Common Pests

A safe food operation is free of insects, birds, and other sources of contamination. Measures must be taken to prevent contamination of food, utensils, equipment and linens by pests. Many pests carry pathogens that can render food unsafe for consumption.

Cockroaches

Cockroaches are common pests in dining services operations and they represent a significant threat. Cockroaches are carriers of disease and can multiply rapidly. Cockroaches are most active at night and in dark areas where there is less disturbance from people. While there are many different species of cockroaches, three types are frequently

Putting It Into Practice

9. In a day care facility, how would you handle refrigerated medicine brought in by parents for their children?

found in dining services operations. German cockroaches, the most abundant species in the U.S., are pale brown with two dark-brown stripes behind the head. They seem to prefer warm places in the dining services operation. American cockroaches are the largest in size and are reddish brown. They prefer open, wet areas and spaces that are slightly cooler than the favorite spots of German cockroaches. Oriental cockroaches are shiny and dark brown to black. They prefer conditions similar to those of the American cockroach.

Housefly

The common housefly is a great threat to food safety. Flies feed on animal and human waste and then transmit pathogenic organisms as they travel from item to item. Houseflies are numerous during late summer and early fall, since the population has been growing during the warmer weather.

Rats and Mice

Rats and mice can force their entry into a building through small openings. Both rats and mice are skilled swimmers and can enter a building through floor drains and toilet bowl traps. Rats and mice are both nocturnal creatures, being most active at night. One indication of an infestation is the presence of fecal droppings in dining services areas. Another sign is the presence of gnaw marks on food and food containers in storage.

Birds

Birds, such as pigeons, sparrows, and starlings, are another pest of concern. Birds can enter a building through doors and windows that do not have screens and through ventilation openings. Birds can be carriers of mites and harmful microorganisms such as Salmonella.

Pest Control

Pest control is the reduction or eradication of pests. Due to the variety and prevalence of pests in and around foodservice operations, a pest service is recommended, and in some jurisdictions, required. There are a number of interventions available.

One of the safest and most effective methods of fly control is the use of insect light traps. Light traps must be enclosed so that pests entering the trap are contained within and cannot fall out into the dining services operation. Mechanical traps can be used with birds and rodents.

Pesticides, insecticides and repellents are other control techniques. Extreme caution should be exercised when using chemical control methods to prevent contamination of food. Only chemicals approved for application in dining services operations may be used. Further, only individuals with the proper training and knowledge should apply pesticides. In addition, pesticide application must not occur during food preparation or service. Check local regulations for further restrictions on the use of pest control devices.

Pest control cannot be accomplished effectively unless proper cleaning has occurred. One method of pest control alone is not often effective. For this reason, many dining services operations use an approach called **integrated pest management (IPM)**. IPM uses a variety of techniques and focuses on prevention. Certified Dietary Managers should implement an IPM including these elements:

- Routine inspection of incoming supplies and inspection of the premises for evidence of pests.
- Restrict access into the facility with screens and building maintenance.

Glossary

Integrated Pest Management (IPM)
A coordinated approach to pest control, food production and dining services to manage pests

- Reduce food sources for pests through good cleaning and sanitization practices.
- Control pests by working with a licensed pest control operator (PCO), someone who is trained and licensed in pest management and use of pest control chemicals and devices.

All openings to the outside of the building must be closed to restrict access to the rodents. Screens in doors and windows can help to restrict the access of insects. Self-closing doors and proper seals around doors also reduce the accessibility of the dining services operation to pests. Some facilities are required to use fly fans or air curtains.

Check all deliveries for signs of pest infestation prior to accepting the delivery. All food storage and preparation areas must be kept in a clean and sanitary condition. Food spills are a source of food for pests. Food stored against the wall creates places for pests to hide, nest and multiply. Proper garbage management can reduce the risk of pest infestation.

Live Animals

Generally, live animals are prohibited from dining services establishments. The FDA Food Code makes an exception for the following, if food, equipment, utensils, linens, and unwrapped single-service articles are kept sanitary:

- Decorative fish in an aquarium.
- Patrol dogs accompanying police or security officers.
- In areas that are not used for food preparation .
- Pets in the common dining areas of facilities such as nursing homes, assisted living group homes, or residential care facilities at times other than during meals if the following conditions are met:
  > Doors separate the common dining areas from food storage or food preparation areas
  > Condiments, equipment, and utensils are stored in enclosed cabinets or removed from the dining areas when pets are present
  > Dining areas, including tables and countertops are cleaned and sanitized before the next meal service.

Summary

Maintaining a safe food supply from purchase to time of service depends upon established policies, employee awareness, and well maintained physical spaces. The Certified Dietary Manager has a shopping list of regulations, inspections and laws to help guide their policy development and validate their expectations and restrictions. Ultimately, the goal is a safe and sanitary dining service for employees and clients.

Manage the Operating Budget

Overview and Objectives

Most Certified Dietary Managers are expected to manage costs and revenues as part of their job. That includes making sure that a budget is monitored. Certified Dietary Managers have an increasingly important role in helping their facility maintain the bottom line. This is the first chapter that focuses on financial control techniques—specifically, you will review menu pricing, prepare a simple budget and calculate costs per client patient day. After completing this chapter, you should be able to:

✓ Prepare a department budget

✓ Compute cost of menus (including supplements)

✓ Conduct a product price comparison study

✓ Calculate daily cost (e.g., food, labor, supplies, i.e., PPD)

✓ Calculate minutes per meal (Chapter 12 addresses productivity)

✓ Calculate meals per labor hour

✓ Compare actual costs to budget costs

✓ Monitor expenses

✓ Prepare an estimate of personnel costs for a dining services department (e.g., salary scales and merit increases)

From the previous information on forecasting, purchasing, and inventory, the Certified Dietary Manager's job is to manage the cost of food coming in and going out. Budgeting is a tool to help manage those costs. Knowing how to calculate raw food costs, and in some cases menu costs, is essential to development food budget.

Review of Financial Terms

This information is the basis of a Professional Practice Standard for Certified Dietary Managers. See the full standard in the *Supplemental Textbook Material—Foodservice.* Two very important tools for planning, monitoring, and adjusting the financial performance of a dining services department are calculating raw food costs and calculating labor costs. A Certified Dietary Manager may determine a cost per meal based on total cost divided by the total number of meals. Managers also talk about cost per client day or cost per patient day (cost/ppd).

(Note: For purposes of this textbook, the word client is being used rather than patient, resident, inmate, or child. However, the industry measure for food costs in healthcare is referred to as cost per patient day. For this measure, patient also means client).

As you begin this chapter, review the financial terms in Figure 21.1.

Budgeting

In any business, sound management dictates that there is a plan for financial performance. This is an essential component that protects an organization against suddenly running out of money. A budget helps a Certified Dietary Manager plan and make decisions about purchasing food and equipment, hiring workers, scheduling overtime, and much more. In essence, a budget provides a road map for the accounting department.

What is a Budget?

The two most basic components of a budget are:

- Revenue: Money coming in or income.
- Expenses: Money going out or costs.

A **budget** is a written plan for income and expenses. Typically, it covers a one-year period. This period may follow a calendar year, such as January through December, or it may follow a different 12-month period, such as July through June. The 12-month period for which a budget applies is called a **fiscal year**. A fiscal year is set by the financial managers of the facility and applies to the entire facility.

In any organization, the budget is arranged according to a hierarchy, or set of categories. Each department or section of the organization has its own set of numbers. A composite of all the individual department financial projections becomes the budget for the facility as a whole. Thus, a dining services budget feeds into the comprehensive plan for the facility.

As an aid in both planning and implementing a budget, financial planners break it into smaller pieces, called categories. A budget for a dining services operation, for example, may list expenses as an annual total and then also list specific groups of expenses with a projected dollar figure for each. The same concept applies to revenues. Figure 21.2 illustrates how budget categories may be presented.

Figure 21.1 Financial Terminology*

TERM	DEFINITION	COMMENT/EXAMPLE
FTE—Full Time Equivalent	The equivalent of one person working full time at 40 hours per week. Or it may mean two or more people whose hours together add up to 40 hrs./wk. Labor budgets are usually based on FTEs.	To determine FTEs per year for one full time person: 8 hrs./day x 5 days/wk. x 52 wks./yr. = 2,080 hr./yr. or one FTE.
Pay Period	A defined cycle for documenting hours worked and processing the payroll to issue paychecks.	If you are paid every other week, your pay period is two weeks long.
Overtime	The time an employee works beyond a regularly scheduled work day or pay period.	An employee who works 83 hours in one pay period (40 hrs./wk. for 2 weeks) would be entitled to three hours of overtime.
Exempt Employee	An employee who is exempt from overtime pay. This person is on salary and receives a standard rate of pay.	In most organizations, managers are classified as exempt.
Non-Exempt Employee	An employee who is *not* exempt from overtime pay.	Most foodservice staff positions.
Census	The number of clients or client count on a given day. How this is determined depends upon the type of foodservice.	Healthcare, Corrections/Schools: Managers will receive a daily census count. Cafeteria or Restaurant: Census is determined from the point of sale (POS) records.
Cost Per Meal	The calculated total food, supply and labor cost divided by the number of meals served.	Often, comparisons of food cost per day or meal are used between facilities.
Food Cost Percentage	Used to calculate the percent of food cost compared to the revenue of a retail operation (cafeteria). The food cost for a specified period such as a month divided by the total sales for the same month.	In Figure 21.,2 the total sales or revenues are $33,245. The total food cost is all of the food costs added up: meat, produce, dairy, Staples = $12,500. To calculate the food cost percentage: $12,500 ÷ 33,245 = .3759 or 37.6%
Gross Versus Net	Gross means a sum of money, as in, before any deductions are applied. Net is the amount of money that remains after all needed expenses have been deducted.	$1,220/month: Net incomes might be $875 after all of the deductions.
Break-Even	When revenues and expenses are equal.	There is no loss or profit.
Subsidies	External funding for foodservice activities.	School Foodservice: Usually refers to funding and/or food received from the USDA. Healthcare & University: Meals for staff may be subsidized as a planned benefit that may be transferred back to Human Resources as a labor cost. More frequently the cost is left as an unreimbursed in dining services.

* Some of these terms have been defined in preceding chapters.

Figure 21.2 Sample Budget Categories

REVENUES		
101	$1,200	Outpatient
102	$120,000	Cafeteria Revenue
	$121,200	**TOTAL OPERATING REVENUE**

OPERATING EXPENSE		

Labor

301	$571,985	Salaries
302	$131,557	Employee Benefits
	$703,542	**LABOR**

Supplies

701	$275,213	Supplies: Meat, Fish, Poultry
702	$234,521	Supplies: Other Food
703	$27,854	Supplies: Supplements
704	$9,853	Supplies: Cleaning Products
705	$5,733	Supplies: Office and Admin.
	$553,174	**SUPPLIES**

Supplies

801	**$15,000**	**REPAIRS AND MAINTENANCE**

Total Expenses

	$1,271,716	**TOTAL OPERATING EXPENSE**

NET OPERATING BUDGET (EXPENSES, REVENUES)		
	($1,150,516)	**NET REVENUE OVER EXPENSES**

Putting It Into Practice

1. Calculate the monthly food cost and the cost per patient day given the following data:

   Beginning Inventory: $15,000

   Purchases: $25,000

   Ending Inventory: $17,500

   Average Daily Census for the Month of April: 118

This is a simplified example of a dining services budget. In this example, revenues come from sales in two categories: a cafeteria and for outpatient education. The budget represents a projection or estimate of the income the operation expects to receive from each of these. Meanwhile, expenses are grouped by: labor, food, supplies and repairs.

Note that in this example, each category in the budget has a number. Meat purchases, for example are in category #701. Numbering of categories is commonly referred to as subaccounts and helps financial planners identify categories clearly.

Types of Budgets

The two most common budgets that Certified Dietary Managers may use are an operating and a capital budget.

Operating Budget. This is an estimate of costs incurred in the process of generating meals. So it would be an estimate of the food costs, beverage costs, and labor costs. The operating budget is a financial plan for the period of time it covers. That time period might be one month, six months, or one year.

Another common practice is to break expenses and revenues down into smaller time increments, which makes it easier to monitor. In a dining services operation, a typical unit of time is one month. There are two ways to determine a monthly budget. If expected revenues and expenses are to accumulate evenly throughout the year, prorate all the figures. This means adjusting each figure according to a specified increment of time. So, to determine a one-month budget, divide each figure of an annual projected dollar amount by 12. In the example in Figure 21.2, wages paid to employees in a one-month period should be approximately: $571,985 ÷ 12 = $47,665.

A more complex budgeting model says that revenues and/or expenses will not be the same from month to month. Imagine operating a dining service for students in a university. Knowing that the client/customer counts or numbers receiving meals will drop sharply for the summer months, when student enrollment is very low, results in lower revenues from student meal plans. At the same time, there will be less spending on food and labor in the dining rooms. In a budget such as this one, a specific figure is planned for each category for each month.

Capital Budget. A capital budget is a plan for building improvements and additions or replacement of equipment. In order to complete a facility capital budget, each department will need to submit their capitol requests. Figures 21.3 A and B show an actual operation budget for a public school system that includes the capital budget line.

Developing a Budget

The budget is an estimate for the future financial performance of the operation. In almost any facility, managers in their respective areas are called upon to submit budgets for an upcoming fiscal year, often months in advance. How much of the process is done by financial managers, versus how much is done by department managers, varies from one operation to another. In some situations, the department manager is not actively involved in the budget process. The manager should always seek to be a participant in the planning and development of the budget they are going to be responsible for managing.

In general, though, the following steps are useful in budget preparation:

1. **Clarify the objectives within the framework of the facility.** Is the aim to operate at break-even or at a profit? If it is a profit, how great? What revenues are expected from the operation?

2. **Break the budget into sections.** For example, if a dining room is intended to operate at a profit, separate it into its own budget. It is easier to track the performance as a unique cost center for accounting purposes. This way, estimated costs and revenues for this area are independent of other department areas. Work with the financial officer to establish appropriate sub-account categories.

3. **Estimate the revenues.** Compare current performance to the existing budget and examine each source of revenue. What changes are anticipated? Estimate revenues from any new services or any predicted changes in volume or pricing of existing services.

4. **Estimate operating costs.** This can be one of the most time-consuming aspects of budget preparation. In this step, examine food and labor costs. For food costs, most Certified Dietary Managers plan for a modest increase. How much this should be varies by product, by season, by market conditions, and by revisions in the purchasing agreements. Speak with vendors, research food price trends, and examine the prime vendor agreement to gain further information.

Figure 21.3a Metro Nashville Public Schools Food Service Fund 2010-2011

ESTIMATED CASH RESERVES JULY 1, 2010	$ 8,170,934
2010-2011 Budgeted Revenue	
USDA Meal Reimbursements	$ 26,566,154
Lunch Sales	2,696,082
Breakfast Sales	252,852
Breakfast Sales	252,852
A la Carte Sales	4,578,351
State Matching	320,130
Interest & Miscellaneous	70,862
Estimated Commodities	1,753,920
TOTAL BUDGETED REVENUE	**$ 36,238,351**
FUNDS AVAILABLE FOR 2010-2011	**$44,409,285**
2010-2011 Budgeted Expenditures	
Salaries	$ 12,271,362
Social Security & Medicare Match	858,995
Retirement Match	1,671,003
Employee Insurance Match	3,697,783
Food Purchases	11,946,237
Warehouse and Vendor Supplies	952,933
Other Supplies	104,976
Equipment	757,674
Equipment Maintenance	393,501
Freight and Storage	367,839
Uniform Rental & Laundry Services	166,270
Mileage	85,995
Other Expenses	255,263
Utilities	954.600
Estimated Commodities	1,753,920
TOTAL BUDGETED EXPENDITURES	**$ 36,238,351**
2011 ESTIMATED CHANGE IN CASH RESERVES	**$ —**

Metro Nashville Public Schools. Used with permission.

Figure 21.3b Metro Nashville Public Schools Fiscal Year 2010-2011 Budget

Account Number		Account Name	2009-2010 Positions	2009-2010 Budget	2010-2011 Position Changes	2010-2011 Budget Changes	2010-2011 Proposed Positions	2010-2011 Proposed Budget	Remarks
1440					FOOD SERVICE				
1440	0	Salaries, Certifications	3.0	$ 237,638		$ (2,731)	3.0	$ 234,907	Food Service Certified Coordinators
1440	1	Salaries, Clerical	10.0	343,575	1.0	(12,364)	11.0	331,211	Senior Secretary, Senior Account Clerks, Account Clerks
1440	2	Salaries, Support	768.0	11,972,206		(266,962)	768.0	11,705,244	Director, Coordinators, Field Managers, FS Managers and FS Workers
1440	3	Food		11,781,619		164,618		11,946,237	Dairy, Produce, Frozen Food and Food Staples
1440	4	Supplies and Materials		1,097,352		(39,773)		1,057,579	Vendor & Warehouse Purchases, Fuel, Truck Repairs, Office Supplies
1440	5	Other Expenses		2,215,539		(77736)		2,137,803	Equipment Repair, Telephone, Commodity Freight, Uniforms, Laundry, Training Permits, Utilities, Technology Vendor Support
1440	6	FICA, Pension & Insurance		5,698,978		528,803		6,227,781	Pension, Insurance, FICA
1440	7	Equipment		739,038		18,636		757,674	Large Equipment, Smallwares, Technology Hardware
1440	8	Travel/ Mileage		78,583		7,412		85,995	Mileage
Function Total			781.0	$ 34,164,528	1.0	$ 319,903	782.0	$34,484,431	
USDA Commodities				1,369,545		384,375		1,753,920	
Total Budget and Commodities			781.0	$ 35,534,073	1.0	704,278	782.0	$38,238,351	

Meal Prices	2009-2010	2010-2011
BREAKFAST		
Elementary and Secondary Adult Priced by A la Carte Item	$ 1.25	$ 1.25
LUNCH		
Elementary	$ 2.00	$2.00
Secondary	2.25	2.25
Adult (MNPS staff or working volunteer)	3.00	3.00
Adult (parent visitor)	3.50	3.50
Adult (parent/visitor holiday meal)	4.00	4.00

Metro Nashville Public Schools. Used with permission.

Most operating costs relate directly to client counts or census. Consult with others in the organization to obtain census estimates for the coming year. Identify time periods where segments of the facility may be closed for renovation, new units may be coming online, service may be added to the campus or reductions in scope are anticipated. Scale operating costs accordingly.

In healthcare, college and universities, corrections, and K-12 schools, often a defined amount per person per day is budgeted. In this situation, it is especially critical to control cost per meal to fit within the parameters defined. The meal counts may be set and the income per meal defined.

In a typical dining services operation there is a level of unreimbursed catering or revenue to include in the operating budget. Using a cost per meal or cost per day method to develop a budget that includes these services is less predictive. Consider this example related to food cost:

- Senior Leadership has given a budget of:
  > $6.75 Food Cost per client day
  > $1.20 Supply Cost per client day
  > $12.67 Labor Cost per client day

- The Food Cost per Client Day helps define the client menu only:
  > Annualizing the Food Cost based on a client count of 100 the Food Budget calculates to: $6.75 x 100 x 365 = $246,375
  > The problem is that this calculation does not adjust for services in non-client activity such as:
    - An increase in the meals served internally through catering that is not part of the client count but increases food cost
    - An increase in cafeteria meals (which may generate revenue) which is not part of the client count but increases food cost
    - Addition of a service, i.e., adding meals for a daycare, which is not part of the client count but increases food cost

Figure 21.4 illustrates some of the calculations that may be required to project changes for a new food budget based on projected changes. The method of simply adding an inflation factor assumes that the current budget is appropriate and does not need to change other than to reflect price adjustments. If, however, the current food cost per client day is high, then senior leadership may define a percentage or dollar amount to by which to reduce the budget. Major adjustments during the budget process directly affects the operating plan for the department and impacts the menu, purchasing options and the use of labor (more scratch less convenience).

For labor, consider any major changes that may have an impact, such as an upcoming contract negotiation with the union, an across-the-board pay increase for employees, the opening of a new restaurant across the street and similar information. Also consider the FTEs. Is there any change in services planned that might affect this number?

Although supplies are only about 5-8% of the total spend in the department, significant changes in the budget can impact the supply costs as well. If the organization decides to cut 1.5 FTE's from the dishroom and use all disposables in the cafeteria, the supply cost for chemicals will go down but the supply cost for paper goods will dramatically increase.

Putting It Into Practice

2. Using the sample budget in Figure 21.5, did the department have a loss in revenue, a profit, or break even?

Figure 21.4 Annual Budget Preparation

CATEGORY	CURRENT BUDGET	PROJECTED CHANGES	NEW BUDGET
Staples	$ 146,000	+1.5% (multiply by 1.015)	$ 148,190
Meals	132,000	+2% (multiply by 1.02)	134,640
Bakery	12,000	no change	12,000
Dairy	27,000	+0.5% (multiply by 1.005)	27,135
Produce	69,000	+3% (multiply by 1.03)	71,070

5. **Estimate capital expenses.** Capital expenses may include new equipment, a different meal delivery system, or renovations and supporting supplies that fall into unique categories for budgeting purposes. The financial decision making around capital expenses are determined by different processes and will be discussed further in Chapter 22.

Calculating Costs

Calculating the cost of food can be simple math that provides a basic figure or it can be a more analyzed calculation that is a better "documented" number. In the most straightforward terms: How much money was spent on food last month? However, that sum total of purchases does not account for what was already in the storeroom at the first of the month nor what was left on the shelves at the end of the month. Adding up the invoice cost of food purchased is the food cost but that is not just the client food cost. The invoices also include the unusual purchases for the annual medical staff gala or the turkeys bought as an employee "gift" each November. For budgeting purposes, a more detailed food cost is needed that divides out client meals from staff meals, catering and guests.

Inventory Method

This method requires a month-end physical inventory each month with the dollar value extension for each item. It is the most accurate method of determining monthly raw food costs. The formula for calculating monthly raw food costs using this method is:

Beginning Inventory Value (the ending inventory value from the previous month)

+ Purchases (for the month)

- Ending inventory

= Monthly Food Costs (what was actually used during the month)

See Figure 21.5 for an example of calculating monthly food costs and the cost/ppd. Computerized inventory systems have made calculating monthly food costs much easier because purchases are recorded automatically. A physical inventory will still need to be completed monthly in order to calculate the ending inventory.

Putting It Into Practice

3. What would the operating budget for food be if the current budget is $147,560 and the cost of living is expected to increase by 2.3%?

Figure 21.5 Sample Food Cost Calculations

MEASUREMENT	FORMULA	EXAMPLE
Monthly Numbers • Beginning Food Inventory $18,345 • Purchases Food $15,267 • Ending Food Inventory $21,112	• Total Patient Days, 3,000 • Total Meals 9,000	
Monthly Food Cost	Beginning Inventory **PLUS** Purchases **MINUS** Ending Inventory	18,345.00 + 15,267.00 - 21,112.00 = **$12,500.00**
Food Cost as a Percent of Sales	Monthly Food Cost **DIVIDED** by Sales	12,500.00 ÷ 33,245.00 = **.3759 or 37.6%**
Raw Food Cost Per Patient Day (PPD)	Monthly Food Cost **DIVIDED** by Total Patient Days (Patient Days = number of patients x number of days in the month)	12,500.00 ÷ 3,000 = **$4.17** (Total Patient Days = 100 patients x 30 days)
Raw Food Cost per Meal	Monthly Food Cost **DIVIDED** by Total Meals Served	12,500.00 ÷ 9,000 = **$1.3888 or $1.39**

Meal Equivalents. Getting the daily census from administration makes the Raw Food Cost Per Patient Day an easy calculation. The Cost Per Meal is not as simple. There are many considerations when defining what is a meal. Is it simply the number of people served or the number of dinner plates used? Is it three times the number of clients listed for the day? What about between meal snacks or how do you count clients that are out of the building or NPO? Is the meal count for toast and coffee the same as a meal count for a full turkey dinner? How do you count food served for banquets, catering functions, guest meals and employee or cafeteria meals?

There are several different systems for counting the number of meals served. Each calculation has its benefits and supporters, as well as potential errors. The patient (or client) day has a more widely accepted standard definition of the midnight count of clients "in house" while a meal has a variety of different definitions. Due to these various definitions, Total Meal Counts are hard to track and verify.

If the facility uses a Meal Count (known as a **Meal Equivalent**, a calculation to estimate a meal) for tracking food costs, budget performance or other Key Performance Indicators, always use the same calculation. Be consistent so the comparison from one point in time to another is valid. Also, be aware that other facilities and organizations probably do not use the exact same calculation for meals, so comparisons between facilities is highly questionable.

When using a meal equivalent, it is important to include the cafeteria service, floor stock (food taken to other locations for clients), catering to outside groups, staff meals, tube feedings, coffee and snack times, and nourishments. Total the food cost for each of these activities and divide this figure by a market basket price (average price for a typical cafeteria meal). Add these meal equivalents to counted meals served directly to the clients and then refigure the food cost per meal.

Requisition Method

If the facility uses storeroom requisitions, then total up all of the cost extended requisitions. The accuracy of this method assumes that every item, down to the salt shakers, is issued *only* with a requisition on file.

Recipe Method

This method is based on determining the total cost of food for each standardized recipe. The cost of each ingredient is added together and divided by the number of servings to calculate the cost per client of the recipe. Recipes must be used exactly as written (ingredients carefully measured and recipe portioned exactly). Most facilities need computer software to assist in this method. (The Recipe Cost versus the Menu Cost was discussed in Chapter 3, along with the impact of the yield factor.)

Record of Purchases Method

This method uses a simple tabulation of the current month purchase invoices to give the total cost of purchases for a specified time period. This represents an estimate of costs and does not take into account the cost of food in storage.

Menu Cost Report

A menu cost report is another very valuable tool. This report shows what it costs to produce a particular menu. A menu may be pre-costed, which means its costs are calculated during the planning phase. A tool such as this ensures that menu planning realistically meets the budget.

In addition to a pre-cost report, some operations run a post-cost report, or one that shows what the menu actually cost when production and service have been completed. This helps to identify operational variances. It shows where the planning may have fallen short, where food is unaccounted for, or where other factors need better control.

There are many formats and options for a menu cost report. An example of a menu pre-cost report appears in Figure 21.6. This report indicates that, as planned, the menu for regular diets served on day 1 of a cycle breakfast menu costs $1.32 per client. The cost of each item has been calculated based on the portion size used and actual food costs. Some of these costs have come directly from purchasing records. For example, a Certified Dietary Manager examining pricing for skim milk has determined that the facility pays $0.17 per four ounce carton of skim milk. Other numbers for a report such as this one come from a calculation of costs for each serving of each standardized recipe.

A manager may also extend a report such as this for additional meals and (if applicable) additional special diets. A more complete costing report for the cycle day also indicates how many clients are actually being served on each diet. A sample menu cost report showing these extensions appears in Figure 21.7.

What is the impact on the budget compliance if one diet costs more or less to serve than anticipated? Based on a report such as this one, the answer depends on how many clients receive this particular diet. In this example, a variation in meal cost for regular diets will have the greatest bottom line impact because there are more clients receiving this meal.

(Notice that the food cost for the Pureed Diet is higher than the other meals. This is due to the increased cost of thickened liquids which are a part of the diet.)

Figure 21.6 Menu Pre-Cost Report for One Meal

MEAL: Breakfast Menu, Cycle Day 1, Regular Diet		
Menu Item	Portion Size	Cost per Portion
Orange Juice	6 oz.	$ 0.31
Cheese Omelet	1 each	0.35
English Muffin	2 halves	0.12
Margarine	2 pats	0.05
Jelly	1 pack	0.04
Coffee	12 oz.	0.19
Skim Milk	4 oz.	0.17
Condiment Pack	1 each	0.09
	TOTAL	$ 1.32

Figure 21.7 Menu Cost Report for All Diets, One Day

Diet	PER CLIENT FOOD COST					Number of Clients	Total Food
	Breakfast	Lunch	Dinner	Snacks	Total Cost		
Regular	$ 1.32	$ 1.77	$ 2.14	$ 0.32	$ 5.55	100	$ 555.00
Diabetic	1.36	1.65	2.11	0.35	5.47	43	235.21
Heart Healthy	1.47	1.55	2.08	0.19	5.29	23	121.67
Pureed	1.38	2.11	2.70	0.61	6.80	13	88.40
Tube Feeding					6.12	21	128.52
					DAILY TOTAL	200	$ 1,128.80

Labor Costs

In a Food Production and Dining Services department, there is an assumption that food purchases are the majority of the budget. However, labor costs, especially employee benefit costs, have increased dramatically. Employees are the greatest assets and greatest expense. Food costs typically run around 40%, while labor costs are closer to 55% of the total department budget (before benefits).

Estimating Labor Costs for Budget Purposes

For facilities that have a daily census (hospital, long-term care, corrections, schools, universities), it is a useful planning tool for estimating personnel costs. Use the average census, since it may drive labor costs, to help estimate personnel expenses for the operational budget. The human resources department might be able to provide the necessary salary information to assist in this calculation.

There are other factors that impact the labor hours in a dining services department. When planning the labor budget, consider the following:

- Number of menu items.
- Type of menu.
- Type and extent of services offered.
- Type of equipment.
- Layout of equipment and department in relation to dining rooms.
- Seasonal variations in staffing.
- Number of hours the dining services department is open for business.

Once the factors affecting labor have been identified, begin estimating the costs. Review Chapter 9 for information on calculating staffing positions, labor hours, and FTE's. Figure 21.8 shows a sample budget with salary and employee benefit categories.

Figure 21.8 Sample Budget With Salary Categories

SALARIES	2016	Year-to-Date	2017
Administrative	$ 53,257	$ 45,001	
Managers	84,412	78,581	
Employees (includes waitstaff, kitchen staff, sanitation staff)	183,645	165,247	
Call-in Staff	2,780	2,649	
TOTAL SALARIES	**$ 324,094**	**$ 291,478**	
EMPLOYEE BENEFITS	**2016**	**Year-to-Date**	**2017**
Health/Life/Dental	$ 139,360	$ 139,760	
Retirement	18,797	19,001	
FICA	20,418	20,067	
Unemployment	3,214	2,978	
Workers Compensation	6,482	5,189	
TOTAL EMPLOYEE BENEFITS	**$ 188,271**	**$ 186,995**	
TOTAL LABOR COSTS	**$ 512,365**		

Managing labor expenses means monitoring it on a very regular basis. Overtime hours can quickly get out of hand if not monitored consistently. When first starting, monitor the labor usage to budget every week to understand the ups and downs. If the budget is computerized access the financial reports with the year-to-date figures. Be sure and review Keeping Labor Hours in Check, in the *Supplemental Textbook Material—Foodservice* online to see additional tips on controlling the labor budgets.

Labor Financial Measurements Used In Foodservice Operations

Labor Costs Per Meal. Just as in calculating food costs PPD or per meal, you should also calculate labor costs per meal. Use the formula listed below:

> **Example:** Use the Total Labor Costs from Figure 21.8 and a sample Total Meals Served of 191,118
>
> $512,365 ÷ 191,118 = $2.68 Labor Cost per Meal

Labor Costs per Meal Served = Labor Costs ÷ Total Meals Served

Labor Costs per FTE = Labor Costs ÷ Total FTEs. Some facilities also track labor costs per FTE.

See the example in Figure 21.9 for a sample calculation of Labor Cost per Meal.

Figure 21.9 Including Meal Equivalents In Labor Cost per Meal

Total Meal Equivalents Costs for March:

Other Meals

Cafeteria Sales for the Month of March	$18,562.00
Floor Stock Requisitions for March	415.00
Catering for Coffee, Snacks, Activities	219.00
Staff Meals for March	1,405.00
Tube Feedings and Nourishments	5,637.00
TOTAL	**$26,238.00**

Average Price for a Typical Cafeteria Meal (Market Basket Method) $3.21

Meal Equivalents for March: $26,238 ÷ $3.21 = $8,174 Meal Equivalents

Recalculate the Labor Cost per Meal from the Example in Figure 21.8
    Total Labor Cost for March: $152,365 (from Figure 21.8)
    Total Meals 191,118 ÷ Meal Equivalents 8,174 = 199,292

Divide the Labor Cost by the Total Meals Served: $512,352 ÷ 199,292 = $2.57

Note: While a decrease in labor cost per meal by 10 cents may not seem dramatic, it can make a huge difference in your overall labor costs. What if your administration said your labor cost per meal could not be more than $2.50 per meal? You could lower the cost by 10 cents per meal just by counting all of the meals you are producing.

It is important to control both food cost and labor cost per meal to meet the fiscal objectives of the facility.

Other Labor Cost Considerations

Part-time Staff. Another way to lower costs in foodservice is through the use of part-time employees. The use of part-time staff to replace full-timers has increased significantly in the past 10 years. Often part-time staff can dramatically decrease labor cost. How much savings is dependent upon the wage differential from full-time staff and the benefit package offered to part-time employees. Let's look at an example of a university foodservice that currently employs 10 full-time cooks over 14 shifts per week. The university employees receive an average wage of $16/hr. plus employee benefits equivalent to an additional 30%.

Wages:	10 cooks x 40 hrs. x $16 per hr.	= $6,400
Benefits:	$6,400 x 30%	= $1,920
	Total Labor Cost	**= $8,320/wk.**

If the university decides to cover some of the shifts with LTEs or Limited Term Employees who work only part-time for $10/hr. and qualify for only 20% benefits.

Full-time Cooks:

Wages:	6 cooks x 40 hrs. x $16/hr.	= $3,840
Benefits:	$3,840 x 30%	= $1,152
	Total Labor Costs	= $4,992

Part-time Cooks:

Wages:	8 cooks x 20 hrs. x $14/hr.	= $2,240
Benefits:	$2,240 x 20%	= $448
	Total Labor Costs	= $2,688
	New Total Labor Costs	**= $7,680/wk.**

If the organization decides to increase the number of part-time employees, make sure they feel a part of the department and are included in all of the training.

Labor Legislation. The effect of labor legislation can be significant when considering the staffing budget. Unfortunately, labor legislation varies from state to state. There are some general terms that apply to all states: minimum wage and provisions for overtime. Both of these are set by the Fair Labor Standards laws that were discussed in Chapter 10.

Working With Human Resources (HR) Department

If the Certified Dietary Manager is fortunate enough to have an HR department, many of the tasks regarding labor will be completed by that department. For instance, HR personnel will help determine where to place an employee on the salary schedule. HR will keep all employee records. They will provide the insurance, tax, and other forms for personnel.

If there is no HR department, the manager may be expected to maintain salary records. Insurance and tax forms along with other information may also need to be provided to personnel. Work with administration to determine what forms are required and what salary should be offered.

Working With Labor Unions

Labor contracts will always be an important factor affecting staff costs. Labor contracts impact wages, benefits, and other aspects of human resources management. Unionization provides certain advantages to employees. It also imposes certain requirements on the Certified Dietary Manager who must comply with a union agreement.

The decision for employees to form or join a union is made through a voting process. A **union** forms an agreement with an organization on behalf of the group of employees. Employees may form or join unions in order to attain better working conditions, improved safety, better pay, or specific benefits. However, membership in a union is not a guarantee that employees will receive everything they want or expect.

Reasons for an employee desiring to join a union sometimes relate directly to relationships with management. Following sound management practices may minimize the employee's perceived need for a union. Implementation of procedures to address employee concerns and a manager who keeps in touch with employees' needs and wants helps create a collaborative environment. Some techniques used to do this include a suggestion box, employee survey(s), employee relations rounds conducted by the HR department (or by the manager in small facilities), employee meetings, and effectively conducted employee appraisal programs. Whenever these or other techniques are used to assess employee concerns, management needs to then act on the concerns and suggestions seriously and attempt to make improvements.

Other reasons for joining a union include a desire to be heard, the appeal of a formal means of expressing concerns to administrators, and a feeling that group attachment brings security. A formal group of employees is perceived as stronger than an informal group.

Impact of Unions On Administration

Once employees are represented by a union, administration will probably have to alter some operations. Follow the contract for salary rather than decide at what level to place a new employee. Regardless of an employee's ability or skills, each must be treated equally if he or she is in the same (or similar) job classification. Frequently, seniority—rather than other factors which might distinguish employees' qualifications and performance—may become the most important factor in matters affecting personnel-related decisions.

There can be advantages to unionization. The presence of a union prompts development and/or improvement of policies or procedures that affect relationships with employees. A facility that does not have well-developed policies and management tools is likely to benefit. On certain issues, administrators will also be able to deal with only one representative of unionized employees rather than with various individual staff members. Finally, top levels of administration may need to recover much decision-making responsibility that had previously been delegated to supervisors, since the actions of a single supervisor may have facility-wide implications in a unionized environment. To the extent that centralized decision-making is beneficial, it is another advantage to union affiliation.

Glossary

Union
An organization of workers intended to represent their co-workers in labor agreements

The Collective Bargaining Process

Many people define collective bargaining as negotiations between union and facility representatives leading to a contract. More generally, however, the term **collective bargaining** applies to routine communications and negotiations involving contract agreements, interpreting contract clauses, and resolving disputes (grievances) between union and administrative officials. A great deal of time can be spent in negotiating a union agreement. It is common for union contracts to apply for a period of three or more years. To prepare for the negotiation, administrative officials in a facility must obtain information about prevailing wage and salary rates and fringe benefit provisions. They must also assess the facility's financial position, resources, and ability to commit to specific wages and other terms. Furthermore, they must analyze existing contracts, communicate with union representatives, and consider probable union concerns.

Through discussion and negotiation, the union, representing the employee and the facility administration reach a final agreement about relevant issues, including wages and salary. This agreement is signed and formalized, with each party committing to honor it for the time period specified.

How can the Certified Dietary Manager prepare and budget for increasing labor contract costs? When administration is negotiating a new contract, a manager should make sure that the labor costs provided by the administration are accurate. If possible, have the HR department survey other union foodservice departments to determine recent changes in their wage scale. This information will also be helpful.

Utilize Guidelines for Salary Scales and Merit Raises

Every facility should have a salary schedule. If the staff is represented by a union the facility is bound by the contract to follow that salary schedule. If there is no union in the facility, there should still be a salary schedule and policies about merit increases. The HR department should maintain a database or have access to a regional database of salary guidelines for the industry. They may have access to local wage rates for positions similar to those in the dining services department. This will help determine the prevailing local rate for cooks, dining room attendants, storeroom clerks and other positions in the department.

Another resource that might help with salary guidelines is The Association of Nutrition & Foodservice Professionals/Dietary Managers Association Annual Salary Survey. Figure 21.4 shows the 2012 Salary Survey results. While this information focuses on salaries for Certified Dietary Managers, it can still be a reference for your facility because it contains benefit information and represents the entire United States. The most recent survey results are available online in the *Supplemental Textbook Material—Foodservice.*

Glossary

Collective Bargaining
Generally refers to communication between administrative officials and union representatives

Figure 21.10 ANFP Salary Survey 2012

		SAMPLE SIZE	2012	2010	2008	2006	2005
					AVERAGE VALUE		
As of October 1, 2012, what was the annual salary or wage for this position?							
POSITION	ALL	3,630	$ 47,201	$ 45,423	$ 42,786	$ 40,374	$ 39,201
CDM, CFPP	Yes	3,480	47,348	45,342	42,733	40,420	39,321
	No	150	43,383	48,575	44,220	39,690	36,956
Education	Associate Degree	748	50,426	49,504	46,855	44,197	43,477
	Bachelor's Degree	649	57,596	56,561	53,685	47,914	46,653
	Dietary Managers Course Completion	2,920	45,826	55,291	38,807	36,741	35,617
	Culinary Arts	394	54,561	44,344	53,488	47,511	48.425
	Technical School	345	47,883	40,975	42,384	38,496	36,362
	Other	299	54,845	53,389	48,749	47,597	44,516
Years of Experience	0-5	265	36,401	34,464	31,591	30,992	30,307
	6-10	387	40,950	37,958	35,777	35,716	34,029
	11-15	457	42,540	41,561	40,438	39,270	37,563
	16-20	570	46,221	44,963	43,473	40,440	39,640
	21-25	591	49,740	47,682	44,723	42,414	41,275
	26-30	583	51,654	49,832	46,647	43,274	41,762
	Over 31	771	52,094	51,805	48,566	45,426	44,432
Type of Facility	Long Term Care/Nursing Home	1,510	42,652	41,382	38,690	37,890	36,581
	Long Term Care/Assisted Living	214	44,661	42,607	42,107	38,957	38,207
	Long Term Care/Hospital	130	45,490	43,946	41,634	38,526	36,222
	Hospital	869	53,123	51,013	46,605	42,885	42,393
	Continuous Care Retirement Community	271	58,264	54,713	53,498	48,654	47,809
	Assisted Living Facility	86	45,368	43,265	40,442	39,378	36,028
	School	114	42,110	40,982	39,214	34,314	32,785
	Correctional Facility	45	46,147	47,929	43,751	38,644	35,828
	Military	10	59,833	60,470	50,052	45,099	48,315
	Other	354	48,311	46,344	44,450	41,803	40,067

Manage the Capital Budget

Overview and Objectives

The Certified Dietary Managers are expected to know their department space and equipment to anticipate the needs for replacements or renovations. They also have to present the case for large dollar investments for the future. The Capital Equipment Budget planning process is significantly different from the operations budget and often includes a more difficult approval process. After completing this chapter, you should be able to:

✓ Review capital equipment needs and requirements

✓ Evaluate existing capital equipment condition and life expectancy

✓ Evaluate options for replacement of capital equipment

✓ Write budget justification for new capital equipment

✓ Recommend specifications for new capital equipment

The Capital Budget

In most organizations, the Finance Department has set a maximum spending level for any one purchase item. Often the top price the manager can spend without additional authorization is $1,000 and up to $5,000 in some facilities. Purchases larger than that amount for a single item are considered to be **Capital Expense** with an expected use, or life, longer the general operating budget. To control large ticket purchases and manage the depreciation of equipment from an accounting perspective, capital budgets are developed using a totally different process.

Often the Capital Budgeting Process includes an estimate of items that will be needed in the next year, 2-5 years and even out 5-10 years. The estimates help senior leadership to project the need for investment funds in the coming years and to spread out the cost of replacement purchases. The annual capital budget is essentially an estimate of the equipment that will be needed in the next twelve months.

In food production and dining services, capital expenses are typically related to the large kitchen equipment or meal delivery systems. Replacement of the dishmachine is often a $75,000 to $250,000 expense and has a lifetime use of many years. Updating the dishmachine may seem obvious but without thorough documentation and justification kitchen updates are typically the result of irreparable equipment failure instead of planned replacement. Often the need for new operating room equipment takes priority over the purchase of a stove or replacement of the walk-in compressor.

Glossary

Capital Expense
The cost of a single item that exceeds a finance defined limit with an expected use, or life, longer than the general operating budget

Managing the capital equipment process starts with maintaining a complete list of all items within the department. Frequently, Engineering has a comprehensive list that they use for preventive maintenance (PM's) on major pieces of machinery. The Information systems department keeps track of all the computers, printers and software systems. The finance department should have a list of all items within the department that are considered to be Capital Equipment and the current depreciation status of each. Compare the respective lists to make sure all items are covered, and add to it any equipment that needs to be monitored such as food processors, meat slicers, and utility carts. (See example of an Equipment Log in Fig. 22.1. An Equipment Log is located in the *Supplemental Textbook Materials—Foodservice.*)

Figure 22.1 Sample Equipment Log

Equipment	Year Purchased	Price	Manufacturer	Model #	Years of Depreciation	How Often PM Conducted (Yr/Qtr/M/Wk)

Use the list of equipment to monitor the repairs and service expenses related to the equipment, see in Figure 22.2, an Equipment Repair Log. (An Equipment Repair Log is located in the *Supplemental Textbook Materials—Foodservice.*) Note the frequency of down time and the cost of repairs, including substitute process expenses (the use of disposable serviceware when the dishmachine is down) and the cost of the company rep service calls. Each year, when preparing the capital budget, review and update the status of every piece of equipment on the list including the estimated remaining "life". Add items that have been purchased and remove items as they are disposed of or retired. Note that the equipment purchased today will likely have a shorter "life-cycle" than older, more heavily designed pieces.

Often, contacting the local equipment company for recommendations of models and features will be enough information for the overall forecasting process. Most vendors will provide a "reasonable" estimate (usually fairly high to cover all costs) of the purchase price, along with the likely cost of installation. Typically, the capital budget requires or recommends that a copy of the product cut sheet be included as a reference. This is also available from the equipment vendor or online.

Figure 22.2 Sample Equipment Repair Log

Equipment	Date	Repair	Cost

What Goes Into the Capital Budget

The list of items that fit into the capital budget can be endless. Common food production and dining services items include:

- Stoves, ovens, fryers, grills, steamers: cooking equipment
- Grinders, food processors, mixers, slicers: preparation equipment
- Coolers, walk-ins, freezers, reach-in: cold food holding
- Hot box, warmer, Bain Marie, steam tables, conduction tables: hot food holding
- Soft Serve, coffee machines, beverages: dispensers
- Prep tables, utility carts, speed racks storage racks, racks: work space
- Serving line, plate warmers, induction systems and pellets, delivery carts, trays, dishware and silverware (as part of the initial line purchase, replacement pieces are considered operating expenses)
- Software systems, computers, printers, cash registers, many pieces of office furniture
- Dishroom equipment, pot and pan sinks and equipment, carts, racks
- Ice machines
- Dining room tables and chairs
- Design and build out of new space or renovations

This is not an all-inclusive list, and some organizations may not include everything that is here, but this is representative of the items that fall under the capital budget versus the operating budget.

What Goes Into the Capital Budget Request

Once a piece of equipment has been identified for purchase, the manager needs to organize the supporting material to justify the expense which may not be obvious when the piece of equipment is limping along. Let's use a dishmachine as an example to demonstrate what information is needed.

- The current equipment is 20 years old.
- The repair record shows that in the past year it has been down 4 different times from 1-6 days.
- The service rep has been in for repairs 3 of those times ($1,500 plus travel expense of $800).
- The chemical service rep has commented that the use of detergent and drying agent is unexpectedly high because the wash and rinse tanks have a continuous leak of water (estimated added cost of $2,200 annually).
- The engineering department has been monitoring the water usage and is concerned about the energy cost of the hot water used and lost (estimated add cost of water and gas of $2,700 annually).
- The labor cost associated with the downtime was 45 hours above budget in the last year (an estimated $1,000).
- The cost of disposables used to provide serviceware during downtime was $2,750.
- Patient survey results during the months affected in the last year all reflect comments regarding cold food and poor presentation, which in turn could impact the facility's reimbursements from Medicare.

- In recent years the dishmachine design has been upgraded to use far less water than previously, run faster and to be more economical in the chemical usage
  - > Replacement of the current unit would save more in water, gas for heating the water, drying agents and chemicals through newer technology than even the amount lost through the leaks
  - > Often the newer machines also use less floor space allowing for better access

The annual cost of repairs and overrun expenses is almost $11,000 a year. Suddenly replacing the poorly functioning dishmachine becomes more financially reasonable.

Using the information collected, the capital request becomes easier to complete. The request form generally requires detailed information about the piece of equipment and installation including the following:

- Specification cut sheets for one or more models
- Competitive price quotes from one to three vendors
  - > The Materials Management (Purchasing) department can help source this information
- Delivery costs and timetables
- Installation costs
  - > Verify with Engineering the availability and accessibility to needed utilities.
  - > Estimated costs of utility upgrades if needed.
  - > Space needs and access (will it fit through the door and under the hood)?
  - > How much downtime of the current equipment will be needed and how will needs be met in the interim?
- Removal and disposal cost of the old equipment.
- What is the need for potential space re-design and cost to accommodate the new equipment?
  - > For example, a new garbage disposal, new scrapping tables, a heat booster for the hot water, water softening equipment, new racks and drying table...

Often, the equipment vendor can assist with organizing the printed materials needed to support a capital request. They have access to materials developed by the manufacturers to calculate replacement costs, benefits and features of different equipment and data to complete the **Return On Investment (ROI)** forms that are part of the request. The ROI is the length of time it takes to get your money back for an investment in the future.

Developing the Capital Budget forces the Certified Dietary Manager to look annually at all of the equipment and supporting systems within the department that are needed on a daily basis. The manager has to assess the current status and estimated useful life of the equipment and decide if replacement is needed this year, next year or sometime further out.

Glossary

Return on Investment (ROI)
The length of time it takes to get your money back for an investment in the future

Putting It Into Practice

1. One of two oven units is not holding temperature. The service rep has been out three times in the last six months. What information would you use to justify the purchase of a new combi-oven?

Equipment Replacement Decisions

Eventually every manager is expected to recommend equipment for replacement or addition as department needs change. The equipment maintenance record will assist in deciding when to repair or purchase new, what to purchase, and why. The steps in replacing or purchasing new equipment include:

1. Develop Equipment Specifications: When the decision is being made to repair or replace equipment, the Certified Dietary Manager should develop a specification for the equipment. Considerations for purchase specifications include:

   - Will the equipment provide the time and temperature control that is necessary for safe food?

   - Is the equipment properly sized for the volume of food that is prepared?

   - Is the equipment reliable or is it prone to frequent breakdowns?

   - Is the equipment designed so that it can be easily cleaned and sanitized?

   - Is the equipment easy to use?

   - Will the equipment fit into the assigned space?

   - Further discussion of equipment specifications is explored in Chapter 23.

2. Conducting **Cost Benefit Analysis**: A cost benefit analysis compares the relative value (quality and expense) of upgrading a piece of equipment with the downtime and cost of repairs.

   - A repair log can provide you with the history of breakdowns, lost time and expenses.

   - Consider the current features that would be lost versus the new capabilities:

     > Will the cost of replacement allow for an upgrade, exact match or maybe a reduction in features?

   - Consider the repairability of any new equipment including

     > Access to moving parts, electrical panels/gas lines/water pipes...

     > Availability of manufacturer's repair reps (a three-day lead time for repair parts may disqualify a potential purchase for "mission critical" equipment).

   - When the cost of materials and labor to repair equipment is near to or greater than the cost of replacement, the equipment should be replaced.

3. When writing a cost benefit analysis or justification for replacement, estimate repair costs by comparing the warranty information against the life of the equipment. Consult with equipment representatives and other food operators who have had experience with the equipment and/or the brand.

4. Installation and Staff Training: Often, the manufacturer or supplier will assist in ensuring that the new equipment is properly installed and provide training to staff. Vendors may charge an additional fee for hardcopy equipment manuals, particularly if the online version of the manual is readily available. Managers and other purchasers should attempt to negotiate the price of equipment operation manuals, staff training, and other support into the purchase price of the equipment.

5. Typically, purchasing requires three competitive bids to compare purchase costs, delivery and installation charges, timeliness of delivery, and service warranty options.

Glossary

Cost Benefit Analysis
Compares the relative value (quality and expense) of upgrading a piece of equipment with the downtime and cost of repairs

Alternatives

The purchase of major equipment is expensive and can be time consuming. Often, manufacturers or distributors offer the option for long-term leasing of the equipment for a fee. Coffee equipment is readily available for an upcharge of a few cents per pound of coffee purchased. Dishwashers can be leased from the manufacturer or sometimes the chemical supply company has leasing agreements.

The downside of leasing is the lack of ownership, therefore, no equity value of the equipment, the commitment to purchase their products exclusively, and the ongoing cost no matter how long the item is in use. The upside of leasing is little or no out-of-pocket cost, since the manufacturer or distributor is responsible for all repair costs, and quicker access to newer technology than what is in current use.

Summary

Capital budgets are very different processes than the typical operations budget. The planning and preparation for capital investments requires different types of information and usually depends upon a well-documented, persuasive presentation to gain approval. When a piece of needed equipment is broken, repair or replacement is obvious. However, when the piece of equipment is not beyond the point of repair, often replacement is seen as discretionary spending—that can wait.

When money is tight and funding for new equipment and projects is limited, plan to prepare a formal presentation with a slide show, statistics to back up the recommendations, cost projections and the value of implementing the proposal. Keep the needs of the clients, and the safety of staff and clients in focus when preparing the proposal and presentation. Review the suggestions in Chapter 15 for effective speaking and design a presentation to convince senior leadership of the need to approve not just the capital budget, but also to release the funds for purchase.

Department Design and Layout

Overview and Objectives

One of the basic management functions is planning. At some point, most Certified Dietary Managers are asked to plan a kitchen redesign of some scale. The manager is expected to justify the department design and layout. This chapter helps prepare for those tasks. After completing this chapter, you should be able to:

✓ Maintain records of suggestions and complaints received

✓ Conduct department improvement discussion session with staff

✓ Evaluate work flow, essential equipment relative to new department designs or construction

✓ Research concepts/products related to department facility design

✓ Prepare proposals, specifications for new construction or renovation in layout/design changes

Both design and equipment have a direct impact on the efficiencies of a food production and dining services operation. Effective design and equipment choices allow for operational objectives related to the menu, customer/client service, quality, schedules, budget, and safety. Whether planning a new operation or remodeling an existing operation, designing the physical layout is a critical step. Any change to menus or service models can trigger a need to revise design, equipment, or both.

Physical Layout

The layout of a facility can impact food quality and the ability to produce meals according to established timetables. It can also affect labor efficiency and staffing schedules. Several factors that influence, or are influenced by, the layout of the facility are:

The menu. The relationship between the menu and the production equipment is a "push me—pull me" one. Menu items such as "fry only" french fries are ill-advised in a production kitchen with no fryers. The menu defines the types of food products to be prepared, and the equipment needed. The equipment present defines what can be written into the menu.

The space available has to accommodate the inventory, pre-prep, preparation, holding, and service defined by the menu. Limited storage space requires either a limited menu or daily deliveries.

Use of convenience foods. As the number and quality of convenience items increases, the need for food production space and equipment decreases. However, requirements for refrigerated and/or freezer storage space will typically increase. Conversely, if many items are being made from scratch, on-site needs for preparation space and equipment increase.

Quantity of food to prepare. Equipment and work space must be sized to accommodate the number of meals being produced for on-site as well as any off-site feeding and catering.

Production and service systems. Both production and service models influence the need for space and the use of space over time. In a decentralized system, much of the required work space and equipment shifts to remote units, such as serving pantries. In a centralized system there is a much greater need for work space and equipment in the central location. In a cook-chill system, there may be greater opportunity to control scheduling of work; it is important to use space and labor time efficiently since food preparation is not intended for immediate service.

Each system also dictates varying needs for storage. For example, a cook-chill system requires large refrigerated storage areas along with blast chillers and rethermalization equipment. A decentralized service system needs refrigerated storage, transport equipment, and rethermalization units. Space for equipment and a layout that supports efficient work flow are essential.

Space. Space allocated for food production and dining services affects both the facility layout and the amount, and type, of equipment that can be considered. Based on the needs of a facility, compromises in space, design, and budget are common. Square footage limitations or unusual layout may drive decisions to select space-efficient equipment options, and/or to choose single pieces of equipment that can perform multiple functions.

Funds. Budget funds allocated for equipment have an impact on plans. Food production and dining services often need to compete with other departments for limited space and budgetary resources for remodeling and/or new building activities.

Design Principles

Efficient flow of products through the food production area and work stations that maximize employee work activity is central to a well-designed work space. The flow of work varies from one operation to another.

Typically, facilities are designed by considering workload requirements. Then, work centers are developed based on logical groupings of menu items and tasks. Generally, the layout of a food production and dining services area should enable a logical, economical flow of foods from receiving through storage, production, additional storage (if required), and service. It should support separation of clean, sanitized products from soiled products.

Over time, an established design and layout may need to be adjusted. For example, any of the following could occur:

- A 30-year baker is retiring, and the Certified Dietary Manager might determine it would be more economical and better for quality control to purchase more convenience items for the bakery.
- A replacement oven may have different space requirements than the existing oven or different electrical service requirements.
- A new service may require the operation to double its production of salad and soup products.

These are just a few examples of how change can generate new challenges in physical design and equipment needs. In selecting equipment, it is often possible to choose equipment that serves multiple uses for the greatest flexibility in responding to future needs and changes. For example, a convection oven/steamer can produce a variety of foods, applying a variety of cooking methods, such as steaming or roasting. It can be a versatile replacement for outdated equipment.

Factors to Consider

The task of designing a food production and dining services department is complex and should involve the team effort of a Certified Dietary Manager along with a project architect, foodservice design consultant, in-house engineering expert, and staff who use the equipment. Concerns that must be considered include:

Energy Efficiency. Over the lifetime of a piece of equipment, operating costs related to gas or electricity usage can be staggering. The food production and dining services department makes up a large percentage of a facility's energy bill. In 2001, an energy efficient program called Energy Star® was launched to designate equipment that is highly efficient. An Energy Star® rating meets the minimum efficiency criteria.

Two research organizations, Foodservice Technology Center (FSTC), http://www.fishnick.com/saveenergy/rebates, and the Consortium for Energy Efficiency (CEE), http://www.cee1.org, also have energy efficiency equipment ratings. Their ratings are more stringent than the Energy Star®. All commercial kitchen equipment will soon be manufactured with both energy and water efficiency. See the Management in the News article in the *Supplemental Textbook Materials—Foodservice* online for Energy Star® equipment examples and suggestions for how to find energy savings in the department.

Sustainable and green building concepts are becoming more common in the industry. An emerging certification called LEED (Leadership in Energy and Environmental Design), developed by the U.S. Green Building Council, is encouraging buildings that are "designed and built using strategies aimed at improving performance across all the metrics that matter most. Some of these strategies are: energy savings, water efficiency, carbon dioxide emissions reduction, improved indoor environmental quality, and stewardship of resources and sensitivity to their impacts." Many facilities are adding composting, rooftop gardens, and herb gardens to further support the green initiative.

Water efficiency is also an aspect of green buildings. A number of facilities are looking at saving and reusing water. One example of water efficiency is a water-cooled ice machine. Other facilities are utilizing biotechnology. One university is using food scraps for bioenergy.

Incorporating energy efficiency in the capital planning for equipment replacement is looking ahead. Perhaps the state or local utility has a rebate program to help cover the cost. Or maybe when the freezer needs to be replaced a larger Energy Star® model will provide more storage and better efficiency. As with any plan, review it annually to update with the latest information on efficient commercial kitchen equipment.

Ergonomic Factors. Ergonomic factors influence the comfort, efficiency, and safety of a work environment, and are of great concern in food production and dining services. Designs that control physical fatigue and help prevent injury related to repetitive motion are important. These concerns are recognized as designers reduce distances employees must travel, adjust heights of work areas to fit the needs of employees, and develop comfortable (thickened) handles for small utensils. See Figure 23.1 for examples of ergonomic factors.

Putting It Into Practice

1. When considering design factors, how would your considerations for temperature and humidity be different for a kitchen versus a dining room?

Noise. There can be a great deal of noise in food preparation areas. Use of soundproofing materials and the selection of less noisy equipment can help reduce these problems. This can distract employees leading to accidents and injuries. Likewise, when noisy equipment carries into the dining space, clients and guests are affected.

Lighting. Adequate lighting is critical for safety as well as for managing the quality of work of a food production and dining services department. Lighting is separated into ambient, task and accent lighting.

- Ambient or general lighting provides overall illumination—often, florescent ceiling bulbs are used in food production areas. The level of brightness is intended to provide light without glare or significant shadows.
- Task lighting is intended to provide illumination for specific work areas. Often, pendant drop lights or ceiling spot lights are used in dining areas to provide focused light.
- Accent lighting adds drama or interest in a space. The light is focused on a design point of interest, such as artwork or architectural features.

Lighting is another area where energy savings can be realized. For instance, check out LED lighting for commercial freezers.

Heating, Ventilating and Air Conditioning (HVAC). Work in food preparation areas can be very hot with high levels of humidity. Concerns about temperature are appropriate as air conditioning needs are considered, and as cooking and cleaning equipment selection decisions are made. Today, most food preparation kitchens have a level of air conditioning to maintain an appropriate work environment.

Typically, the food production and preparation area is a large open space with large volumes of air that need to be continuously circulated (the ventilation component of HVAC). Access to "make-up air" directly relates to how much equipment, particularly heat producing items like grills and fryers, can be designed into a space.

Safety and Sanitation. Health regulations dictate cleanability of equipment, temperature and humidity requirements for dry storage and lighting requirements, along with the design and venting of heat, ventilation, and air conditioning systems, and much more. These concerns are important and must meet all applicable federal, state and local codes.

Local Construction Codes. Building codes may stipulate many aspects of design. In some locales, special regulations apply to healthcare facilities. Working with a foodservice kitchen designer, for major projects in particular, will ensure compliance to the building codes that are different for kitchen construction. The general construction designers often are not aware of the specific codes related to dining rooms and kitchens.

Security. Security concerns are always a top priority in the design. For example:

- Should storage areas be located close to the back door? No, because this may increase the opportunity for theft.
- Should receiving and preparation areas be under the view of the Certified Dietary Manager? Yes. Thus, an office design may use glass partitions that allow a manager to monitor operations from a desk.

While the list of questions can continue, the point is that the control of food and materials during production and service is influenced by the amount of security built into the facility.

Design of Receiving and Storage Areas

Receiving areas should typically be as close as practical to storage areas. They should also be large enough to house incoming deliveries, so that employees can follow effective receiving practices. Additional space should be available for related equipment, such as scales and dollies.

To limit access by unauthorized persons, storerooms should be designed with walls that extend from the floor to the ceiling and with ceilings that cannot be entered from an adjoining room through a drop ceiling, pipe chase area or other connecting area access points. Locked doors are usually required. If an ingredient room is used, it should be planned close to dry storage areas and to the food preparation areas.

Design of Food Preparation and Service Areas

In production areas, cooks need storage space for pre-preparation items, aisles to accommodate carts and space for small equipment, such as scales, slicers, and food processors. To organize work efficiently, they need counter space and prep areas close to their production equipment (stoves, steamers, grills, etc.).

For decentralized service in which products are prepared in a remote location and re-heated or finished close to the point of service, consider what additional equipment and space requirements are needed. Service needs may require less space but more specialized equipment and utility service.

In a cafeteria, it's important to structure a design that fits the service model. For example, a design for a straight-line service is much different from one used for a scramble service. In addition, it's important to consider client's entry and exit points, and to allow space for clients to move around comfortably while serving themselves, without getting in each other's way.

If food items are to be prepared on an as-ordered basis, utility connections, ventilation systems, and space to house cook-to-order equipment in service areas must be considered. Equipment to hold hot and cold food items near the point of service will be needed. Sometimes cafeteria operations use a hot and/or cold food pass-through so that production staff can make items readily available for service without having to go into public food production and dining services areas. A pass-through is a connecting area between the kitchen and the service area.

If cafeteria operations are to collect cash, space for cashiers, point-of-sale equipment, and other necessary items must be included. Electrical and computer networking requirements are part of this planning component.

Dining area planners must consider not only the number of persons to be served at one time, but also the flow of soiled dishes back to dishwashing areas and the removal of trash from the public spaces. Commonly, food production and dining services operations use a conveyor system to transport soiled dishes. The servery and dining space needs to be practical for the clients being served, comply with sanitation guidelines, and also be aesthetically comfortable.

Dining areas greatly influence the clients' impression of an establishment. The atmosphere of the facility itself, the cleanliness and condition of dining room furniture, fixtures and equipment, lighting, and a wide range of other concerns are important to these impressions. Planning a dining area requires consideration of questions such as:

Putting It Into Practice

2. You are considering a culture change and plan to move away from a trayline and implement restaurant service in the dining room. What design considerations do you need to consider when planning for this change?

- How many clients must be fed at one time?
- How much space should be allocated for each diner?
- Does space for walkers or wheel chairs need to be planned?
- Who else will be present (service staff, nursing staff, family, etc.), and how much additional space will be needed?
- What other activities besides dining services will occur in dining areas? (In many skilled nursing facilities, dining areas become multi-purpose rooms at other times of day.)
- What specialized equipment is needed to ensure client comfort?
- How will food be served in the dining area such as a salad bar or food cart?

Design of Other Food Production and Dining Services Areas

In addition to food storage, production, assembly, serving, and dining areas, other spaces also merit planning. Consider the need for:

- Office space for the manager and supervisors.
- Space for dish and pot washing, holding of refuse until pickup, space for washing carts and shelving equipment, and so on.
- Cleaning and other chemicals storage.
- Refrigeration equipment for walk-in units.
- Space for mobile transport equipment.
- Location of handwashing and prep sinks consistent with local, state or federal codes.

Many healthcare facilities provide snacks for unit based nourishment centers. The Certified Dietary Manager should lend expertise about how nourishments are stored, rotated and protected until the time of service.

Space Allocation

The proportions of space used for receiving, storage, production, service, and clean-up can vary depending on menus and service models. Figure 23.1 is an example of the breakdown and space allocations for a traditional 6,000-square-foot kitchen. This is one that essentially cooks food and then serves it.

How might this allocation vary for other kitchens? A cook-chill kitchen would require much more refrigerated storage space. A kitchen relying intensively on convenience foods or a no-cook kitchen might require a great deal of storage space, but very little production space.

Design Principles and Employees

A great source for getting input into redesigning or building a new kitchen will come from the current employees. They are the experts who use the equipment and the current kitchen design every day. Allow them to provide suggestions about work flow and essential equipment relative to new department designs or construction. Involve employees with each step of the redesign/design project for valuable, insightful information for planning meetings.

Keep a record each time an employee complains about a piece of equipment or a design element in the kitchen. When ready for the redesign/design process simply access the history of issues already documented. An easy way to document these complaints/suggestions is to have an email file labeled Kitchen Design and send yourself a quick email each time an employee provides a suggestion or a complaint.

Remember to include needs such as wiring for computers. More areas of the food production and plating services need network connectivity, docking stations and remote printing capability.

Figure 23.1 Space Allocation for a Traditional Kitchen

Subsystem	Space Allocation (sq. ft.)	
Receiving	120	3.00%
Storage	1,120	28.00%
Preparation	1,100	27.50%
Cooking	470	11.75%
Serving	800	20.00%
Clean-up	390	9.75%
Subtotal	4,000	100.00%
Fixed Space*	2,000	
Subtotal	6,000	

Includes janitorial storage, restrooms, lounge areas, etc. Source: John B. Knight, Ph.D,. Purdue University

Specifying and Purchasing Equipment

In many facilities, a Certified Dietary Manager has direct purchasing authority for ongoing supplies and small purchases but must seek approval to purchase capital equipment, so the purchasing procedure may be different. As discussed in Chapter 22, a capital budget justification is likely required. In addition, a manager may need to review plans and specifications with a maintenance or engineering expert to plan installation and to assure compliance with all relevant codes and regulations. Because capital equipment does require significant investment and will become a part of the operation for a long time, purchasing decisions are very important.

Before making a purchasing recommendation for capital items, follow these basic background procedures:

Step 1: Determine a need.

Step 2: Consider the capital budget (Review Chapter 22 for information regarding the Capital Budget).

Step 3: Investigate options.

Step 4: Consult with others (Engineering, Information Systems, Purchasing...) in the organization.

Step 5: Obtain price quotations.

- For very large purchases, a Certified Dietary Manager may use a process called **request for proposal (RFP)**. This is a formal document stating the requirements for the purchase. It is distributed to potential suppliers, each of whom indicates ability to meet each requirement along with a price. In some facilities, purchasing staff may be involved in requesting price quotations from suppliers, comparing quotations, and undertaking supplier negotiations.

Step 6: Prepare a capital budget request.

Step 7: Make a decisions.

Step 8: Award the bid and schedule delivery.

Keep senior management updated regarding issues or concerns during the purchasing process.

Finding a Supplier for Equipment

To find a supplier use any of the following resources:

Local Equipment Suppliers

A local supplier may be able to identify options and explain the differences among them. In some locales, there may be a showroom where the various models of the equipment can be examined and tested.

Trade Shows

An industry trade show provides the opportunity to see and try equipment in person and discuss needs with a representative.

Trade Magazines

Food production and dining services magazines offer ongoing coverage and advertising related to capital equipment. In addition, there are special (complimentary) magazines devoted solely to food production and dining services equipment. Some carry complete buyers guides or directories of sources, as well as informational articles about equipment designs and specifications.

The Internet

Major manufacturers of food production and dining services equipment offer considerable product information on websites. Many also offer contact information for a dealer or representative in the area who may be able to help. In addition, a number of foodservice equipment websites catalog products from various suppliers. Interactive tools may provide a specifications by fax or directly from the website.

Colleagues

It is also valuable to discuss equipment needs with colleagues, and obtain feedback and ideas about both specifications and products. A list serve is a good place to ask questions to seek opinions.

Glossary

Request for Proposal (RFP)
A written description of large dollar items that is then sent to a supplier to obtain a competitive bid

Selecting Food Production and Dining Services Equipment

To make a decision about an equipment purchase, review a number of factors:

Suitability for Intended Use

Since a wide range of equipment products is available for almost any purpose, it is important to consider the suitability of each product. Suitability issues include how well the equipment can perform the required job in the intended setting. The volume of output a piece of equipment can handle may not match the need.

Consider a pizza oven for an example. How many pizzas will need to cook at a time to meet service requirements and how long it will take to cook them? Specified equipment must accommodate the load, as well as any anticipated increases in volume. Some equipment is described in terms of a duty cycle, or how many operations it can perform within a specified period of time.

Ease of Operation

Equipment should be as easy to use as possible, requiring minimal steps for operation, and providing a user-friendly design. To evaluate this, it is wise to test equipment while involving any employees who will be responsible for using it.

Durability and Warranty

It is necessary to confirm that the product will stand up to its intended use. A warranty provides some indication of durability, as well as financial protection if the product cannot withstand use. Study a warranty carefully to determine any conditions that apply. Review what is and what is not, covered by the warranty and whether service charges may apply.

Construction and Safety

Closely aligned with durability is the integrity of the equipment's construction. Equipment must be easy to clean and safe to operate. Compliance with established standards for safety and sanitation are indicated by seals and certifications from various organizations, such as NSF and UL. (See Figure 23.2 for a summary.) Many pieces of food production and dining services equipment today are treated with antimicrobial protective compounds that discourage growth of bacteria and mold. These products are incorporated into construction materials and last the lifetime of the equipment.

Compatibility With Existing Equipment

It is important that equipment be compatible with existing systems. For example, trays being purchased must fit into the current carts, and attachments for electric mixers must fit existing equipment. As applicable, be sure equipment being purchased will fit into available space, integrate into existing structures and utility systems, move through doorways, and is compatible with current wiring. Is equipment compatible with ADA regulations?

Assistance Provided Before and After Purchase

Before a purchase, some suppliers provide design analysis, technical analysis, creative suggestions, and a plan for operational integration. After a purchase, suppliers may provide delivery, installation, on-site testing, demonstration, training, and maintenance. Evaluate and clarify tasks such as these. In cases where a supplier is not supplying these services, it is also important to determine how each will be accomplished, and what costs will be incurred.

Figure 23.2 Approval Agencies for Foodservice Equipment

National Sanitation Foundation *(approval designated by the NSF seal)*: Provides standards for materials, design, construction, performance, cleanability, and foodservice sanitation.

Underwriters Laboratories *(approval designated by the UL mark)*: Provides testing and certification to verify that electrical or gas equipment is safe to operate. Appliances are tested to ensure they comply with fire safety requirements and won't emit shock.

American Gas Association *(AGA certification)*: Provides safety testing services for gas appliances through the International Approval Service.

International Standards Organization *(ISO)*: ISO standards address quality in manufacturing. Through compliance with established standards, a manufacturer can become ISO certified.

Agencies providing energy information for foodservice equipment Energy Star®: Provides a listing of Energy Star® commercial equipment. www.energystar.gov/products

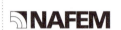

North American Association of Food Equipment Manufactorers *(NAFEM)*: A trade organization that provides links to equipment companies. www.nafem.org

The Food Service Technology Center *(FSTC)*: Provides fact sheets and other publications such as energy efficiency calculators on commercial equipment.

Federal Energy Management Program *(FEMP)*: Provides up-to-date information on energy efficient federal procurement, including the latest recommendations. www.energy.gov/femp

Price

A detailed clarification of price incorporates the items above. In comparing prices from alternate suppliers, be sure to compare the bottom-line figure that reflects all associated costs and discounts.

Operating Cost

This is different from price but is critical in the evaluation of what a piece of equipment will cost. Operating expenses include the cost of energy to use the equipment, as well as the cost of supplies. Some equipment uses proprietary, disposable supplies available only from the manufacturer. Pricing for such supplies must be evaluated carefully. To evaluate costs, it can be useful to project supply costs over a period of one year.

Service and Reputation

As with food purchasing decisions, ultimate success with a purchase depends on a supplier's reliability in meeting commitments and the quality of services and repairs provided.

Types of Equipment

The menu served, the style of service, and the number of meals served daily will have the greatest impact on the types of equipment needed. Figure 23.3 summarizes equipment options for preparing a variety of menu items. Each type of food production and dining services will need different equipment.

Figure 23.4 outlines preparation equipment suitable for a school food production and dining services operation based on number of meals served daily. Additional information, with a full listing and description of types of equipment, is available in the online *Supplemental Textbook Material—Foodservice*.

Equipment Specifications

Any piece of equipment chosen for a food production and dining services department is available with alternatives and options. In preparing a capital budget or even making a small equipment purchase, develop an **equipment specification**. This is a detailed description of the product. When multiple suppliers are asked to quote equipment prices, as in an RFP, the specification is important for ensuring that the same features are referenced in each quote. The specification nails down what is essential for ensuring that what is purchased will meet the defined needs precisely.

Glossary

Equipment Specification
A detailed description providing information needed to purchase a piece of equipment

Figure 23.3 Food Preparation Equipment for School Foodservice

PREPARATION EQUIPMENT	MEALS PREPARED PER DAY		
	<400	401-700	701-1000
Convection Ovens	(1) double	(2) double	(3) double
Tilting Braising Pans	(1) 23 or 30 gallon	(1) 23 or 30 gallon & (1) 40 gallon	(2) 40 gallon
Kettles	(1) 10 gallon	(1) 20 gallon	(1) 10 gallon & (1) 20 gallon
Steamers	(1) 2-compartment	(1) 2-compartment	(2) 2 compartment
Ranges	(1) 2-burner	(1) 2-burner	(1) 2-burner
Mixers	(1) 60 qt. with 30 qt. attachments	(1) 60 qt. with 30 qt. attachments	(1) 30 qt & (1) 60 qt.
Slicers	(1) automatic	(1) automatic	(2) automatic
Food Processors	(1) tabletop	(1) tabletop	(1) tabletop
Heated Cabinets: Pass-thru or Reach-in	1 section	2 section	3 section
Refrigerators: Pass-thru or Reach-in	1 section	2 section	2 section

Source: Adapted from National Food Service Management Institute. University of Mississippi. Guidelines for Equipment to Healthy Meals. NFSMI-R-25-96. Used with permission.

To develop a specification, it helps to do some product research first to identify what are realistic expectations. Answer questions about the product needs, such as:

- What size or capacity is required?
- What time constraints must the product meet, e.g., cooking time for a particular product, number of dishes per hour, etc.?
- What construction materials, e.g., stainless steel (___ gauge), glass, aluminum, antimicrobial treatment, etc.?
- What exterior finish is needed?
- For power equipment, gas or electric, and to what specifications (e.g., 220 volt, single phase or 3-phase)?
- What size motor is needed (e.g., ___ HP)?
- What technologies should the equipment use, e.g., convection, conduction, pressure-less steam, etc.?
- What water treatment systems or filtering systems are required?
- What safety seals are required (UL, NSF, etc.)?
- Where will this unit reside—floor model, countertop, under counter, etc.? Does it need legs or wheels?
- What space dimensions are available (specify length, width, depth, and height)? What door size or hood height does it need to fit into?
- If the unit has doors that open, in what direction will they open, and what amount of space is available?
- What pan or tray sizes should this equipment use (if applicable)?
- What user features are needed, e.g., control panel features, manual or automatic functioning, multiple speed options, etc.?
- What special features are needed, e.g., HACCP data logging, programmable memory, optional accessories, etc.? (A range is typically sold with one oven rack or no oven rack—do you need more?)
- What features will enhance cleanability, e.g., easy disassembly, self-cleaning options, etc.?
- What safety and ergonomic features are required, such as auto shut-off when not in use, guards for sharp components, etc.?
- How will equipment be installed and by whom?
- Where should utility connections be provided (back, side, etc.)?
- What are the warranty requirements (parts and/or service, for what period of time)?
- What energy-saving or energy efficiency requirements are required (KW or BTU usage)?
- What training needs are specified?

A sample equipment specification appears in Figure 23.5. Consult with suppliers for information, and with in-house engineering staff to be sure of the specific power requirements and installation needs are correct. Once the specification is complete, provide it to suppliers and ask them for a quote. While a specification needs to be detailed enough to ensure expectations are met, leave some space for flexibility with qualifiers like "equal to or better than…" In the final analysis, the specification should be realistic and attainable for a number of competing products in the marketplace.

Figure 23.4 Equipment and the Menu

	OVENS			STEAM EQUIPMENT					BROILERS	
	Ranges	Convection	Cook & Hold	Steamers	Kettles	Braising Pans	Fryers	Griddles	Cheese-melters	Char-Broilers
Breakfast										
Eggs	•	•		•	•	•		•		
Pancakes	•					•		•		
Biscuits	•	•	•							
Bacon	•	•	•			•		•		
Hash Browns	•	•	•			•		•		
Appetizers										
Soups	•				•	•				
Pizza	•									
Shrimp	•	•		•	•	•	•		•	•
Fish	•	•		•	•	•	•	•		•
Scallop Gratin	•	•	•							
Potato Skins	•	•	•						•	
Entrées										
Steak	•	•				•		•		•
Roast Beef	•	•								
Whole Chicken	•	•				•				
Meatloaf	•	•				•				
Lamb	•	•				•		•		•
Veal	•	•				•		•		
Burgers (4 oz.)	•							•		•
Ribs	•	•		•		•				•
Chicken Parts	•	•		•		•	•			•
Shellfish	•	•		•		•	•			•
Salmon	•	•		•	•	•		•	•	•
Vegetables										
Grilled	•							•		•
Steamed	•			•	•	•				
Boiled	•				•	•				
In cream sauce	•	•			•	•				
Au Gratin	•	•	•						•	
Sautéed	•					•				
Sides										
Sauces	•				•	•				
Gratin Potatoes	•	•							•	
Baked Potatoes	•	•								
Mashed Potatoes	•	•		•	•	•				
Fries							•			
Rice	•	•		•	•	•				
Desserts & Bakery										
Breads	•	•								
Soufflés	•	•								
Pastries	•	•								
Cakes	•	•								
Crème brûlée	•	•	•						•	

Figure 23.5 Sample Specification—Convection Oven

Equipment Name	Convection oven, floor model, double stack
Location	Main kitchen, floor
Intended Use	Hot food preparation for muffins, roasts, casseroles, potatoes, and similar products
Dimensions	Must fit in area 5' x 5' x 5', maximum 70" in height
Power and Motor	Gas, rear connection with auto shut-off valve; 44,000 BTU/hour; 115 volt electrical connection; 1/2 HP motor
Capacity	(10) 10" x 26" pans with adjustable rack guides
Instruction Details	Stainless steel front, sides, and top; porcelain enamel on interior; glass windows on doors; wheels and casters
Other Features	Auto-ignition, interior oven light; cook and hold cycle; minimum 5 programmable cooking settings
Approval	UL listed, NSF seal, AGA certified, Energy Star®
Warranty	3 years parts and labor (minimum)
Delivery & Installation	To be provided
Training	On-site training required (one-time)

Financing Capital Equipment Purchases

Financing may be a special concern, especially if adequate funds are not immediately available. In some situations, a facility may lease equipment. Leasing can also be a way to test feasibility of a new idea. For example, a facility desiring to test a satellite delivery program may use leased equipment for a short-term trial.

In another payment scenario, the supplier may finance the purchase. With a typical financing arrangement, an initial down payment is necessary at the time equipment is ordered to protect the supplier against costs incurred if the order is canceled. Another payment may be required at the time of delivery and the remaining balance may be financed by the supplier at a defined interest rate.

Sometimes suppliers offer special deals related to equipment in conjunction with food purchases. For example, a supplier of waffle batter may offer the specialized iron required to make waffles on a free-use basis for as long as the operation is purchasing the batter. This can be helpful with cash flow. However, it's important to evaluate a decision to bring in this equipment by all established criteria and to evaluate the overall costs of using the supplier's products.

When a capital budget is tight, another option is to purchase used equipment. This can be an alternative when funds are not available, when compatibility with other, older equipment is an issue, and/or when a facility does not need equipment that has a long life. Used equipment can become available as equipment suppliers receive trade-ins, as discontinued businesses hold auctions, as government agencies offer sales of surplus items, or as contracts expire on leased equipment and leasing companies sell the equipment. There are even used-equipment dealers in some large municipalities.

While availability may exist, there are some disadvantages to purchasing used equipment. Typically, used equipment does not include a warranty. The equipment may be sold on a cash-only basis. Responsibilities for moving and installing the equipment may rest with the buyer. The life expectancy of used equipment is typically shorter than that of new equipment, and used equipment may not have newer, preferred energy-saving design qualities. Maintenance requirements may be greater when compared with new equipment, and it is unlikely that competitive bids are possible. It may also be difficult to match required specifications with used equipment. It will be difficult to determine the level of previous use, and the Certified Dietary Manager may need to deal with unfamiliar supplier sources and may have difficulty securing required service or parts.

A Certified Dietary Manager needs to work closely with the business office to consider financing options.

Equipment Maintenance

The best way to maintain equipment is through in-depth training on the use and upkeep of the piece of equipment. (See Figure 23.6 for a list of common equipment training needs.) Initial training for use, cleaning and maintenance for complex equipment is typically provided by the supplier. Some equipment bears clear labels with instructions and safety precautions. A Certified Dietary Manager may also create a simple cheat sheet or poster outlining operational steps.

Maintain operating manuals and associated literature such as purchase price, vendor, and maintenance records in organized equipment files, accessible to all who may need it.

All equipment requires basic care such as routine cleaning and sanitizing after use. On another level, many pieces of equipment require periodic preventative work to limit breakdowns and ensure maximum lifetime. Even well maintained equipment can experience breakdowns that require immediate repair.

Putting It Into Practice

3. When developing a specification for a commercial food processor, what information would you need to consider?

Figure 23.6 Common Equipment Training Needs

Overview—what this equipment is for

How to turn equipment on and off

Basic operational steps

Safety precautions

Protective equipment to use if required

How to identify and use special attachments and what each is for

Procedures for cleaning and sanitizing

Auto shut-off features

Routine disassembly/reassembly (for cleaning)

Procedures for cleaning and sanitizing (and what products to use)

Food safety precautions (e.g., how to avoid cross-contamination when using a slicer)

Use of self-cleaning features

Use of programmable controls

How to ensure adequate functioning

Use of data logging, temperature monitoring, or related systems

How to add consumable supplies

Preventative maintenance

Signs of trouble and reporting procedures

Preventative Maintenance

Beyond cleaning, a Certified Dietary Manager should plan a preventative maintenance schedule for all equipment. **Preventative maintenance**, an organized routine of cleaning, inspecting, and maintaining equipment, is essential to ensure that:

- Equipment operates at maximum efficiency, often with savings in energy costs.
- Equipment works correctly.
- Equipment attains its maximum life expectancy.
- Unscheduled downtime is minimized.

Several basic steps can be used to develop preventative maintenance programs.

1. Identify and list all equipment in the food production and dining services facility that need periodic inspection and maintenance. This includes equipment not only in the kitchen, but also in serving areas, clean-up areas, decentralized kitchens or pantries, and other areas.

2. Set up a schedule of preventative maintenance. Depending upon the equipment item, maintenance work may be necessary on a weekly, semi-annual, or other basis. Figure 23.7 illustrates a preventative maintenance schedule used for this purpose. This sample summarizes required preventative maintenance activities for a six-month period. Some operators track preventative maintenance activities through computerized systems—with a simple spreadsheet, or a software application designed expressly for equipment management.

Glossary

Preventative Maintenance
An organized routine of cleaning, inspecting and maintaining equipment

3. Review maintenance requirements. Typically, this information is developed by the manufacturer and provided with the equipment at the time of purchase. You can incorporate manufacturer's recommendations about equipment maintenance into a preventative maintenance and repair log, as illustrated in Figure 23.8. The log should identify routine maintenance functions and how often they need to be completed. This may include items such as oiling a motor or replacing a fluid. The form should also identify the equipment name, model, manufacturer, serial number, and purchase date. As routine maintenance and/or repairs are conducted, the log should document each activity.

4. Maintain complete documentation of all maintenance and repair activity. More than just paperwork, this documentation helps in identifying and justifying decisions to replace equipment. A piece of equipment whose repair overhead becomes excessive is often a candidate for replacement. With documentation, a Certified Dietary Manager can determine when replacement will be cost-effective.

Certain preventative maintenance tasks may require the work of individuals outside the food production and dining services department. For example, in-house engineering or maintenance staff may handle maintenance on a conveyor system, a small engine, or ventilation hoods and fans. Some facilities make use of maintenance or service contracts with suppliers. Under this plan, eligible suppliers bid on the facility's maintenance needs. Quotations may be based upon time and materials, which means the client pays for labor and supplies each time he or she orders repair service. Or, a contract may be structured to provide any needed services and parts for a set monthly fee. Arrangements such as these may apply to repairs as well as preventative maintenance, and often the two are bundled into a service agreement.

Regardless of the players involved, a Certified Dietary Manager has responsibility for ensuring that all preventative maintenance tasks are defined and tracked. In addition, it is important to ensure that preventative maintenance meets manufacturers' recommendations, both to ensure effectiveness and to preserve the validity of any equipment warranty.

Putting It Into Practice

4. Over the past month, a repair service has been called four times for your high-temp dishmachine that is 10 years old. What should you be documenting?

Figure 23.7 Preventative Maintenance Schedule

Equipment Item	Work Necessary	JANUARY				FEBRUARY				MARCH				APRIL				MAY				JUNE			
		1	2	3	4	1	2	3	4	1	2	3	4	1	2	3	4	1	2	3	4	1	2	3	4

Figure 23.8 Equipment Maintenance and Repair Log

Service _____   Type Machine _____   Equipment No. _____

Location _____   Serial No. _____   Model No. _____

Make _____   Date Purchased _____   Purchase Cost_____

Preventative Maintenance Procedure

Function	Interval

Special Instructions

Specifications

Voltage		Drive	
Amperage		Belts	
Phase		Fuse	
Pressure		Lubrication	
Horsepower		Filter	
RPM		Fluids	

Spare Parts Required

Part	Mfr. Part No.	Hotel Stock No.	Quantity

Date	By	Work Performed	Hours	Material	Labor	Cost to Date

Cleaning Schedule

Part of a Certified Dietary Manager's responsibility is to manage all phases of maintenance. The first step is to define a cleaning schedule and assign tasks to employees. A cleaning schedule must flow from the production and service timelines, so that cleaning takes place when equipment is not in use, and is completed before a cook needs to use equipment. To make cleaning timely and effective, prepare a schedule and hold employees accountable. Most operations ask employees to sign off on cleaning tasks. On a daily basis, it's important to inspect this work and talk with employees about their responsibilities. Employees should also be encouraged to report any problems or concerns about equipment to their supervisor or the manager.

Specific cleaning procedures vary greatly from one piece of equipment to another, so it is important to develop guidelines from the manufacturers' instructions. As cleaning products are required, it is also important to name them specifically by product name for employees, rather than using generic terms. Cleaning instructions should be readily available to the assigned employees and the subject of employee training and periodic review. An example of a cleaning procedure appears in Figure 23.9.

Figure 23.9 Sample Policy and Procedure: Equipment Cleaning

Department: Foodservice

Date: 06/15/16

Approval By: Joe Jones, Certified Dietary Manager

Subject or Title: Cleaning Electric Mixers

Policy: It is the policy of ABC Nursing Home that electric mixers be properly cleaned after each use according to the following procedure.

PROCEDURE:

1. **Removable Parts:**
   a. Immediately after use, take bowls, beaters, and all removable parts to pot sink for washing and sanitizing according to manual pot-washing instructions.
   b. Fill both compartments of pail with warm water. To the wash compartment, add Cream Suds in the ratio of 2 oz. per gallon of water; to the rinse side, add Mikroklene in the ratio of 1 oz. per gallon. Use separate sponges for wash and rinse compartments.
   c. Rinse thoroughly with sponge dipped in sanitizing rinse solution and squeezed nearly dry. Dip and wring sponge frequently so all parts are sanitized.
   d. Allow removable parts to air dry on sanitary drying rack.
   e. Replace removable parts.
   f. Return cleaning equipment to proper storage.

2. **Stationary Parts:**
   a. Fill both compartments of pail with warm water. To the wash compartment, add Cream Suds in the ratio of 2 oz. per gallon of water; to the rinse side, add Mikroklene in the ratio of 1 oz. per gallon. Use separate sponges for wash and rinse compartments.
   b. Use sponge and detergent solution to thoroughly scrub all stationary parts of mixer. Pay particular attention to underside of head, corners, handles, and underneath rolled rims.
   c. Rinse thoroughly with sponge dipped in sanitizing rinse solution and squeezed nearly dry. Dip and wring sponge frequently so all parts are sanitized.
   d. Return cleaning equipment to proper storage.

Managing the Cost of Supplies

Chemical products are needed to clean dishes, pots and pans, and work areas. A wide range of products are available. Check with suppliers for ideas about available items and recommended uses, and use the supplier representative as a partner to help resolve cleaning and sanitation problems in the operation.

Cleaning supplies should be kept in non-food storage areas. As is true with other food production and dining services inventory, cleaning supplies must be properly controlled. Since these products are expensive, a formal issuing system similar to that used to control expensive food products may be in order. The rate of product usage, particularly for dishmachine chemical, is frequently tracked by managers as a controllable expense.

Product selection also plays a role in supply cost management. Sometimes, a cost-benefit study is necessary to confirm which product is the most potentially useful. To undertake this study, first define what the product is to do. Then, ask suppliers for suggestions about and samples of products that they believe will be useful. Using the instructions provided by the manufacturer, test each product. Then, objectively determine which meet your requirements. Keep in mind that the recommended chemicals for one facility may be different from another due to the equipment in use and the hardness of water quality available.

From that group of products, next examine cost. For example, one gallon of a cleaning agent may cost $50 but clean twice as many square feet, compared with a less expensive product. Calculate the defined cost per square foot, rack of dishes, load of laundry, and so on, to make a fair comparison. This boils down to a usage cost, rather than a purchase price.

Another cost control consideration relates to how employees use products. Sometimes, employees are tempted to over-use cleaning products, in a belief that more is better. This not only costs money; it may also pose safety concerns. Training and ongoing supervision are in order. As applicable, also assure that the correct measuring or portioning devices are on hand to eliminate guesswork.

For certain equipment, supply usage is largely controlled by the equipment itself for self-cleaning. High-pressure cleaning systems with applicable chemicals are also used for cleaning many items. Monitoring supply usage can help identify when there is a malfunction. Prompt service, in turn, can get supply usage under control.

The need for selecting a reputable supplier is just as important for the purchase of chemicals as it is for the purchase of food products, capital equipment items, and other purchases. The supplier may be included in the purchasing program and vetted by the GPO. Chemicals are a unique segment of the department requiring a vendor that is knowledgeable about the product needs of food production and dining services. Access to competitive pricing consistent quality and quantity, and timely delivery of the needed supplies are essential characteristics of a good chemical supplier.

The Purchasing Process

Overview and Objectives

While Certified Dietary Managers may not have to write purchase specifications, they will spend valuable time purchasing food and supplies for their facility, and must be able to differentiate between products when ordering. Once purchasing is completed, the purchasing process continues with receiving and inventory. This chapter reviews all aspects of the purchasing process. After completing this chapter, you should be able to:

✓ Identify purchasing policies and procedures of department

✓ Examine vendor product/selection

✓ Establish purchasing specifications

✓ Use the ordering and bidding process

✓ Evaluate facility needs, budget restrictions, and products available

✓ Gather and evaluate product information

✓ Be familiar with computer applications and create a purchase order

✓ Check inventory and identify purchase needs

✓ Complete purchase order requisition forms

✓ Maintain inventory records

✓ Recognize inventory management practices (FIFO, par stock, physical, perpetual)

Purchasing is a highly specialized process and the topic alone is the subject of many books. This chapter covers only a few of the decisions in the process. Purchasing has changed significantly in the past 20 years, with most facilities completing the process online through a computerized ordering system with their prime vendor. Often, smaller healthcare facilities belong to multi-unit purchasing co-ops and have enjoyed the benefits of cooperative purchasing to leverage better prices.

The main focus of purchasing is to buy the products needed at the best cost and appropriate quality—and get them delivered when (and where) they are needed. Through effective purchasing, a Certified Dietary Manager achieves objectives related to quality, quantity, price, supplier, and schedule.

Quality. The purchaser must obtain the right quality products and services. This is not always the highest quality available. Instead, it matches the needs and budget of the facility. The relationship between quality and price is called value.

Quantity. Products must be purchased in the right quantity. Otherwise, the operation can run out of products, delaying or altering food production and service. Or, the operation can carry excess inventory, with resulting cash flow and loss implications.

Price. The buyer has a responsibility to obtain required quality products at the best overall price. Price shopping individual items across multiple vendors consumes time and rarely results in a lower net cost. Typically, a prime vendor relationship leads to a better total invoice bottom line.

Supplier. It is important to select product sources with thought, analysis, and comparison, rather than simply to select a supplier based on random factors.

Schedule. Delivery times should be coordinated with the vendor so needed staffing is available when deliveries are made. While occasional problems must be anticipated, supplier selection should include reliability of delivery schedules.

In large facilities, purchasing may be the responsibility of a specialized food buyer or purchasing agent. In smaller facilities, it is often the responsibility of the Certified Dietary Manager, supervisor, or food production and dining service director.

The purchasing task is ongoing. Through experience with suppliers, products, and services, the Certified Dietary Manager can develop a very effective system to help control costs and to assure that quality requirements are met.

Specifications for Equipment

As discussed in Chapter 23, specifications are also written for equipment and disposable items such as paper and plastic. Equipment manufacturers usually provide a spec sheet with their equipment that details the specific features of the equipment such as equipment type, model number, standard features, etc.

This information can be very helpful when writing equipment specifications for the purchase of new equipment. The specs should be as generic as possible and include what the equipment needs to do, and not so tightly written that only one item can meet the stated specs.

Specifications for Food

Management of the purchasing process begins with a specification for each product. A **specification (spec)** is a quality statement that spells out what requirements must be met in order for a product to be acceptable. It really describes the suitability of a product for its intended use in the operation. There may be multiple specs for the same general product depending upon the intended use. For example, if olives are used for garnishes as well as for the salad bar, two different products may be needed. Large olives that are perfectly shaped and are of uniform size (and also expensive) are not necessary if the olives will be chopped for a salad.

The purpose of a specification is quality control. "You get what you ask for. If you don't ask for it, you are not likely to get it!" A product spec is used when requesting prices or bids from a list of possible suppliers. A spec helps assure a comparison of apples to apples, so to speak. In turn, this helps to compare prices meaningfully. It also defines a clear, mutual expectation of what will be received at delivery.

Glossary

Specification (Spec)
A quality statement lists what requirements must be met in order for a product to be acceptable

Writing specs comes after the decision about what general products will be needed for the menu as planned. Once the recipes are selected and the ingredients defined the specific quality characteristics can be written.

Specifications should be:

- Accurate and objectively describe quality aspects.
- Realistic.
  - > Quality definitions cannot be so strict that few or no products will be acceptable.
- Stated in clear terms.
- Provide some flexibility for both the supplier and the buyer.

To write a product spec, begin with a product name (not the brand name but the product identifier). Include an intended use descriptor if it affects the choice of product, i.e. sliced olives for the salad bar. Provide a description of the product with quality information. Note any special requirements. An example of a specification format appears in Figure 24.1. Along with these details, identify required food safety controls, such as delivery temperatures, acceptable product dating, and any other essential characteristics.

What characteristics can be listed in a specs? These vary by product. For certain

Figure 24.1 Product Specification Format

[Name of Foodservice Operation]

1. **Product Name:** _____

2. **Product Used For:** Clearly indicate product use, such as olive for garnish, hamburger patty for grilling, etc.

3. **Product General Description:** Provide quality information about desired product. For example, "iceberg lettuce; heads to be green and firm without spoilage, no excessive dirt or damage. No more than 10 outer leaves; packed 24 heads per case."

4. **Detailed Description:** State other factors that clearly identify the desired product. Examples of specific factors, which vary by product being described include:

• Geographic Origin	• Grade	• Brand Name	• Container Size
• Variety	• Size	• Density	• Edible Yield, Trim
• Type	• Portion Size	• Specific Gravity	• Inspection
• Style			

5. **Check-In Procedures:** Describe what a receiving clerk will do to verify acceptability of the product. For example, products to be delivered at or below 41°F will be tested with a thermometer. Portioned meat patties will be randomly weighed. Lettuce packed 24 heads per case will be counted.

6. **Special Instructions and Requirements:** Any additional information needed to clearly indicate quality expectations can be included here. Examples include bidding procedures, if applicable, labeling and/or packaging requirements, and delivery and service requirements.

agricultural products, a USDA grade is an essential tool. A **grade** describes the quality of the product. A grade may describe uniformity, texture, fat content, flavor, maturity, and/or other quality factors. Grade assignments are based on standards established by the USDA for each applicable food. They provide an objective measure or standard which can be used for comparison. For example, a Fancy grade of canned vegetables indicates the best flavor, color, and tenderness. It also indicates the product is uniform in size.

In addition, portion and count can be critical. For fish filets, decide what weight is required for each fillet in order to match the needs of the recipes and menus. As another example, canned pear halves may be packed with varying counts in a #10 can. Container size may vary slightly from one vendor to another. However, if requirements are rigid due to space or usage quantities, specify them. For example, if a product will only be used in very small amounts for individual orders on demand, do not accept products in large units. Common can sizes appear in Figure 24.2. For ideas about other factors to include in specifications for particular products, search for the USDA Commercial Item Descriptions, available on the Web at http://www.ams.usda.gov.

In some facilities, the packaging itself is also specified. For example, glass may be prohibited for safety reasons. Today, processing methods may be important as well. Some facilities are also developing specifications that relate to food additives and allergens (factors likely to cause allergic reactions in sensitive individuals). If specific factors are important to the client group, include them.

Examples of factors that may be included in a quality statement appear in Figure 24.3.

Figure 24.2 Common Can Sizes

SIZE	NET WEIGHT	MEASURE	COMMON PACK	PRINCIPAL PRODUCTS
#10	6 lbs. 9 oz.	12 - 13 cups	6 per case	Fruits, vegetables, some other foods
No. 3 Cyl	2.9 - 3.2 lbs.	5-1/4 cups	12 per case	Condensed soups, some vegetables, meat and poultry products, fruit and vegetable juices
#2-1/2	1 lb. 13 oz.	3-1/2 cups	24 per case	Fruits, some vegetables
#2	1 lb. 4 oz.	2-1/2 cups	24 per case	Juices, ready-to-serve soups, some fruits
#300	14 - 16 oz.	1-3/4 cups	24 per case	Some fruits and meat products
#1 (Picnic)	10-1/2 - 12 oz.	1-1/4 cups	48 per case	Condensed soups, some fruits, vegetables, meat, fish
8 oz.	8 oz.	1 cup	48 or 72 per case	Ready-to-serve soups, fruits, vegetables

Source: Food for Fifty

Figure 24.3 Purchase Specification Factors

MEATS	SEAFOOD	POULTRY	FRESH FRUITS & VEGETABLES	PROCESSED FRUITS & VEGETABLES
• Inspection (mandatory) • Grading (if desired) • IMPS/MBG Descriptions • Weight/Thickness Limitations • Fat Limitations • State of Refrigeration • Miscellaneous (tying, boning, packaging, etc.)	• Type (fin fish or shellfish) • Market Form (whole, eviscerated fin fish, alive, whole, shucked, etc.) • Quality Requirements (describe flesh, eyes, skin, gills, etc.) • Grade (if desired) • Inspection (voluntary) • Processing Requirements	• Kind (chicken, turkey, duck, goose) • Class (typed by age) • Grade (if desired) • Size (weight limitations) • Style (weight limitations) • Inspection (mandatory) • Style (whole, breasts, breasts with ribs, etc.) • State of Refrigeration	• Grade (if desired) • Variety • Size • Type of Pack • Count per Container • Growing Area	• Grade (if desired • Drain Weight • Packing Medium • Can (container) Size

To identify additional details and options, talk with several suppliers. Many food distributors can provide a specifications manual. Some may also provide their own quality ratings that will help match products to needs. Realize that using known brand-name ingredients is not essential. A distributor's house brand may prove more economical, and may even be the very same product under a different label.

Use of branded menu items is a growing trend. A school system may serve French fries produced by a recognized fast food chain or chocolate chip cookies manufactured by a well-known company. A cafeteria may serve doughnuts, pizzas, or tacos that have national brand-name recognition.

When using branded menu items, a food production and dining service operation enjoys marketing clout as well as quality control. Costs may be higher, but sales may be too. Thus, a facility needs to base decisions to use branded products on value, impact on the financial bottom line and where the product name will be seen. When offering unlabeled bulk salad dressing on a salad bar, a house branded dressing will likely be more economical and of equal quality (and flavor profile) to the nationally branded item.

Usually the specification should not include the brand of the food or equipment item. However, in some cases where the chef may want specific products such as ABC ketchup, the brand would be included in the specs. If specifying a brand, be prepared to defend why that brand must be purchased. Ready-to-use pasta sauce may seem like a standard item. However, flavor profiles differ significantly from one brand to another. In one university setting, the pasta sauce that had been purchased had a tomato paste aftertaste. The product did not meet the expected flavor profile. That data was used to justify a change in product brand.

Finally, if writing specs for specialized dietary products, involve a Registered Dietitian in developing specifications. Simple product names for low-sodium soup, heart healthy convenience entrées, or enteral nutritional supplements do not tell all. A dietitian can specify nutritional content for these products.

This has been a fairly detailed discussion about the writing of specifications and what to include. In today's marketplace, the writing of food specs is rarely so detailed for each item in the inventory. Typically the standards have been defined by the broadline vendor purchasing managers through what they bring into inventory, the Group Purchasing Organizations, through what they spec for contract pricing and industry standards, through what similar facilities are willing to buy. Organizations driven primarily by budget concerns may choose to purchase lower grade products and, as such, may need to define their specs.

Evaluating Products

As suppliers suggest products to match the needs, the next step is to taste and test the products. It is important to taste products under consideration. Sometimes, it is also important to test it through the recipe production process, in order to verify quality and taste. When relevant, ask the supplier to deliver samples of several products that meet the specification for comparison. If the standard has been XYZ Peanut Butter, and the same product is available from a new vendor, then a sample is not necessary. However, when the recommendation is for a different brand, a taste and performance comparison is advised.

Some operations use the term **can-cutting** to describe the process of sampling products for possible purchase. To perform a successful taste test, involve several key members of the operation. At least one person involved in food production should attend—a manager, chief chef, or head cook. In addition, the person responsible for purchasing should be involved, and should review the product carefully. Use a simple rating card to allow panelists to rate taste, appearance, texture, and other pertinent characteristics. After each person has made an independent evaluation, ask panelists to compare notes and discuss the products. Can-cutting can be done for one product and multiple vendors or multiple grades and products from one vendor.

Comparing product yield and waste is part of the evaluation process. Generally, there is a difference between package weight and net weight for products. Net weight is the weight of the food product itself, after all packaging is removed. For canned products, consider the drain weight, or how much usable product is present after draining away the liquid. Ultimately, it affects both yield and price. Figure 24.4 shows an example of how this can make a difference.

Glossary

Can-Cutting
A procedure for sampling products for possible purchase

Figure 24.4 Impact of Drain Weight

You are comparing two different products for canned peach slices, each packed in #10 cans.

Product #1: Minimum drain weight = 63 oz.
Price: $3.00 per can

Product #2: Minimum drain weight = 75 oz.
Price: $3.10 per can

All other factors being equal, which product represents a better value? To determine this, calculate the price per ounce of usable product:

Product #1: $3.00 ÷ 63 oz. = $0.0476 per oz.
Product #2: $3.00 ÷ 75 oz. = $0.0413 per oz.

In this example, Product #2 is actually a better value if the quality is equal.

Purchasing Decisions

The person responsible for purchasing is expected to purchase the required products for the best price. There are several buying techniques that may help the purchaser: using bid pricing, purchasing groups and cooperatives, manufacturer's rebates, valuing inventory, and make or buy decisions.

There are essentially four styles of purchasing systems commonly in use: Group Purchasing Organization (GPO) contracts, multi-vendor bid process, independent specialty product vendors and the local grocery store. Facility need and access to the various services will determine which system, or combination of processes, is best for the facility.

Local Grocery Store

The local grocery store offers the advantage of "keeping it local" and supporting community businesses. Often facilities need smaller amounts of a limited number of items such as single served vegetarian items or a variety of single served baby foods, that are easiest to acquire from the grocery store. In remote communities where grocery deliveries are available once a week, the local grocery store may be the backup source for last-minute items or fresh produce.

Typically the cost of products purchased at the local grocery are significantly higher than purchasing through a major distributor, but the ease of access, ready availability and community goodwill can offset the cost. Frequently, the grocery store will setup a charge account so petty cash funds are not necessary, and often they are willing to order products in smaller pack size specifically for the facility.

Independent Specialty Products Vendor

The **Independent Specialty Products Vendor** is the source of a narrow scope of products or items not commonly found through the larger vendors. The niche these vendors serve is commonly related to dairy products, fresh bakery goods, hand-cut meats, fresh seafood, locally grown produce or fresh produce. The Certified Dietary Manager

Putting It Into Practice

2. Your facility is deciding whether to change from one cola company to offering a different brand of cola products. Your clientele is requesting this change. The brand you currently use is part of the prime vendor contract. What process should you use to make this change?

needs to carefully manage the purchasing through the specialty vendors to ensure that the specialty nature of the products being purchased, often at a specialty based cost, delivers the value for the price paid.

Multi-Vendor Bid Process

The multi-vendor bid process goes back to a time when group buying contracts were not readily available. The concept behind a multi-vendor bid process is to obtain price quotes from a number of different vendors for each item being purchased. Requests for pricing on a list of items may be monthly or quarterly. Expecting vendors to "lock in" pricing for a year denies the vendor the ability to react to market variability.

To obtain price quotations from any supplier, a Certified Dietary Manager can use a competitive bidding process. **Competitive bidding** allows multiple vendors to submit bids or price quotations for products based on defined specifications. The manager can then accept the lowest approriate quoted price resulting in cost savings to the facility.

Competitive bidding will help the manager in getting a lower price when:

- The volume of purchases is large enough to justify the time and expense involved for the vendor.
- Specifications are clearly known by all suppliers.
- Several suppliers desire to quote prices on the order.

Competitive bidding can be done through an informal or formal process. In an informal process, the terms of the bid may be discussed or agreed upon by phone, email or other form of open communication. In a formal process, the Certified Dietary Manager or purchasing agent invites suppliers to submit sealed bids on a detailed, written prospective order. The manager reviews written responses and makes a selection.

Keys to success for a bid purchasing system include:

- The quoted price and other terms of the agreement must be clearly understood.
- The price quoted by the supplier must remain firm for the length of time needed by the purchaser to make a decision.
- All suppliers must quote according to the same specifications for any given product.
- All eligible suppliers should be allowed to quote on the order.
- Parties document the agreed-upon price and all other terms.

The multi-vendor bid process is often related to a concept called **cherry picking**. In this model, a Certified Dietary Manager purchases each individual product from the vendor with the lowest price. Thus, one facility may place a relatively small number of purchase orders with many different suppliers. An advantage of this method is that the manager presumably obtains the lowest possible price for each item. However, normally the disadvantages outweigh the possible saving:

- The manager forms weaker relationships with vendors and may dilute the facility's clout with suppliers.
- The time and administrative commitment to monitor each bid, assess the pricing options and hold numerous vendors accountable to their price quotes is significant.
- Time is spent with multiple vendor reps resolving issues, reviewing new products, processing invoices and multiple checks.
- The workload for receiving staff to deal with multiple deliveries also increases.

Glossary

Competitive Bidding
Asking multiple vendors to submit price quotes for products or equipment based on defined specifications

Cherry Picking
A purchasing concept where individual products are purchased from individual vendors, usually based on price alone

Group Purchasing Organizations (GPOs)

The **Group Purchasing Organizations (GPOs)** are typically groups of facilities banded together to negotiate both prime vendor contracts and manufacturers rebate agreements. In one model, the facilities work together through a separate organization called a purchasing group, representing multiple clients. The GPOs generally represent a market segment of similar facilities: healthcare, schools, resorts and casinos, hotels and hospitality.

The GPO is often organized around committees of operators representing a common service such as Pharmacy, Housekeeping, or Food Production and Dining Services. The operators bring to the committees their knowledge and experience in products and purchasing. The group defines or approves the specs for products to be included in the bid process, standardizes use of many products, reviews bid quotes, conducts product evaluations and selects vendors. The group uses its volume to exert buying power and obtain preferred pricing. A purchasing group may involve all supplies to the facility, not just food.

In another model, Certified Dietary Managers work together through a purchasing cooperative (co-op) to achieve volume and buying power. Generally, members of the group work together to specify and select products and suppliers.

If the facility belongs to a purchasing group or cooperative, it is important to participate as fully as possible, buying products on the contract. Otherwise, the clout of the group is diluted. It is equally important to participate in selection of products and vendors to assure they meet the needs.

Figure 24.5 Purchasing Options—Pros

GROUP PURCHASING	MULTI-VENDOR	LOCAL GROCERY	SPECIALTY PRODUCTS
• Easy access to pricing • The greater the purchases, the better the pricing • Less work for the manager • Specs are set by "the committee" • Rebates and incentives typically available • Someone else manages the contracts and vendor compliance • Value-added services are often available	• More product and branding options available • More delivery options • Rebates and incentives may be available • May have some value-added services	• Keeps the business local • Able to purchase items in smaller quantities • Able to purchase items in smaller pack size • Local access with immediate availability • Often has specialty items needed on an occasional basis	• Each vendor has a specific list of products • Product listings may be very deep for a limited scope • May provide rotation onsite of product for freshness • May provide locally grown items

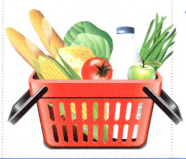

The Bid Process

Whether at the GPO or multi-vendor level, once specifications are ready, the next step is to obtain bids from suppliers. The key purpose of this process is to obtain the best value (the cost-quality relationship) and selection of products based on the needs of the buying group.

Commonly, a food production and dining service operation will select one main vendor for the majority of its food items. This primary supplier is referred to as the **prime vendor.** In a prime vendor arrangement, an operation agrees to purchase the majority of its products from a given supplier in exchange for guaranteed pricing for a defined period of time. Typically, this is about 80-percent.

Today, a prime vendor agreement is usually managed beyond the level of individual facilities. Instead, it is negotiated at a corporate level and passed on to the Certified Dietary Manager. The parties responsible for negotiating a prime vendor contract may be the corporate purchasing agents of a healthcare chain, a contract management company, or other organization. Meanwhile, a corporation or individual operation may select additional vendors, often locally based suppliers, for certain perishable items like fresh meats, produce, and dairy products.

Note that in a competitive bid process for a prime vendor, it is important to provide vendors with projected usage figures for each product because they will base quotations on the total volume. Then, as bids are received, examine the bottom line of each vendor. Prices for individual products may vary, with one lower or higher from one bidder or another. However, the real price comparison is made based on the sum total of all items. This figure helps drive the decision of which vendor to select.

Prime vendor purchasing offers a number of advantages:

- It improves the consistency of food purchased.
- It locks in predictable pricing.
- It makes the receiving process more efficient.
- It often generates improved vendor performance because of the value of the contract and the commitment of the client.
- It may provide an opportunity to enjoy value-added services. These are services a distributor adds to its line at a free or reduced cost for customers. Examples include, computer software for ordering, inventory tracking, leveraged purchasing, or training materials.
  - > Provision of standardized menus, computer hardware or menu software, at no cost to a facility, could be considered an **Anti-Kickback Safe Harbors** violation and could result in charges by Health and Human Services.

Prime vendor purchasing can have some disadvantages too, including:

- The loss of a reliable backup vendor.
- A limited variety of products.
- An increase in prices of specific products or brands that are not under preferred contract pricing.

While price is important, it is not wise to base vendor selection entirely on price. Here are some additional questions to ask before selecting a vendor:

- Does the vendor carry the majority of products needed, including any specialized items for modified diets?

Glossary

Prime Vendor
A primary supplier who usually provides about 80% of the products purchased

Putting It Into Practice

3. Your clients are complaining about the quality of the muffin product. Your administrator is asking you to recommend a higher quality product. You are considering making the muffins rather than purchasing them. What steps would you take to make the decision?

- What is the vendor's ability to meet scheduling needs for delivery?

- What ordering procedures or technology does the vendor provide (such as interfaces with a computer system, or online ordering)?

- How reliable is the vendor's service? Can references be checked among other customers?

- How willing is the vendor to commit to established food safety guidelines?

- What access will be available to a service representative or sales person to assist with any problems that arise?

Manufacturer Rebates

In today's food production and dining service environment, many Certified Dietary Managers have been pressing the limits of budget cuts. As a result, the margin of profit enjoyed by food distributors has decreased to a very minimal level. As managers continue to look for price breaks, a new avenue has evolved—manufacturers' rebates. A manufacturers' rebate is a refund offered directly from the producer of the product. For example, if purchasing ABC brand coffee: The manufacturer of ABC coffee gives a refund of $5 for every case purchased. Typically, the relationship between the manufacturer and the GPO or buying group identifies the potential for a product-specific rebate.

This opportunity can provide a significant impact on operating expenses. However, it also requires tracking commitments to see that purchasing levels are met and rebate checks are received. Often, the GPO, or buying group, works with the distributor to track the qualifying purchases through an online ordering systems and automatically claim rebates.

Distributor Incentives

In an effort to secure purchasing commitments, many distributors have included access to discounts and incentives based upon reaching purchasing or payment targets. Although, discounts vary from distributor to distributor they often include:

- Drop Size—based on the average dollar value of the deliveries:
  > Total dollars divided by the number of deliveries
  > Reducing deliveries to one, two or three times a week can increase the average drop size

- Early Payment—based on how quickly the invoices are paid.

- House Brand Percentage—based on the percent of purchases that are from the distributors house brands.

Additional discounts may be available or customized to the buying group.

As noted, there are many factors that need to be balanced when deciding which distributor to align with as a primary vendor that go beyond individual product price or local convenience.

What Is On the Shelf—Inventory Management

Valuing Inventory

An essential tool for financial management in food production and dining services is an inventory valuation. This is a dollar figure representing the value of all inventory on hand at the moment. This figure is not only useful in completing operating statements

Glossary

Anti-Kickback Safe Harbors
A Health and Human Services regulation to prevent a kickback or bribe for providing a service

reflecting the department's financial performance; it can also provide useful information to use in managing the purchasing process. Based on accounting procedures in the facility, an **inventory valuation** may be required at the end of each month, or at other defined intervals.

To calculate value, track food prices (what was paid) for each product, per purchase unit. Multiply the number of purchase units on hand by the price for that product. Then, add all product values together. An example of a form for valuing inventory appears in Figure 24.6. Note that in computer-based systems, purchase prices are often maintained in the system. Then, a user enters a physical count for each product, and allows the computer to calculate value.

Inventory Management Tools

Some items are needed only for immediate and one-time use. However, most inventory products for a food production and dining service operation tend to repeat themselves. Planning what to purchase for each of these needs requires a different process.

For example, planning a Volunteer's Dinner for next week calls for beef tenderloin. This is an item not routinely use in any menu cycles. Hence, the filet mignon is a one-time need. To determine requirements, count the expected number of clients, pad this figure as appropriate, and then order according to the needs dictated by the recipe to be used.

Routinely, though, the vast majority of products on hand are used over and over, based on the menu cycle. There are several ways to manage ongoing inventory needs, including the minimum/maximum system, the par level system, the perpetual inventory system, and just-in-time purchasing. Each of these is described below.

Glossary

Inventory Valuation
The dollar figure or value of all inventory on hand at a given time

Figure 24.6 Physical Inventory—Valuation Form

Date: _____

PRODUCT	UNIT TYPE	QTY. IN STORAGE	UNIT PURCHASE PRICE	TOTAL PRICE

Total Value:_____

Minimum/Maximum system. A minimum/maximum inventory system is one in which inventory levels are maintained within established ranges for each product. It is based on two reference points for each product in the inventory:

1. The minimum quantity for the product is the least amount that should be available; inventory levels should not fall below this figure.

2. The maximum quantity of the product is the most amount of this product that should be carried in stock at any given time; inventory levels should not rise above this figure.

Quantities for inventory products are expressed in purchase units. To determine how much to order, take a current count of purchase units on hand for an item in inventory (physical inventory). Then subtract the current count from the maximum quantity. Here is a simple example:

- The maximum level for canned peaches is four cases.
- The operation currently has two cases on hand.
- The order would be: 4 - 2 = 2 cases.
- Order two cases.

However, the system can become a bit more complex, based on how long it will take an order to arrive, and how much product may be used in the interim. In the above example, what happens, if while waiting for the two cases of peaches just ordered, an additional two cases are used? Now, there are no peaches available. Whether this is a serious issue for any given product depends on:

> Lead time: how long it takes from the time an order is placed until it actually arrives, and

> Usage rate: how much product is typically used during a defined time interval.

To account for these factors, calculate the lead units. Lead units are a special factor representing the number of units needed to subtract from current inventory to determine how much to order.

Each time the inventory is counted, subtract the number of lead units from the amount on hand. If the answer is below the minimum, order more. If it is not, re-evaluate at the next order date. Figure 24.7 illustrates how several key terms relate to each other, and Figure 24.8 illustrates how to calculate lead units and purchase quantity.

Figure 24.7 Terminology In a Minimum/Maximum System

The following terms and established values apply to each product you manage in a minimum/maximum system.

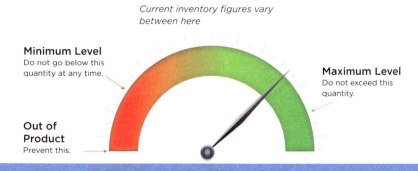

Current inventory figures vary between here

Minimum Level
Do not go below this quantity at any time.

Maximum Level
Do not exceed this quantity.

Out of Product
Prevent this.

Figure 24.8 Calculating Lead Units and Purchase Quantity

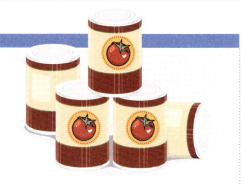

Background: You are setting values for canned, stewed tomatoes in a minimum/maximum inventory system. Tomatoes are purchased in #10 cans, 6 cans per case.

Purchase Unit: Case

Based on predictions, volume of usage, and experience, you have set the following figures:

Maximum Quantity	6 cases. Do not want to carry more than this amount at any time.
Minimum Quantity	4 cases. Do not want to fall below this minimum, or you may risk running out.
Lead Time	3 days. It takes 3 days to receive the product.
Usage Rate	1 case per day. General use is about 1 case of stewed tomatoes every day.
Lead Units	This is lead time multiplied by usage rate or 3 days x 1 case/day = 3 cases If the order for stewed tomatoes is placed today, expect to use another 3 cases of stewed tomatoes while waiting for the order to arrive.
Purchase Quantity	Take an inventory count today. If there are 5 cases of stewed tomatoes in stock, calculate purchase quantity as follows: Maximum Quantity: (Current Quantity - Lead Units) = Quantity to order, or 6 cases - (5 cases - 3) = 6 - 2 = 4 cases Order 4 cases of stewed tomatoes today.

A minimum/maximum system of inventory management works well for non-perishable products, or products that can remain in storage for extended periods of time. Examples of such products include canned goods, dry goods, spices, condiments, and the like. In addition, it is appropriate for items routinely kept in stock, not for an occasional item ordered for a special event.

Notice that in this system, how the minimum and maximum quantities are set can have a great impact. If the minimum quantity is set too low, there is a risk of running out of products. If the maximum quantity is set too high, excess inventory may be on the shelf. Excess inventory poses several disadvantages. It incurs storage costs, ties up cash flow, and increases the risk of losses through spoilage, theft or product expirations.

Today, most Certified Dietary Managers attempt to maintain the smallest quantities of inventory products feasible, while still assuring that supplies will be adequate to produce and serve food reliably. Look carefully at lead units and also consider the reliability of the supplier. Sometimes, a supplier runs out of products, fulfillment of orders may be delayed, or a weather emergency may prevent deliveries. As with menu forecasting, inventory forecasting requires ongoing monitoring and refinement. The minimum level is set too low if product runs out when there are no unusual delays or other circumstances.

Par Level System

A simpler inventory management concept is the **par level** concept. Par levels, or minimum quantities, are set for each inventory item. Take physical inventory on a scheduled basis. After each count, compare the amounts on hand with the established par. If the on-hand figure is lower, order more to bring it up to par. This system can work for facilities with very stable menus and forecasts. For example:

- The green beans are packed 6/#10 cans to a case.
- The par for canned green beans is 10 #10 cans (or 1 case and 4 cans).
- Inventory count is 3 cans.
- The amount to order is 7 cans (1 case and 1 can).
- Due to pack size (6 cans /case), order 2 cases.

The par level needs to reflect the typical usage rate between deliveries and account for any needed lead time on special order or unique products. In the example of the green beans, a product always available from the distributor the par is set at the amount needed through the next delivery. However, if an item is a special order and requires a three week lead time, then the par level needs to include the usage over a longer period of time.

Typically, the par system sets both the minimum amount to be on hand and the maximum amount is basically the par level plus one case or unit of purchase. The Par Level System is probably the most commonly used inventory ordering process.

Perpetual Inventory System

While minimum/maximum and par systems require a frequent **physical inventory**, a perpetual inventory system, in theory, does not. A **perpetual inventory** represents a running count of products on hand. In many respects, it operates just like a bank checkbook. The process works like this:

- Begin the system with a balance for each product. The balance is how many purchase units are on hand.
- When product is purchased and received, add this to the balance.
- When product is issued for use, subtract them from the balance.
- At any given time, a review of the balance will determine purchases required to replenish supplies. Generally, the total withdrawals over the period since the last order, are used to order for re-supply.
- Periodically, reconcile the perpetual balance by taking a physical inventory. Compare the actual figures for amounts on hand with what the perpetual inventory calculates should be on hand for each item.

This is just like balancing a checkbook. An example of a form for maintaining perpetual inventory appears in Figure 24.9.

Good practice dictates that one person take responsibility for maintaining the balance sheet, while someone else conducts the physical inventory for reconciliation. Just as in an accounting system, a reconciliation is a type of audit. Involving different people imposes control and helps prevent the opportunity for theft.

An advantage to the perpetual inventory system is control. Based on orders received and units issued, you know what should be in stores. If the figures do not match, you may have valuable information that can help control inventory shrinkage.

Glossary

Par Level
A minimum quantity to maintain in inventory

Perpetual Inventory
A running count of inventory that is updated continuously

Physical Inventory
A physical count of items in inventory that occurs weekly, monthly, quarterly or annually

Figure 24.9 Perpetual Inventory Form

Product Name: _____

Purchase Unit Size: _____

DATE	STARTING BALANCE	IN	OUT	ENDING BALANCE	PRODUCT USAGE (Starting Balance + Qty In -Qty Out - Ending Balance)

Shrinkage

Shrinkage is a decline in inventory counts through anything other than withdrawals that have been accounted for. What can cause shrinkage? Here are some examples:

- A cook is opening a jar of pickles and drops it. The product is cleaned up and discarded.
- A visitor or employee walks through a storage area and pockets a product for personal use.
- A storage clerk does not rotate product effectively, following a first-in, first-out (FIFO) system. A case of sandwich meat becomes outdated and is thrown away.
- A purchaser buys food in excess quantities, and again, food expires and is thrown away.
- The salad maker decides that the fruited gelatin salad needs more fruit cocktail than what the recipe calls for, so she grabs another can off the shelf.

Furthermore, discrepancies may arise from documentation errors in the receiving process. For example:

- A purchase order specifies 40 pounds of ground beef.
- The delivery is only 38 pounds, but no one notices and documents this fact.
- The figure of 40 pounds is added to the perpetual balance. In fact, though, only 38 pounds have been added to the physical inventory. The running balance for ground beef is now incorrect.

In a related example, the distributor runs out of a product and is unable to supply it. If no one documents this error, the anticipated delivery may be added to the perpetual balance. In fact, though, no product was added to the physical inventory.

Glossary

Shrinkage
A decline or loss in inventory counts through anything other than withdrawals

Any discrepancy discovered through reconciliation merits investigation. Often, by following up on discrepancies, a Certified Dietary Manager can pinpoint problems, make improvements, and better control inventory. Through this process, the manager may contain unnecessary expenditures as well.

A perpetual inventory system is most effective in a setting where the storeroom and walk-ins are closed, locked and access is limited to the Storeroom Clerk. This usually includes staffing to pre-measure, tray up and prep all items requisitioned by the production team, thereby, controlling access to the inventory. Just like managing the checkbook, when one person is responsible for writing the checks and keeping the numbers up-to-date it works quite well. However, when 15 people are in and out of the checkbook every day it is hard to keep the numbers accurate. Control and limited access is key to a successful perpetual inventory.

Just-In-Time Purchasing

As mentioned above, there are many advantages to limiting supplies on hand for each product. The challenge though, is to keep inventory totals low while assuring adequate supplies are available as they are needed. A growing trend today is to shorten the timetable from purchase order to use. This is called **just-in-time purchasing (JIT)**. In this concept, a Certified Dietary Manager purchases products just in time for use.

How does this work? When frequent deliveries are available or menus are planned with specialty or fresh product usage within hours of delivery, JIT purchasing can be beneficial. Items such as hand cut steaks, custom vegetable mixes for stir-fry or fresh ground beef can be ordered one day and delivered the next morning for use at lunch or supper that day. This allows for reduction in the inventory held on hand since the product delivery and usage are so close together.

Some large volume production centers have established JIT ordering so the products needed for everything made on Tuesday afternoon are delivered Tuesday morning. This requires a highly stable menu in terms of items and quantities and tight coordination between the distributor and the production center. This concept also functions best when the production site is close to the distributor in the event a back-up item is needed.

Inventory Control Tools

The Receiving Process

It is essential that the right products, in the right quantity, at the right price, and from the right supplier be received at the right time. Thus, attention to the receiving process is critical to controlling inventory. (Review Chapter 18 for the food safety indicators in the receiving process.)

There are several components in an effective system. Trained staff must be available to perform required tasks. Employees with receiving duties must:

- Know quality specifications for each product.
- Recognize required quality.
- Recognize food safety indicators to assure food received is wholesome.
- Know how to handle discrepancies in quality or quantity.
- Know how to complete receiving records.

Glossary

Just-in-Time Purchasing (JIT)
Purchasing items as needed just in time

In small facilities, the Certified Dietary Manager may perform the receiving tasks. In larger facilities, there may be one or more employees whose duties are devoted to receiving and storage. A basic receiving process follows the steps described below.

Step 1: Check against purchase records:

- The quantity of all items must be verified against what was purchased; count items that come by count and weigh items that are ordered by weight.

Step 2: Inspect against specifications:

- Compare products against written specifications, especially meat products.

Step 3: Accept or reject products and contact the manager for the following:

- Wrong product is delivered or product does not meet specifications.
- Product was not ordered.
- The supplier has made an unacceptable substitute.
- Food safety indicators are unacceptable.
- Product was not delivered on time.

Step 4: Requests or receives a credit memo if necessary:

- This occurs if only a partial order is delivered, *OR*
- The required items are not available (see Figure 24.10 for a credit memo example).

Step 5: Inspect against delivery invoice before signing it:

- It is important that items appear on the delivery invoice in the correct quantity and the correct price.
- Contact the Certified Dietary Manager if an unauthorized substitution is made or corrections are needed.

Step 6: Complete the receiving report:

- Large facilities that have a designated person receiving the products will require a signed, completed receiving report.

Prompt storage secures the inventory and keeps cold or frozen foods out of the danger zone. Conversely, deliveries left standing in hallways become invitations to theft. Depending on the layout of the facility, a delivery may be stored in an area where many people are walking, some may not even be food production and dining service employees.

Equipment for Receiving

A receiving area must have adequate space for completion of the steps outlined above. In a large facility, there may be a receiving dock connected with a special entrance for trucks. Generally, the receiving area should be located near the delivery door.

Necessary equipment may include: tools to open containers, an accurate scale, carts or dollies, containers to hold ice removed from fresh poultry or seafood, a thermometer, a calculator, marking and tagging equipment, and any needed office equipment (computer, file cabinet, clipboard, etc.).

Putting It Into Practice

4. The assistant manager is the person who checks in deliveries in your facility. She is in a hurry today because she is short one staff person in the kitchen. The following day, there aren't enough chicken breasts for the production of the noon meal. What might have happened?

Figure 24.10 Credit Memorandum

To: _____ Number: _____

Address: _____

City: _____ State: _____

Please send credit for the following:

Invoice	Item	Quantity	Unit of Sale	Unit Price	Extension

Reason:

Delivery Person: _____ Authorizing Signature: _____

Inventory

To be effective in placing an order, you have to understand the items in the inventory. From Chapter 4 (Standards and Specifications for Preparing Foods), the quality of the products to use was discussed. Earlier in this chapter, the specific standards (specifications) for the products were identified. Understanding the items in the inventory also means knowing the amount of items in inventory and what the par levels are.

Inventory Basics

To understand inventory, it's helpful to know a few basic terms:

- **Inventory item.** This is any product routinely supplied to the facility. Both food and non-food products can be inventory items. The food products are generally ingredients for recipes, or items that will be served directly to clients, such as individual cartons of milk or pats of margarine. Just as with a recipe, each inventory item has a unique identity or its own title. In computerized inventory or menu systems, each inventory item also has a unique number or identifier.

- **Inventory category.** Inventory may also be managed under categories just as recipes are. A category is a grouping that is logical and useful to the food production and dining service operation. For example, some Certified Dietary Managers categorize items according to where they are stored. Thus, a category called frozen foods may refer to foods stored in the freezer. Sub-categories may include names like: frozen foods—chicken, frozen foods—ice cream, and others.

- **Purchase unit.** A purchase unit is the package, container, or unit in which a product is purchased. For example, canned peaches may be purchased by the case of 6/#10 cans. Each case contains six cans. The purchase unit is a case. Other purchase units include: pounds (as in pounds of meat), bags (as in large bags of flour), drums (as in drums of fat for deep-fat frying), and others.

- **Issue unit.** An issue unit is the package, container, or amount in which a product is issued from the inventory storage area. Sometimes the issue unit is identical to the purchase unit. Other times, it is different. For example, the canned peaches purchased in whole cases of six cans each are issued by single #10 cans to food production staff. So, the issue unit for this example is: #10 can.

- **Storage areas.** Storage areas are defined locations where products are stored. Each product in an inventory list should have a defined storage area or location for easier control. Storage areas include freezers, refrigerators, deep-chill units, pantries, storerooms, and small supply carts kept in the kitchen or serving areas.

- **Inventory list.** A complete and up-to-date list of inventory is recommended. The inventory list defines the products specified as ingredients for recipes and direct-serve products for menus. A typical inventory list identifies: name, inventory number, inventory category, storage location, purchase unit, issue unit, and source (supplier from whom it is ordered).

- **Physical inventory.** A physical inventory is an actual count of products on hand at the current time. Counting products is often called taking inventory. A physical inventory is an essential control tool. How often a physical inventory is completed depends on the method used and the guidelines set by the finance department, which is often only at the end of the fiscal year. For tight control of inventory and purchasing dollars, once a week may be indicated. If theft is suspected, a nightly inventory of high-ticket items (roasts, shrimp, barbecue ribs, turkey, hams, etc.) should be re-checked every morning and throughout the day. In general, a good target for a price extended inventory is once a month.

Most distributors also offer a downloadable spreadsheet with the listing of all items purchased and the most current pricing. Often, the spreadsheets can be edited to add items from other vendors so all inventory is tracked in one file. The sheets can be printed for use during inventory or the count can be entered directly into the computer for quick calculations. Review the sample form in Figure 24.6 if access to a distributor's version is not available. In a physical inventory, each item on the shelf (this does not include opened items in the production area like flour in the bin or spices on the rack) is counted by the whole and partial purchase unit. A count of eight cans of peaches would be 1.3 cases.

One computer-based tool for taking an inventory uses bar codes to identify products. A handheld scanner reads a bar code representing each item on the inventory list and then the user keys in a number to indicate quantity on hand. This can speed up the process of taking inventory. When it is complete, the user can then apply the figures to determine inventory requirements. In addition, a user can typically print a report showing the current physical inventory.

ABC Analysis

Most Certified Dietary Managers recognize that the greatest dollar value of an inventory investment is represented by a relatively small number of items. If a facility purchases 400 products, perhaps only 100 or fewer of these items, such as meats, represent the greatest cost. The concept of **ABC analysis** helps a manager focus inventory controls where they are most needed. In an ABC analysis, follow these steps:

- Study purchases to determine which products are most costly.
  - > Categorize these as "A" items.
  - > Then group products that are next most costly. Categorize these as "B" items.
  - > Finally, identify items that are least costly, and categorize them as "C" items.
  - > Here, the idea of cost refers to the price of an individual item in a typical usage unit, not the total dollars spent on any item during the course of a week or month. In other words, while breads, cereals, and dairy items may represent a significant cost because of the quantity used, it is the use of costly "A" items that is of interest in ABC analysis.
- Categorize items in this manner to set priorities in purchasing, receiving and storing. Costly "A" items must be carefully controlled; less expensive "C" items need less control.

In an ABC approach to managing inventory:

- Expend time and efforts to control the most costly inventory items.
- Minimize inventory investments, carrying smaller quantities of "A" products in inventory.
- Develop specific policies and procedures to control, purchase, receive, and store top-priority items.

How can the concept of ABC analysis be used in storage? Small facilities might designate one section of a reach-in refrigerator or freezer for storage of most expensive items. These units can be kept locked and inventory levels visually checked daily, if needed, to monitor the quantity of "A" items in these areas. The *precious room concept*—locked storage within a locked storage area—can be useful to store the most expensive dry items, including chafing dishes, buffet utensils, alcoholic beverages, and other expensive supplies and materials.

Ways to Reduce Inventory Costs

Cash flow problems can occur when inventory levels are too high. Steps to reduce inventory costs include the following:

- Reduce the quantities of products purchased. To make the transition when stocks are too great, "live on inventory" for some time period and reduce the inventory on the shelf.
- Reduce turnaround time on deliveries. Only purchase what is needed and reduce dead inventory on the shelf. Computerized ordering systems can greatly support this practice.
- Adjust inventory pars when practical.
- Be sure that purchase units are well suited to usage needs. For example, a product used in very small amounts should be purchased in small units, not large ones. For instance, purchase very small amounts at a local grocery store only when needed.
- Streamline the list of products carried. For example, streamline three sizes of ground beef patties. Through critical analysis, reduce this down to one or two sizes of ground beef patties.

Glossary

ABC Analysis
Helps a manager focus inventory controls where they are most needed

- Manage the menu to use each item in the inventory at least two to three times during the menu cycle.

- Examine special dietary products for possible consolidation with regular products. In facilities serving a number of special diets, there may be a tendency to carry two types of each fruit, vegetable, bread, frozen entrée, baked product, and so forth. One product may be for clients requiring modification of salt, sugar, or fat. Another may be for clients with no dietary restrictions. By reviewing dietary needs and product options, you may be able to select one product to serve both needs. Examples are: a juice-packed canned fruit or a healthy convenience food.

- Avoid minimum purchases from specialty or secondary vendors. If a $500 minimum order is required to get the $30 specialty cookie, then skip the cookie.

Food Issuing Practices

A controlled process for withdrawing products from storage for use is called **issuing**. Here, the idea is that not just anyone can go take what is needed. Instead, someone has to issue a product. The active process of issuing denotes control, responsibility, and accountability. An effective food issuing system does three things:

- Matches items removed from storage with those required for actual food production.

- Supports security procedures.

- Documents the quantities of items issued for record-keeping and accounting.

Glossary

Food Requisition
A documented request for specific products and quantities

Issuing
Process for withdrawing products from storage

Clearly, these objectives require basic controls and documentation. Many facilities use a **food requisition**. This form organizes requests for food and non-food items to be dispensed from inventory. The form documents the transactions and assigns responsibility for the cost when items are requisitioned by outside departments. An example appears in Figure 24.11. Unit price and food cost may or may not appear on the form, depending on how the accounting system is structured.

The issuing process is managing the movement of ingredients to production and service areas. Each facility should establish policies about inventory issues. For example, who may complete the requisition and authorize inventory withdrawal? When should products be issued? Are receiving areas charged for the items issued? What items can be requisitioned?

Figure 24.10 Food Requisition Form

Date: _____   Location: _____

Quantity	Description	Unit Price	Extension

Authorized: _____   Received By: _____

A basic plan may be that the cook completes a food requisition for recipes to be prepared for the next meal period. A standardized recipe will indicate the types and quantities of necessary ingredients. In a more comprehensive computerized food production systems, a printout may show what withdrawals will be needed days in advance based on forecasted levels.

After the food requisition is completed, it goes to the storeroom for issuing. An employee assigned to storeroom management pulls the products needed, and delivers them to designated areas. The person who receives the items verifies the delivery and signs off that everything has been received.

In another example, a service employee requisitions ready-to-use products from inventory. For example, a cafeteria employee stocking the cold service area may request cartons of milk, fresh fruit, and other items. The same steps hold—the cafeteria employee completes a requisition, the assigned storeroom employee fills it, and the cafeteria employee checks and signs off on it. In many ways, this process is similar to the initial receiving process. Each person involved in the transaction is responsible for accuracy and verification, and is accountable for the products.

Controlling access to storage areas is a prime concern in security at the time of food distribution. After items are issued and transferred to food production or service areas, the issuing process is complete.

In a very large facility, some food may be stored off-site in a warehouse. Again, the process follows the same principles. However, the requisitions must be organized and communicated well in advance of need. Assigned employees pull products for use and deliver them to the requesting location.

In another scenario, some food production and dining service facilities accommodate issuing systems for areas that maintain par inventory levels. Consider items on nourishment carts in nursing stations or supplies in a decentralized pantry where rethermalization of trays takes place just before meal service. As items in these areas are reduced to a predetermined level, a specified quantity of additional products is issued to build the inventory levels to a predetermined par level.

A modification of this system is the exchange cart process. In this model, an employee stocks a cart with required supplies (following a predetermined list), and wheels it to a pantry. Then, the employee exchanges this cart for an old cart. He takes the old cart back to the kitchen for restocking of remaining inventory.

Some food production and dining service facilities use computerized issuing systems while others use optical reading devices that read information from bar codes and enter it into computerized information systems. Software calculates the quantity of products leaving storage areas and maintains an ongoing count of products in inventory, supporting a perpetual inventory system.

A stockless inventory systems works in some facilities. For example, a satellite unit may have no or little inventory on hand. Products to be prepared/served are brought to the facility daily. Any remaining products are taken back to the central preparation area at the end of the serving period. While not practical in many facilities, this system is useful when satellite facilities have very minimal food storage areas. In this system, very frequent deliveries of necessary products are essential.

Putting It Into Practice

5. Your facility is small and you do not have a formal requisition process. Kitchen staff members just sign a sheet of paper in the storage room when they take products out. Lately, you have noticed that inventory for some products seem to be short. What should you do?

Even small facilities can implement the basic principles of issuing control. Perhaps expensive and/or theft-prone items are kept in locked storage. Management staff can be present for issuing these relatively few items at specific times preceding production. Other items can remain available in storage areas for request on an as-needed basis by production personnel.

Small food production and dining service operations may not find it practical to use a formal food requisition system. However, these facilities might require that a Certified Dietary Manager be physically present at the time withdrawals are made from inventory. Some facilities may use a requisition taped to the wall or door of each storage area. Staff members authorized to withdraw products from storage can then enter information onto the form. Consistently enforced policies regarding storage areas being off-limits to unauthorized personnel can reduce the number of employees who issue products to themselves. Close supervision is necessary to assure that personnel adhere to this procedure.

Requisitions can be used by the Certified Dietary Manager to match the quantity of items withdrawn from inventory with that used in actual food production as a method of monitoring product movement and control. The objective in issuing is to distribute needed items for production efficiently, safely, and economically. Related to this objective is to keep food stocks secure from theft and pilferage. Record-keeping is a supportive service, but not an objective unto itself. The end result is effective food distribution throughout the operation.

Purchase Orders

Once inventory needs have been determined and vendors selected, it is time to place a purchase order. A **purchase order** is a business document that specifies what is being purchased, in what quantity, from whom, for whom, and under what terms. In most facilities, a pre-determined purchase order format and set of related procedures already exist. Additional information that may appear in a purchase order includes: the vendor's item number, an internal inventory number, and the purchase unit (e.g., case).

Typically, a purchasing agent (Storeroom or Purchasing Supervisor) bears responsibility for making purchases. In smaller facilities, the Certified Dietary Manager or designated cook may place the order. In large multi-site facilities, purchasing may be handled by a purchasing department, or a buyer serving a number of food production and dining service operations. Note that it is important to clarify who is authorized to make a purchase order. If the Certified Dietary Manager ordinarily holds the authorization, others should be designated to place an order when the manager is not available, such as during a vacation or an emergency.

There are many methods of placing a purchase order. In a traditional system, a Certified Dietary Manager writes down all needs on purchase order forms, and then calls suppliers to place the orders. Today, managers use web-based ordering systems to connect with a vendor's online order entry process directly. If a computerized menu system is in use, the software may generate a proposed purchase order on screen for review and approval, and then transfer the order electronically to the designated vendor.) See Figure 24.11 for an example of an online purchase order system.)

Most software and web-based options provide detailed reporting of purchasing history. This is valuable for cost analysis, as well as for determining usage history.

Figure 24.11 Purchase Order

These are examples of online tools available for interfacing the inventory and purchasing process. Handheld electronic devices are becoming more common to the foodservice industry, allowing the buyer direct access in the storeroom to complete inventory and purchasing.

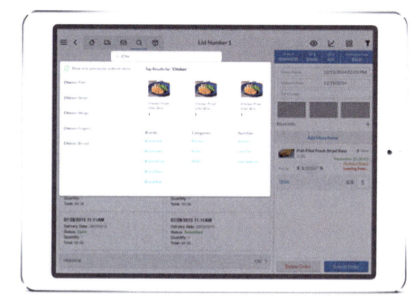
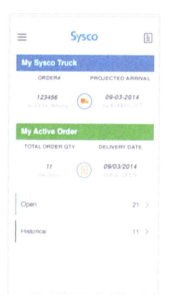

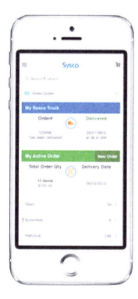
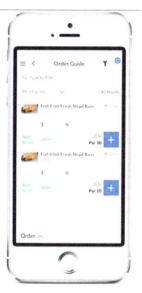
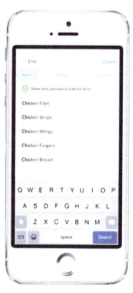

Source: Sysco Corporation, used with permission.

Purchasing Ethics

With the authority of purchasing comes the responsibility of ethical practices. Business ethics identify purchasing decisions based on objectives of the facility and not influenced by personal factors. This is essential to the sound fiscal operation of a facility, as well as professional standing. Most facilities have a policy addressing ethical practices. Become familiar with this policy and follow it.

Broadly recognized ethical practices dictate that a purchasing agent not accept meals, gifts, or favors from suppliers. In addition, treat all suppliers and potential suppliers fairly and equally. For example, in a competitive bid process, include all possible candidates. Final selections of vendors are based on the criteria described above, including price, value, and service. An ethical Certified Dietary Manager continuously evaluates purchasing choices on an objective basis and remains open to new opportunities. Sometimes, the most appropriate business decision is not the personally preferred decision.

From forecast to specification to purchase order, it is clear that there is a great deal of planning, attention to detail, and sound management required to perform effective purchasing.

Deciding How Much to Purchase

Understanding Product Yields

As products are specified and later quantified for purchase, it is essential to consider product yields. Much like the recipe yield discussed in Chapter 3, a product yield tells how much usable food will be obtained from each product purchased. It also helps compare and control costs of competing products.

Calculating the As Purchased quantities to obtain the needed Edible Portion amount of the menu is a daily activity in food production. Knowing that there are approximately 25 ½ cup servings of sliced peaches in every #10 can means that five cans of fruit are needed each time peaches are on the menu in a community of 115 clients. The As Purchased weight of fresh produce may have as much as 60% loss in processing to the Edible Portion of seasonal melon cubes. Product yield significantly impacts the amount of product that needs to be purchased.

Make or Buy?

In developing product specifications and making purchasing decisions, a Certified Dietary Manager often faces the opportunity to use convenience foods. Convenience foods are products that offer ease in preparation and minimal labor. They may be pre-made, such as a frozen entrée, or they may have been processed in a manner that reduces labor, such as grated carrots or diced onions. For macaroni and cheese, the manager could purchase a heat-and-serve frozen product, ready-to-make mix, or make it from scratch. Similarly, for a cake, the manager could purchase a frozen cake, a cake mix, or make the product entirely from scratch. Decisions between convenience and from-scratch products can have broad financial implications.

In determining whether to make or buy, consider both financial and quality factors such as:

- What is the final quality of the convenience food? Is it acceptable for our needs?
- What is the labor requirement of the convenience food versus the product we would make from scratch?
- If you consider both labor and food cost, which product comes out to be least expensive?

If quality is acceptable and total expense is less, convenience foods may be a good choice. A make-or-buy question has become pivotal in food production and dining service operations in which either the operation is experiencing a labor shortage, and/or the cost of labor is very high.

An example of high-cost labor comes into play in some environments. To calculate labor costs for any product:

- Start with an average wage for the production staff who would prepare the product.
- Then, account for the additional expenses of benefits (time off, health insurance, etc.):
  > Typically, benefits run 25-35% of the base wage. Check with the human resources department to obtain the actual factor for benefits.
- From this, set a labor factor, such as 1.30 to reflect a 30% benefit cost:
  > Meaning the real cost of labor is 130% the actual wages.
- Multiply the labor factor times the number of hours required to obtain a labor cost for the product. Here is an example:
  > Chicken soup production from scratch requires 0.25 hours of work by a pre-prep employee, plus 1.5 hours of work from a hot food cook. Total hours = 1.75.
  > The average wage for these employees is about $11.00 per hour, and the benefit factor is 30%.
  > Multiply $11.00 by 1.30 to calculate what the labor really costs per hour:
  $11.00 x 1.30 = $14.30
  > Multiply number of hours required by the true labor cost to total the labor expense:
  1.75 hours x $14.30/hr = $25.03

In this example, every time you make a batch of chicken soup from scratch, it costs $25.03, in addition to the cost of food purchased for the recipe. To make a final comparison, calculate food costs, and then convert the figure to cost per serving. Compare this with cost per serving of the canned or frozen soup, plus the labor cost of producing the convenience product. (This should be minimal.) Finally, evaluate the quality and value for each option.

The decision to purchase a convenience or ready-to-mix product versus making-from-scratch is often a balance between raw costs (ingredients and labor) and the availability of skilled labor to prepare the item. Scratch preparation is almost always less expensive in food cost but often requires more labor, or a higher skill set, than what is available.

The choice between convenience and scratch is usually more complicated than just the labor or food cost. The use of quality convenience items on the menu as alternates may free up skilled labor to make featured or signature items. Consideration of convenience items available from the vendor may deserve more than "we cook everything from scratch".

Don't Cook Off-the-Truck

Distributors offer/provide an order guide of the items they sell. Often the vendor will customize the order guide to the items approved or commonly purchased by the facility. The Certified Dietary Manager does not want to see all 10,000 items in their warehouse. They really want to focus on the 800 items they frequently purchase. Some of the online ordering systems allow the manager to further refine the order guide to the items they purchase for week one of the menu with a separate order G=guide for week two.

An experience manager will arrange the order G=guide and review their purchasing history to order products based on their needs for the day after delivery through the day of the next delivery. If the purchase order is being placed on Monday for a Tuesday delivery, there should be no items needed for Tuesday's menu being delivered on the truck that day. If an item is "shorted" or "mis-picked" on the delivery, then there is time to recover or change the menu.

Receiving and Food Storage Process

Safe receiving and storage procedures were discussed in Chapter 18. The primary concerns to address are:

- The items delivered are the items ordered, in the correct amounts and in the proper condition (frozen foods are frozen, no damaged cases observed, etc.).
- All appropriate inspection stickers, date codes and temperature records are present.
- There are no signs of spoilage, pest infestation or tampering.
- Delivery statements are signed for and any exceptions or credit memos noted.
- Products are promptly moved to the appropriate storage area and shelved based on FIFO.
- All record keeping and documentation are turned into the office for payment processing.

Security and Controls

Throughout the process of purchasing, receiving, storing, and issuing food, there are ongoing security concerns. Many relate to the flow of products from one task to the next. The first concerns come into play in the purchasing process, where a form of theft or error can occur. Here are some of the issues:

- **Kickbacks.** Kickbacks involve the purchaser working in collusion with someone from the supplier's company. In one type of kickback scheme, products are purchased at higher than necessary prices; the two thieves split the difference between the real and inflated price. The payment can be in money or gifts. Either way, the food production and dining service operation is the loser. Routine review of invoices and competitive bids can identify this unethical practice.
- **Padding the invoice.** This means adding items that were not received, and/or increasing the invoice by adding unreasonable "handling" or other charges. This scheme works well when the employee who purchases also does the receiving. The recommended accounting practice encourages separated purchasing and receiving tasks.
- **Fictitious companies.** Personnel who purchase can steal by setting up a "dummy" company to submit invoices for products that were never received. To identify this, periodically review the distribution summary generated by the Finance Department that lists every check cut for the department with the payees' names to ensure that all vendors listed are valid.
- **Duplicate invoices.** Suppliers may send an invoice through twice if the facility does not have an internal system to verify which invoices have not been paid and cancel invoices that have been paid. This type of problem may happen unintentionally and is not necessarily a sign of bad faith or malicious intent. Reconciling the invoice number against the monthly billing statement from the vendor with the distribution summary of checks cut helps identify duplicate invoices and adjustments to the delivery statements caused by credit memos. What's important is to have basic accounting practices in place to address any failures, omissions or errors.

- **Credit memo problems.** Financial loss can occur when products are not delivered and no credit memo is issued to reduce the original delivery invoice accordingly. A similar problem can occur if a product is rejected and the supplier fails to process a credit memo. Certified Dietary Managers can require that a credit memo be issued and attach it to the delivery invoice whenever shortages or related problems occur.

- **Delivery invoice errors.** Intentional or unintentional arithmetic errors, short weight or count, quality deviations, and similar mistakes can cost food production and dining services money. It is important to check the arithmetic on invoices. Regardless of whether these are innocent errors or intentional frauds, the bottom line is the same. The facility loses money.

- **Quality substitutions.** Downgrading a product with the hope that it won't be noticed is a type of theft that can sometimes occur. Paying more for a lower-quality product can be prevented by proper receiving practices.

> Note: In most organizations the Accounts Payable staff do not know or understand what is appropriate or consistent billing for the operation. They see an invoice from an approved vendor for food items with what appears to be the manager's signature of approval, so they pay it. If a someone has figured out how to get around the system and is buying food not delivered to the facility, but hiding the invoice in with legitimate invoices, Accounts Payable will pay it.
>
> Review the invoices carefully before approving for payment. Review the "Distribution Summary" of checks issued to verify that all invoices were valid. Restrict "will call" picks-ups to Manager Approval Required. Invoice fraud is easier than you think because we do not review our own records.

Security concerns become important at time of receiving, too. There are many opportunities for employee and supplier theft. Consider the following examples:

- The facility receives the wrong item, such as ground beef at 30% fat instead of 20% fat. If the employee does not catch this error, the higher price for a lower-quality product is now in the system.

- The facility receives a short weight or count and fails to notice. Now, the food production and dining service operation pays for a product it does not even have (and may not have enough food for scheduled production).

- Delivery of a product containing a filler, such as ground meat to which ground ice has been added.

- A similar scenario is meat that has not been trimmed to specifications. In this case, weight of the product may match the invoice, but edible yield factor is lower, you are paying more per ounce of Edible Portion.

To help guard against loss at the time products are received, focus on some basic principles. First of all, schedule deliveries to allow adequate time for careful check-in of products. Next, make the investment in training for receiving staff. Recognize staff for their role as gatekeepers, and assure they understand the details and mechanics of how to accomplish their mission.

While direct access to the receiving dock is efficient, the receiving doors should not be left open or unsecured. An audio signal can be installed to permit delivery staff to signal when they have arrived. Delivery persons should be under visual supervision of receiving staff during the entire time they are in the facility and access to possible deliveries is controlled.

In storage, yet additional problems can arise. The most common is theft (also called pilferage), either by food production and dining service employees, house staff or outsiders to the facility. Several practices can help reduce pilferage:

- Move deliveries to their storage locations as quickly as possible.
- As an additional control, prohibit access to storage areas.
  - > Locking all storage areas and controlling access to keys is a generally accepted practice.
- Have a clear policy about who may or may not enter the storage areas.
  - > Post signs on storage areas to reinforce the policy.
  - > Enforce the policy and escort non-departmental or outsiders out of any storage areas.
- Manage personal items and access in storage areas, for example, employee lunches or a client's birthday cake.
  - > If allowed by the facility, have a policy that designates a special reach-in cooler away from the general storage areas for outside items.
- Develop policies that prohibit staff from taking "leftovers" from the facility without the managers signed approval stating that the employee is authorized to remove this item from the building. It names the item(s), and contains a date and authorized signature.
  - > If leftovers are available for employee use, at no charge, there will always be "leftovers" of the most popular items.
  - > In some facilities, all employees leaving the building are asked to show their property to a security guard on the way out the door.
- Secure storage during off-hours access:
  - > There may be only one or two employees working, such as a late night clean-up employee or an early morning storeroom employee. When possible, secure areas that do not require access during these times.
  - > In addition, coordinate with a security manager, an evening administrator, or someone else to provide monitored access to the department after hours.

Security of the department is a concern beyond the potential theft of product. It also relates to the safety and wholesomeness of the food items. Intentional or inadvertent contamination of the food supply can affect every client in the dining room. Coolers left slightly open overnight by a distracted aide can result in thousands of dollars in lost food products. The safety of the food supply is the goal.

Paying for Purchased Products

The role of the accounting department deserves special attention in this discussion because all products received must be paid for accordingly. Designing a system that incorporates the accounting function as an integral part of the purchasing task is very important.

In small food production and dining service operations, the owner or Certified Dietary Manager may be both the purchaser and the bill-payer. As facilities become larger, these tasks are split between operations and accounting or office personnel. As food production and dining service operations grow bigger still, purchasing responsibilities may be assumed by the Procurement or Purchasing Department in an increased effort to separate duties. Typically, a flow of documentation is used to help the manager, accountant, and supplier communicate with each other. This documentation may be paper-based, or it may be maintained in a computer system.

One type of document is a source document. This means it is a source of original entry for financial information into the accounting system. For example, a time card may be a source document for payroll. A purchase order is a source document, as is a signed invoice. Figure 24.12 identifies the source documents and flow of accounting information in a small facility, from the time that an order is placed until the supplier is paid.

At the end of the day or shift, purchase orders and delivery invoices are forwarded to the designated manager or bookkeeper. This person is responsible for:

- Ensuring that there are no differences in quantity and/or price between items ordered (purchase order) and received (delivery invoice).

- Verifies that arithmetic extensions on the delivery invoice are correct.

- Submits and files the invoice for payment by accounting.

Procedures may be modified by larger food production and dining service facilities.

Although responsibility for purchasing tasks may vary from one facility to another, it is most common for a food production staff members to bear responsibility for purchasing food. This is because the specification and selection process requires an in-depth knowledge of food and the needs of dining services.

There are generally two methods used to pay suppliers for purchased products. One is managed by invoice, while another is managed by statement. An **invoice** is a document designating what has been purchased, accepted, and at what price. The purchases are totaled as the amount due. A **statement** is an accounting document that summarizes all invoices, credits, and payments for a given time period and provides the bottom line, as the amount due.

Figure 24.12 Source Document Flow In a Small Facility

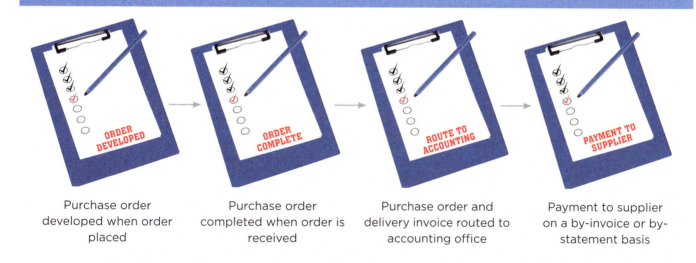

| Purchase order developed when order placed | Purchase order completed when order is received | Purchase order and delivery invoice routed to accounting office | Payment to supplier on a by-invoice or by-statement basis |

With the by-invoice plan, the Certified Dietary Manager takes the following steps:

- Review invoices received daily. Question and correct any matters of concern. Be sure that the final figure on each invoice reflects all discrepancies, credits, or adjustments noted by the receiving clerk.
- Assign dollar amounts to appropriate accounting department codes (food, paper goods, chemicals, etc.), mark the invoice "approved for payment," sign and date them.
- File invoice by due date.
- On a scheduled basis (such as once per week), forward invoices for payment to accounting:
  - > Typically, accounting cuts checks for vendors one day a week so all invoices should be submitted at least 1 day prior for prompt payment.

With the less common by-statement plan, the Certified Dietary Manager begins as above, but then follows a slightly different process. Here are the steps:

- Review invoices from receiving daily. Question and correct any matters of concern. Be sure that the final figure on each invoice reflects all discrepancies, credits, or adjustments noted by the receiving clerk.
- Assign dollar amounts to appropriate accounting department codes (food, paper goods, chemicals, etc.), mark each invoice "approved for payment," sign and date them.
- File invoice by supplier, in an organized date sequence. For example, all invoices from Axl Distributors go into the "Axl" file, with oldest invoices in the front, and newest in the back.
- Wait for a statement from each supplier to arrive.
- When the statement arrives, pull all invoices from this supplier's file. Verify the statement against the invoices. If there are any discrepancies, contact the supplier for clarification or adjustment. Then, process the statement for payment.

In most facilities, documents approved for payment then go to a business office or accounting office, where designated personnel actually cut the checks and mail them. Regardless of whether payments are managed by-invoice or by-statement, similar procedures are necessary to prepare the documents for payment.

Monthly Spend Down Tracker

Managing the purchasing process to stay within budget is often a difficult task. A number of systems have been designed from simple paper and pencil to formal computer systems that control costs to the penny.

The simplest system is to invest in a steno notepad and a calculator.

- Start with the annual budget for all food and for all non-food items.
- Divide the total by 12 for a monthly target or by 52 for a weekly target.
- Enter that amount at the top of the page.
- Write down every invoice received by date, invoice number, vendor, amount and the date the invoice was sent to accounting.
- Subtract that amount from the total and keep track of how much money is left for the week or month.
- If at the end of the month and there is not much left—adjust the purchases.
  - > Or, if it looks like you have a generous amount left in a 30-day month, buy a little extra (insurance) quantity for the 31-day month coming.

A more structured program or computer spreadsheet may be available from the vendor, online, or set one up to meet the facility's needs on the computer. Figure 24.13 is an example of a simple Spend Down Tracker that can be accessed in the online *Supplemental Textbook Materials—Foodservice.*

Figure 24.13 Sample Monthly Spend Down Tracker

Purchases for the Month August 2016

	Food	Non-Food	Total
Annual Budget	$ 365,000	$ 36,500	$ 401,500
YTD Spend	$ 192,142	$ 16,660	$ 208,803
Monthly Budget	$ 31,000	$ 3,100	$ 34,100
MTD Spend	$ 6,831	$ 1,517	$ 8,349
Spend Down			
Remaining	$ 24,169	$ 1,583	$ 25,751

Date	Invoice Number	To Accounting	Vendor	Food	Non-Food	Total Purchases
8/2/2016	1259543	8/6/2016	Good Food Del	$ 3,512.33	$ 251.00	$ 3,763.33
8/4/2016	B26543	8/6/2016	Bread	$ 393.25	$ -	$ 393.25
8/4/2016	62582	8/6/2016	Dairyman	$ 563.11	$ -	$ 563.11
8/6/2016	1259677	8/6/2016	Good Food Del	$ 2,362.80	$ 1,266.03	$ 3,628.83
						$ -
						$ -
						$ -

The Spend Down Tracker closes the purchasing cycle by documenting the approval for payment of products specified, ordered, received, inventoried, and used. Purchasing is a major element of the Certified Dietary Managers responsibilities impacting budget, food quality, menus, and client satisfaction.

Revenue and Cash Handling

Overview and Objectives

Cafeterias and retail operations in most facilities are expected to break-even, or bring in a profit. As a Certified Dietary Manager, you may be expected to find ways to offset operational expenses or enhance profits by increasing revenues through the department. In this chapter, we will examine ideas for generating and managing revenue, including the most common approach, catering. After completing this chapter, you should be able to:

✓ Research revenue generating opportunities

✓ Analyze revenue generating opportunities

✓ Supervise cash activities and reports

✓ Calculate cost and set prices for catered events

✓ Plan foodservice and menus for catered events

✓ Estimate price-per-unit serving for catered events

✓ Use cost-control techniques to balance revenue budget

✓ Prepare business plan and justification for new revenue generating programs

✓ Promote existing and new revenue generating programs

Throughout this textbook, you have read many times about the importance of talking to the clients, surveying the clients, involving the clients in panels, and in general, determining the client needs and wants. In so doing, you are marketing the department services. Marketing is much more than advertising and promoting products; it is also about meeting the client's wants and needs. Marketing is also one aspect of managing revenue generating services.

Money that is coming into the facility is considered revenue. Revenue generating opportunities for the dining services department are activities, such as:

- The meals served every day to clients in the dining room (if a per meal charge is tracked by the organization such as the independent living meal plan).
- Catering activities (paid for in cash).
- The cafeteria.
- Serving meals to community groups.
- Food items offered in a "C-Store".

Revenue Generating Services

The key objective of implementing revenue generating services is to increase gross revenue in the operating statement. Depending on the overall financial plan of the facility, this money may increase profits or fund other activities. Opportunities for generating revenue abound in any foodservice department and generally draw upon the resources in place, such as physical facilities for producing food, a ready client base, culinary talent, and business support services within the facility. Thus, the possibilities are limited only by the imagination and resourcefulness of the Certified Dietary Manager.

Some options may employ special merchandising techniques in a cafeteria, while others may require creating new systems and services. Some may use the existing client base, such as employees of the organization, while others may extend the client reach further into the community.

Here are examples of revenue generating services and opportunities:

- Cafeteria, coffee shop or sit-down restaurant
  > Ice cream sundaes available at break times
  > Point-of-sale merchandising for specialty items (see Figure 25.1 for examples)
  > Home meal replacements for busy employees on their way home
  > Take-out holiday specialties, such as deli trays, pies, holiday cookies, etc.
  > Sunday brunch services in the cafeteria
  > Payroll deduction service for employees to charge meals and take-out (improves sales)
  > Take-out pizzas
  > Gourmet meals (at a price) for clients and their families/friends
- A coffee cart for specialty coffees and espresso service
- Vending machines
- A snack shop or C-Store (convenience store)
- Catering (discussed later in this chapter)
- Providing satellite meal service to other facilities, i.e., day care centers

The Certified Dietary Manager can use a variety of techniques to manage revenue generating services such as: supervising cash activities and reports, business planning including a profitability analysis, calculating costs for services, and promoting revenue generating services.

Figure 25.1 Point-of-Sale Merchandising Ideas

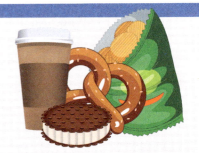

- Freshly baked cookies—small cookie oven
- Ice cream and confectionery frozen products—ice cream freezer
- Hot soft pretzels—pretzel machine
- Chips—chip racks
- Nachos—nacho dispenser
- Coffee—coffee maker
- Instant cappuccino or specialty coffee drinks—specialty beverage machine
- Rice bowls, burritos, etc.—tabletop freezer

Source: Der Garabedian, Carrie. 77 Ways to Increase Revenue. DMA, 2003.

Business Planning

While it is not practical to implement a long list of revenue generating services all at once, a Certified Dietary Manager should carefully weigh the strengths of in-house resources along with the various opportunities. It is important to conduct some financial analysis to decide which option is most likely to meet the revenue objectives.

The simplest approach is to build these services without increasing the operating costs. For example, weave the production of homemade cookies for takeout into the existing routine of the bake shop cook. This means the only added cost is the raw food cost for the cookie ingredients. Work with the food supplier to obtain merchandising equipment at no cost based on purchases of related food products. Then, each sale (if priced appropriately) generates added revenue for the department.

Some revenue generating options pinpoint high-profit menu items. Specialty coffee is an excellent example. Taking the cue from the foodservice marketplace, specialty coffees are very popular, and clients are willing to pay extra for a cup of premium latte, cappuccino, or iced coffee. The added revenue comes from quality ingredients, along with creative merchandising, while the raw food costs are relatively low. Some revenue concepts may require extra labor time along with a boost in raw food expenses. Providing take-out holiday foods is an example. For this idea, some additional staff time may be needed, as well as purchasing additional ingredients.

Any time your idea begins to incur extra costs, a profitability analysis is warranted. A **profitability analysis** is a financial calculation that compares costs with revenues to determine whether an idea is profitable. To create one, detail the costs, set a selling price, project a sales volume, and then calculate the bottom line. Figure 25.2 provides an example for take-out deli trays. Another type of financial calculation is a **break-even analysis**.

For some ideas, an investment may be required, e.g., purchasing new equipment or building a snack shop or purchasing a kiosk for mobile food sales. If there is a significant budget cost to an idea, the next step is to create a **business plan**.

A business plan is a formal document that includes the following:

- Goal.
- Overall description of the revenue generating service, including the proposed products and/or other services.
- Description of the target market (who will purchase the products and/or services).
- Pricing strategy that includes a review of the competition for the products and/or services.
- Detailed timeline, including the management team responsible for each task.
- Financial projections with pricing, sales volume, costs, labor, expenses, payback period, and net revenues.

In essence, a business plan is a blueprint for all aspects of the new business. Thus, the profitability analysis needs to expand to include a more detailed accounting of:

- Capital expenditures.
    - > Building or renovation costs, equipment cost, initial supply acquisitions.
- Advertising costs.
- A timeline of projected sales volumes, pricing and profit or loss.

Glossary

Profitability Analysis
Financial calculation that compares costs with revenues to determine whether an idea is profitable

Break-Even Analysis
Financial calculation that compares costs with revenues to determine if a profit is passable

Business Plan
A formal document that provides details for a proposed revenue generating service

- Project what level of sales will be required to break even, i.e., pay off the investment—and estimate a timeframe to reach this level of sales.

    > It is not unusual for a break-even point to occur 12 or 18 months down the line on a business investment.

- Review the resources available within the facility and ensure the required business support from senior leadership and the finance department to launch the venture.

- Survey of the competition: locations, pricing, traffic levels, customer demands.

- Verify with the legal and finance departments that all needed paperwork (licenses, Certificates of Occupancy, retail tax status, insurance…) will be available.

- Define a new cost center with the finance department with budgetary goals.

Due to the financial risk involved, the business plan needs to provide a realistic estimate of investment costs, the ongoing operating costs, and the potential revenue. Not all good ideas get funded and not all new programs succeed, particularly in retail food operations. Writing a business plan helps expose areas of concern and provides a guideline to success. There are countless books and online assistance in writing a well-documented business plan, and ready to use templates, accessible through an online search.

Figure 25.2 Profitability Analysis: Take-Out Deli Trays

COSTS:		REVENUE:				
1. Food		Selling Price per Tray	$21.95			
Ham	$0.60	Total Production Cost per Tray	$11.01			
Turkey	1.20	Gross Profit per Tray	$10.94			
Soft Cheese	0.72					
Gouda Cheese	0.51	**# Trays Sold**		**Gross Profit**		**Net Revenue**
Jack Cheese	0.37					
Crackers	0.93	5	X $10.94 =	$ 54.70	-$120 =	($65.30)
Garnish	0.14	10	X $10.94 =	109.40	-$120 =	(10.60)
Food Total	*$4.47 per tray*	11	X $10.94 =	120.34	-$120 =	0.34
		15	X $10.94 =	164.10	-$120 =	44.10
2. Packaging		20	X $10.94 =	218.80	-$120 =	98.80
Packaging Materials	*0.19 per tray*	25	X $10.94 =	273.50	-$120 =	153.50
3. Labor		50	X $10.94 =	547.00	-$120 =	427.00
30 minutes—1 employee@ $12.70/hr., including benefits	*$6.35 per tray*	75	X $10.94 =	820.50	-$120 =	700.50
	$11.01 per tray	100	X $10.94 =	$ 1094.00	-$120 =	$974.00
4. Advertising						
Advertising Cost	**$120.00 total**					

Promoting Revenue Generating Services

Let's say that you have chosen to expand catering as a revenue generating service. How will clients, either internal or external, know about the expanded service? **Marketing** is part of doing business today, especially in the foodservice industry.

Marketing and Image

Have you ever been responsible for selecting a nursing home for someone? Many healthcare consumers today follow advice from a number of organizations, such as the American Association of Retired Persons (AARP), the National Council of Senior Citizens, and others when they look for a facility. A specific tip offered by these organizations is simple and consistent: visit the facility during meal time.

This is powerful information. What it tells us is that in a healthcare environment, the dining services department may have significant impact on the decisions of others to use the facility's services. This is just one example of why marketing is important in a dining services operation.

More specifically, marketing activities can have great impact on the immediate sales within an operation, such as sales of the lunch special in an employee cafeteria, or sales of products in a convenience store. Thus, a Certified Dietary Manager needs to consider marketing on two levels: the role of dining services marketing in fulfilling facility objectives, and the role of marketing in fulfilling the objectives of the dining services operation.

Let's take a closer look at the process of marketing. At the highest level, we know that marketing has to do with presenting products or services to persuade people to buy them. There are several components to a marketing plan: advertising, promotion, and direct communications with clients or potential customers.

The basis of marketing relies on the image, which is the view or perception of products and services, as presented in the marketplace. A successful business creates an image of what its products or services represent. Often, this comes directly from the corporate vision. It relates to the idea of identifying (or creating) the client's needs and defining how the business will meet that expectation.

Here is an example: Axl Hospital has a vision to provide state-of-the-art healthcare, blending technology with human compassion to meet clients health needs. From this vision, Axl Hospital would want to build an image in the marketplace that:

- Focuses on caring for people.
- Relates the technical excellence of the hospital's resources.
- Explains the benefits of this combination to potential clients.

Now, any marketing activities Axl conducts are likely to revolve around these ideas. When Axl Hospital produces a billboard for local highways or places a radio advertisement, at least one of the themes listed above will be reflected. Figure 25.3 lists some examples of specific images that might be defined by a dining services operation.

Glossary

Marketing
Presenting products or services to clients (and potential clients) in a way that persuades them to buy

Figure 25.3 Images a Dining Services Department Might Convey In Marketing Efforts

SETTING	EXAMPLE OF AN IMAGE
Employee Dining	Provides the freshest food with quickest service
Hospital	Provides highly personalized meal service with respect for individual needs
Nursing Home	Offers home-style food in a home-like environment
School	Provides the most nutritious meals at the best price with a commitment to the well-being of students

The image is somewhat specific to each facility, and becomes part of its corporate personality. The more consistently a facility uses and supports a cohesive image, the more various campaigns and communications will work together in synergy to generate powerful results. Hence, the Certified Dietary Manager should define the departmental marketing efforts around the facility's mission and image.

Advertising and Promotion

Once image is established, a facility can begin conducting effective advertising and promotion. What do these terms mean? Advertising means placing persuasive announcements in the marketplace to generate sales. These announcements may take the form of newspaper ads, radio ads, television commercials, or even banner ads on the internet. Advertising is also done through direct mail campaigns, email campaigns, and other techniques.

Promotion

Promotion is a little more general, referring to any activity that is designed to publicize a product or service. It may take the form of press releases sent to a local newspaper or even menus posted in a dining area.

Interestingly, promotion can have a secondary effect beyond support for sales. For example, in a healthcare facility where the mission is to promote the nutritional well-being of clients, part of the task may simply be to persuade clients to eat. How the menu and the food are presented may make a big difference. The dining environment and the service provided have an impact too. Hence, the ability to promote food becomes a clinical care concern as well as one of business development.

Following are some examples of advertising and promotion activities a foodservice operation might use.

Posted Menu

One of the most basic tools for promotion in any dining services operation is the menu. This simple document offers a superb opportunity to call attention to the food, to reinforce a defined image, and to build sales and/or acceptance. A menu is always of interest to dining clients. When available, it may be studied far in advance of meal service times.

What makes a menu an effective promotional tool? First of all, it must be easy to read. A clear layout groups offerings by days and meals that are readily identified. It uses a font that is easy to read and adequately sized. Often, it uses clip art, borders, or images to draw attention to its contents.

Glossary

Promotion
Activities designed to publicize a product or service

Here are a few specific tips used by graphic designers:

- Use consistent alignment, generally to the left. Do not center everything, as this is difficult to read.
- Use a consistent design for menu headings that is larger type, bold type, and/or a unique font. Often, a good choice is a sans serif font (one in which the strokes contain no decoration).
- Select and use one font for the remaining contents of the menu.
- Use ALL CAPS sparingly, as it is difficult to read. Generally, it works best only for brief headings.
- Use little or no clip art. It draws attention away from menu contents. Do not let it compete with the words on the menu.
- When used, select pieces of clip art that are compatible with each other in style. They should look like they were all drawn by the same artist, even if they weren't.
- Use colors carefully. Generally, dark type is easiest to read. It should have good contrast. For example, black type printed on dark blue paper will not be very readable. Dark blue type on white paper will.
- Use each design element for a purpose, such as to highlight an important idea. Do not overdecorate, as this actually impairs readability and makes the menu difficult to understand.
- Samples of appropriate and questionable menus are available online in the *Supplemental Textbook Materials—Foodservice* files.

Distributed Menu

In a facility that serves long-term clients, such as a school or a retirement community, Certified Dietary Managers often create a copy of the menu for distribution to clients. Clients may keep this menu as a reference for the time period it covers. The same presentation ideas addressed above apply to this distributed menu. In addition, this menu may include some general information about the facility, such as locations, hours of service, payment options, a phone number or hotline number, a Website address, or other useful reference. This menu also provides an excellent opportunity to relate a clear message about the organizational commitment.

In a healthcare facility where clients complete a selective menu, the promotional opportunity is on the menu form distributed to clients. Once again, readability issues are very important. The type should be large, clear, and dark, with good contrast to the paper on which it is printed.

Catering Menu

If a standard catering menus is offered, consider the appearance of these as well. They are a marketing tool. Some Certified Dietary Managers print them attractively, add photos from real events, and place them in a booklet or notebook for review by potential clients.

Naming Products

What to call the items offered on a menu? This is a subtle but forceful choice. For instance, which of these products would is more tempting to select from a menu—coffee cake or fresh-baked coffee cake? Tossed salad or garden green salad? Vegetable soup or autumn minestrone?

The name is a promotional activity. Furthermore, the name can go a long way in conveying the image defined for the dining venue. Figure 25.4 lists some examples of product names that relate directly to the appearance a foodservice department might wish to convey.

Figure 25.4 Naming Products to Convey an Image

IMAGE	PRODUCT NAMES	
Fresh Food	• Garden Green Salad • Fresh Diced Apples • Harvest Frittata • Wholesome Cornbread	
Home-Style Foods	• Down Home Biscuits • Home-Style Beef Stew • Martha's Apple Pie • Robust Bean Soup	
Upscale Food	• Portabella Pastry Puff • Authentic Bruschetta • Spinach Roulade • Blackened Salmon	

Definitely, the choice of a name builds an image about the food. There is a caution here, however. A name should still be clear and as descriptive as possible. The challenge is to communicate clearly and creatively at the same time. For example, the name double fudge delight sounds interesting, but we don't know what it is—a drink? A cake? A cookie? An ice cream sundae? So, a name should convey enough information to avoid confusion or surprises, which can backfire and disappoint a client. This is especially important in a setting where clients order their food without seeing it, e.g., from a hospital bed. Many Certified Dietary Managers also add brief descriptions to menu listings to tell more about the food.

Where can you go to obtain inspiration for naming products? Cookbooks, restaurant menus, trade magazines, and recipe websites can all be good sources for ideas. Of course, customize the names to the organization, and clearly avoid using the unique product names of other commercial establishments. Avoid overly flowery descriptions that confuse or mislead the client (and may commit you to purchasing product specified by name but not always available):

Sally's Homemade Chicken Pot Pie—A delectable blend of petite peas with garden fresh carrots and Blue Lake green beans, simmered with aromatic garlic and new season pearl onions that complement the diced red potatoes.

Sally's Homemade Chicken Pot Pie—A blend of fresh vegetables simmered with diced white chicken meat in a light cream sauce, topped with flakey pastry dough browned to perfection.

Meal Deals

Special deals or meal packages often constitute a way of promoting food. Many operations have a creative name for a lunch special. The special, dubbed Chef's Choice or Incredible Edibles or something like this, may include a group of menu items and bear a value-oriented price tag. The price tag usually reflects a cost savings. In marketing, this approach is called bundling. It means that a group of products are joined together with one price tag to encourage the sale of all of them. Bundling can increase sales. At the same time, it can often speed up the service in a restaurant or cafeteria, as clients make their choices more quickly.

Discounts and Coupons

Discounts can be a way of encouraging greater volume of sales. An example of a discount in a convenience store might be an offer to purchase one deli sandwich and receive the second one at half price. This type of offer is often short-term, and of course pricing must be calculated to be cost effective for the operation.

For a new product or service, a promotional special or coupon can be a valuable marketing tool. A promotional special at a low price, or a coupon for a free introductory trial, can motivate clients to try something new without feeling that they are taking risks. For example, to advertise a new meal delivery service for clients of an independent living community, you might offer a coupon good for one free home-delivered meal.

Loyalty Programs

Another approach is to reward clients for loyalty or repeat business. A punch card that earns a punch (or stamp) for every cup of specialty coffee or take-out meal purchased and with ten punches earn a free one. For this strategy, select a high-profit item to promote. In debit card systems, a client may earn so many points for every $100 placed on the card. The value is added to the debit balance. There are many possibilities, but the objective is always to encourage a client to continue using the service. Continued business is valuable and can contribute significantly to revenues.

Special Signage

As food is displayed, special signs can draw attention to products and advertise them. A cafeteria offering healthy fare items may develop a special graphic to identify these products throughout the service area. A sign may also be used to highlight a featured item or a special price. A sign should be simple, clear and easy to read. It should be attractive but should not detract from the visual impact of the food itself. It should not block view of the food products.

Newsletter

A newsletter can be a simple tool for telling clients more about the operation. It may also reach people who are closely involved with customers, such as family members of nursing home clients, or visitors to a hospital, or parents of students in a public school. Quite often, the most effective newsletters are very short, such as one page. A set of two or three brief articles can address new offerings, new services, the mechanics of interacting with the foodservice department, the ways in which foodservice staff can be reached to discuss clients' needs, and much more. Here again is an opportunity to support the defined image by including content that tells more about what you do, how you do it, and why you do it.

Some dining services operations offer nutrition tips in a newsletter, too. They may also include a signature recipe from an in-house culinary expert. Ultimately, the emphasis of a newsletter designed for marketing purposes should be to build image, to help clients, and to advertise products or services through editorial content.

Specfic Product Promotions

On a rotating basis, a Certified Dietary Manager may promote specific items on the menu. This can encourage clients to try new fare, and may thus expand sales and establish new loyalties. Branded food items create a ready opportunity for promotion. Brand names should be featured prominently in menus and on signs.

Some operations use self-branding concepts. This means they create their own special product line based on a theme or identity, and create a unique name for this line of products. This can be an excellent way to hone an image and to promote food items.

An operation that offers home meal replacements or take-out items or gift baskets can most certainly promote these products uniquely, too. Signage, fliers, community advertising, and public announcements can all support this effort.

Theme Meals and Events

Particularly in situations in which a client group represents repeat business over extended time periods, there is a genuine need to break up the monotony of cycle menus, and produce renewed excitement in meal service. One way to do this is to present theme meals. Theme meals are built around a theme, such as a holiday, a season, an event, a type of food, a destination, an ethnic cuisine, a cultural custom, a famous character, a cooking style, or almost any idea. Figures 25.5 and 25.6 present ideas for theme celebrations.

Figure 25.5 Theme Example: Halloween Dessert

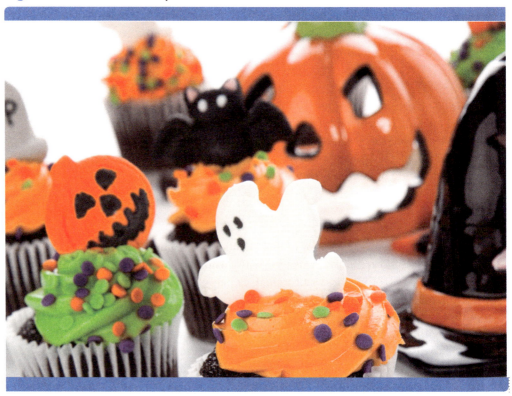

Figure 25.6 Theme Example: Luau Entrée

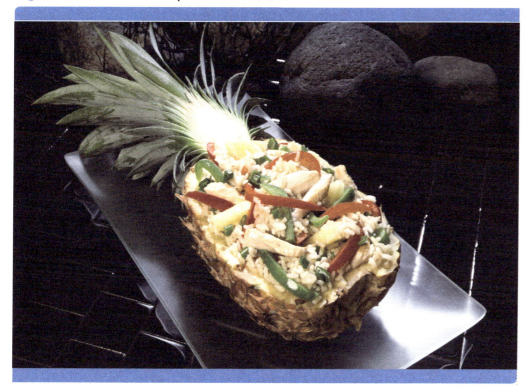

The success of a theme meal is more than food alone. Dining is a sensory experience that encompasses not just flavor, but ambiance, sounds, and sights, too. In a skilled nursing facility, a theme meal is often a full-blown event, and it becomes an interdisciplinary project. Recreation therapists often become very involved and help to plan the themes, the decor, and the activities that will turn a meal into an experience. Some of the details that can make a theme meal successful include:

- Decoration of the dining area.
- Special entertainment.
- Games and activities.
- Background sound or music.
- Theme-related serviceware and napkins.
- Characters/servers dressed in special costumes.

Theme Weeks

A related idea is a theme week, in which a special theme may work its way through an entire week. For example, a holiday season theme may include specialties each day of the week, such as eggnog, holiday cookies, and more. Ideas for full weeks can also piggyback on publicized recognition weeks/months, such as National Nutrition Month, Pride in Food Service Week, or many of the health-related promotional weeks that occur throughout the year.

Needless to say, theme dining ideas require menu creation and advance planning. Some Certified Dietary Managers save their holiday menus, theme menus, and other materials for re-use in the future. Search online for theme day or party ideas. Contact the vendors and food distributors for marketing support and concept meals. Sites, such as http://stylecaster.com/101-theme-party-ideas/ offer clever ideas.

Open Houses

An open house is often a way to help the families and significant others of the clients become more familiar with the service and try the food themselves. In addition, an open house can bring in potential clients.

Press Releases

An inexpensive way to promote products and services is through the use of press releases. For example, an open house may be announced in a press release issued to local newspapers, radio stations, and television stations. A press release is a brief document developed specifically for the media. When writing a release, keep these tips in mind:

- Write a clear headline that tells what this is about.
- Write a lead sentence that gives the key point.
- Add further description about the announcement, followed by more information about the facility.
- Provide contact details for more information, and invite inquiries.
- When possible, provide a photo for print media.
- Clear the announcement with in-house marketing or media relations department, or senior leadership.

Media representatives do not always use a press release as is. They may call to obtain more information or conduct interviews, and write the story according to their own editorial guidelines and needs.

Website

Many dining services operations use a website to communicate with clients and promote products and services. A website may include upcoming menus, a few featured recipes, profiles of the culinary experts, contact information (address, phone, fax, and email), and descriptions of special offerings. Some dining services websites offer online ordering, too.

To make use of this medium, always keep the site fresh and up-to-date. Menus, for example, should always be current. In some facilities, it is appropriate to offer special coupons on a website to promote sales.

Brochure and Fliers

A printed piece can be available to promote special products and services. A flier may also be used to promote catering, home meal delivery, nutritional counseling, or other features. As with printed menus, a promotional brochure should also be neatly designed without excessive decoration. It should be easy to understand, and should always include identity and contact information.

With a desktop publishing program and a color printer, a Certified Dietary Manager may produce many pieces in small runs from a simple computer system. Some managers use pre-printed, specialty papers to make design a little easier.

A basic approach for writing a promotional piece is to follow these steps:

- Identify the audience. Who will read this piece? Make sure that everything written is directed to this group.
- Write a brief sentence describing the concerns or needs the product or service will meet.
- Then tell how the product or service will help.

- Briefly describe the features of the product or service. Bullet points are often effective for this part.

- Summarize the benefits the client will enjoy as a result of using the product or service.

Catering Services

While catering is a service mechanism, it also doubles as a promotional vehicle for many operations. Every time catered food is provided, the food and service is placed in front of potential clients. If the facility caters within the community, there is an ongoing chance to build the image and generate interest in the facility. This can be a superb way to support the broader marketing efforts of the facility, while also generating revenue.

Informal Promotion

This is one of the most effective marketing techniques of all time. It is better known as "word of mouth". A client who enjoys a positive experience tells others about it. This is inexpensive, honest marketing, and it is a natural byproduct of simple, ongoing attention to clients' needs. A personal recommendation for the products or services will likely have a profound impact.

Calculating Costs for Services

Costing and Pricing

Any retail operation has the potential to be a significant revenue generating service or a source of additional cost to the organization. It is important to plan pricing to ensure the retail operation meets the facility's financial objectives. Often, the guideline stated by senior leadership is to break even or make at least a little profit. However, the expectations of menu offerings and the customer willingness to pay rarely result in a profit for the facility.

Pricing a menu item should reflect the cost of the food needed to make the item, the labor to prepare it, serve it and clean up at the end of the meal, plus the supplies like china, detergent, and serving pans. In a true profit environment, the cost of overhead expenses, such as utilities, rent, insurance, and property taxes, also needs to be included in the calculation. Without a magic wand to make food appear, every expense and minute of labor, down to the cost of the individual foil wrap for baked potatoes, is part of the cost.

There are a number of different ways to calculate the cost and determining the price point for each item on the menu.

Detail Cost Analysis

Add up all expenses and set the sell price to cover the cost.

- Based on the cost calculation of a standardized recipe (refer back to Chapter 3 for information on the costing of a standardized recipe), determine the food cost of the portion being sold.

- Add to the food cost the cost of every minute of labor associated with the portion being sold:

  > Remember to include the labor time of the person who took the inventory and added the ingredients to the order from the vendor.

  > And the labor of the dishroom crew to wash the pots.

  > And the Accounts Payable person who wrote the check to the vendor for the food delivery.

> And the finance person who reconciled the bank statement of checks paid against checks written.

> Every minute of labor related to the menu item.

- Add to the food and labor cost the supply expenses related to the menu item:

  > Dishmachine detergent

  > China, silverware, glassware

  > Disposables

  > Office supplies

- Total the expenses (assuming building and overhead expenses are not included) and set the price for the menu.

- If Food Cost is $1.70, Supply Cost is $0.22, and Labor Cost is $3.04 then the total cost is $4.96.

  > $4.96 would be an odd price, so round it to $4.99.

  > Notice—there is no profit in this sell price.

Food Cost as a Percent of Sell Price

Using the recipe food cost and a pre-determined target food cost percentage, calculate the menu selling price.

- Often, a dining service will set their food cost target at 33-40%.

- Based on the cost calculation of a standardized recipe (refer back to Chapter 3 for information on the costing of a standardized recipe), determine the food cost of the portion being sold.

- If the food cost is $1.70 per portion and the target food cost percent is 35%, then (here comes the math):

$$\frac{\$1.70}{35\%} \diagdown \frac{\$?.??}{100\%} = \text{Calculated Sell Price}$$

Cross multiply and divide
1.70 times 100 = 170
170 divided by 35 = $4.86
$4.86 would be an odd price, so round it to $4.85 or $4.89

Food Cost Times a "Factor"

Many menus use a food cost times a factor of 2.5 to 3, as a quick estimate of the food cost percentage. A factor of 2.5 is equal to a 40% food cost, while a factor of 3 is equal to a 33% food cost.

- If the food cost is $1.70 per portion and the factor is 3 then the sell price is 3 times $1.70 or $5.10.

  > $5.10 would be an odd price, so round it to $4.99 or up to $5.29.

  > Notice, there is some profit in this sell price.

The "Wing-It" Pricing Method

This is looking at the cost of the major recipe items plus a little fudge factor for the seasonings and a quick rough calculation of "Let's say somewhere around $5.00".

- Experience and history often allow operators to be very accurate with their estimates.
- The level of profit or loss is an estimate.

Pricing Buckets

Operators and guests do not want to see 50 items with 50 different prices. Streamlining the menu pricing into some similar price points makes the menu easier to read.

- For example, in a cafeteria items may be grouped into three or four price point buckets: $3.29, $3.99, $4.79, and $5.29.
- Using the preferred method to estimate the price point, assign the menu item to the appropriate bucket.
- The level of profit or loss is an estimate.
  - > Some items may even be underpriced because they fit a lower bucket better than the "profitable" bucket.

In general, customers have become accustomed to pricing that is set at five cent or nine cent increments. Products are rarely priced as $4.37. Operators and guests alike would expect that price to be $4.39 or even $4.49. Rounding of the pricing to the five or nine cent points makes the menu more consistent with what the customer expects to see.

> **Warning:** Menu options, costs and pricing are not always within the manager's ability to control. Employees and customers may have a history of a wide variety of their favorite items at money losing price points. Senior leadership may say that they want the cafeteria to break even on food cost but do not want prices to go up. For most managers, setting the pricing to match the cost and quality of the menu items is a long battle. Often, senior leadership does not want to pay the political cost of raising the cafeteria pricing.

Food, supplies and labor costs not covered by money in the register (either cash, payroll deduction or credit card) represents a loss to the organization. In effect, there is a subsidy being provided to the customers for using the cafeteria.

Non-Cash Revenue

Catering represents a specialty service provided based on demand and it can be a revenue generating service. However, often the target market is the clients internal to the facility. A catering service within the community may generate cash revenue for the department, but it may be a loss if the pricing does not cover the expenses.

For in-house clients, the catering transaction typically occurs within the organization's bookkeeping, indicating an expense on one department's budget that becomes a credit in the dining services department's budget. Generally the cost of the catering services that are transferred to another department reflect food cost only and even then are under-valued relative to true cost. Labor and supply costs are often not included so the function is provided at a loss to the department.

Catering charges should not be taken as a reduction in cost to the food expense sub-account on the budget. Food cost is food cost. The only credits that should be taken against the food cost sub-account are vendor credit memos, manufacturer's rebates applied to the food cost account and GPO or prime vendor incentives assigned as a reduction in cost. Inter-department charges for catering should be entered as a credit for dining services in a separate sub-account in the expense section of the budget. Any cash revenue generated by catering should be recorded as income in the revenue section of the budget.

As with the cafeteria, there are different pricing options for catering services; what is used may depend upon the type of services being offered.

Fixed Pricing

If catering activities consist of in-house catering, such as meals for staff, board meetings, and training sessions, fixed pricing may be preferred. Fixed pricing is where a defined cost for a variety of menu items is established in advance. Figure 25.7 is an example of a requisition to be completed by those requesting in-house catering services, followed by a fixed menu for catering items in Figure 25.8.

Custom Pricing

Custom pricing is mainly used for external events where the cost of the catering is determined after all of the details about the event have been defined. Once the basic expenses are tallied, price the event by using a percentage that meets the financial objectives. Some facilities use a food cost percentage method, some use a total cost percentage method, and others use the factor method. Today, many software packages can help determine the menu prices by just entering the menu item and the portion size. The software is set up to calculate cost percentage and determine the selling price.

Factor Method

A less accurate method of determining the markup on menu items is to multiply the food costs by a set number or factor such as three (3). With this markup, there is a 67% margin on the food cost that may or may not represent the real costs.

Again, work with the finance department to establish a costing method and profit percentage. Document every catering, no matter how small, i.e., cookies and coffee for three in the assistant administrator's office, as a cost to the dining services department. Whether or not labor is included in the catering charges depends upon the facility guidelines. For internal purposes, if nothing else, document the labor cost for each catering service provided. (At some time in the future, departmental labor costs may be questioned and the dollars spent on non-patient/resident/student/detainee services suddenly has great importance.)

Extreme care must be taken when providing catering services in the community or as a cash revenue generating activity. Most healthcare facilities, and many educational organizations, are classified as not-for-profit or non-profit for tax purposes. Providing catering services in the community can be viewed as putting that tax status at risk. Rely on the Chief Financial Officer to help navigate the legal and tax implications of providing catering services in the community.

Putting It Into Practice

1. You are establishing the selling price for a catered event. Your Chief Financial Officer (CFO) suggested you use 21% as the profit percentage on top of your costs. Your total costs are $427.00. You are expecting 40 people for this event. What will be the selling price per person?

Figure 25.7 Sample Catering Requisition

Today's Date: _____

Date of Function: _____

Location: _____

Contact Name: _____

Department Charge Code Number:

_____

Number of Guests: _____

Time of Function: _____

Delivery Time: _____

Pick Up Time: _____

Contact Phone Number: _____

Contact Email: _____

Payment by Cash, Check or Credit:

_____

MENU	QUANTITY	PRICE		TOTAL	
Sandwich Buffet	50	$	8.00	$	400.00
				$	—
				$	—
Linen and China Up Charge	1	$	20.00	$	20.00
	Total Requisition	$	**28.00**	$	**420.00**

_____   Date: _____

Requester's Signature

_____   Date: _____

Director/Administrator's Signature

Notice: Without Budget Number, Payment Due Upon Delivery

THIS SECTION FOR FOODSERVICE USE ONLY

○ Department Charged   ○ Bill Submitted

○ Payment Received   ○ Payment Attached

Time Delivered: _____

Who Delivered: _____

Dining Service Contact Information:

Name: _____

Email: _____

Phone: _____

Figure 25.8 ABC HealthCenter Sample Catering Menu

Breakfast Bundles		Price Per Person
1	**Continental Breakfast:** Includes pasteries, muffins, bagels, butter, cream cheese and jellies, juice, water, and coffee	$ 4.00
2	**Full Breakfast:** Includes scrambled eggs, bacon or sausage, pastries, muffins, butter, cream cheese and jellies, juice, water and coffee	$ 9.50
3	**Simplified Breakfast:** Includes coffee, water, and assorted muffins with butter	$ 2.50

Lunch and Dinner Bundles		Price Per Person
1	**Sandwich Buffet:** Includes assorted breads, meats, cheeses, and toppings, choice of potato or pasta salad, chips, cookie or dessert bar, coffee water, soda, or lemonade	$ 12.00
2	**Salad Buffet:** Includes mixed greens, standard salad toppings/dressings and grilled chicken, cookie or dessert bar, coffee, water, soda, or lemonade	$ 12.50
3	**Pasta Bar:** Includes two types of pasta with red and white sauce, grilled chicken and parmesan cheese, mixed green salad, bread, cookie or dessert bar, coffee, water, soda, or lemonade	$ 14.00
4	**Taco Bar:** Includes grilled chicken and ground beef, soft and hard shells, taco toppings, cookie or dessert bar, coffee, water, soda, or lemonade	$ 10.50
5	**Soup and Sandwich:** Includes soup, assorted sandwich, chips, potato, coleslaw or pasta salad, cookie or dessert bar, coffee, water, soda, or lemonade	$ 9.50

Upscale Dinner (Menu customization available—prices may change accordingly		Price Per Person
1	**Steak Dinner:** Includes steak, potato, vegetable, salad and dessert, coffee, water, soda, or lemonade	$ 18.00
2	**Chicken Dinner:** Includes chicken kiev, rice pilaf, vegetable, salad, dessert, coffee, water, soda, or lemonade	$ 15.00
	Seafood Dinner: Includes seafood determined by client, starch, vegetable, salad, dessert, coffee, water, soda, or lemonade	Market Price

Al a Carte	Quantity	Price
Coffee	Gallon	$ 16.00
Assorted Soda/ Bottled Water	Gallon	$ 15.00
Lemonade	12 oz. Container	$ 1.50
Assorted Pasteries	Per Each	$ 1.00
Cinnamon or Caramel Rolls	Per Each	$ 1.50
Cookies	Per Dozen	$ 8.00
Dessert Bar	Per Dozen	$ 10.00
Cheese and Fruit Tray	Per Person	$ 2.00
Fruit Platter (in season fruit)	Per Person	$ 1.50
Raw Vegetables and Dip	Per Person	$ 1.50
Chips and Salsa	Per Person	$ 1.50
Chips and Dip	Per Person	$ 1.50

NOTE: All catering will be served on disposable dishes unless linen/china requested at a $20.00 upcharge fee.

Source: dk Foodservice Solutions, LLC

Planning a Catered Event

First, confirm that the date, time and location are available. Consider the size and style of service being requested. Select the menu. Most dining services departments develop a set of catering menus to suit various occasions. For example:

- Breakfast
    - > A simple coffee and breakfast pastry bar
    - > A continental self-serve breakfast
    - > A full service buffet breakfast
- Luncheons
    - > A casual soup and sandwich
    - > A more elegant luncheon
- Dinner
    - > A quick pizza and salad buffet
    - > A formal annual Board of Directors white linen dinner

The Certified Dietary Manager or catering coordinator should meet with the client to review menu choices and select a specific menu or design a custom meal for the event.

The advantage of working with pre-defined catering menus is that the planning process is significantly streamlined. Using catering menus (with minor adjustments and customization) will minimize managerial time in working out pricing, recipes, purchasing needs, production plans, and service needs. A specialty menu for high-end events takes considerably more resources, as each step has to be planned and tested down to the point of placing special orders for food items not normally purchased.

All catering events should be documented either as an in-house catering request or as a formal business contract for external clients. A written document is important for confirming the order and related details. Later, it is also used for invoicing or accounting.

- Confirm date, time, and location of the event.
- Determine the number of people to be served.
- Define service expectations. Is this for a fine dining event or a casual snack? Is this for a buffet or tabled-waited service?
- Plan the work schedule, responsibilities, supervision, and staffing to include adequate time before, after, and during the event to cover setup, preparation, service, and clean-up.
- Plan and request the physical support required, such as room setup.
- Plan the ambiance, food presentation, and table setting (if applicable).
- As relevant, plan and order flowers, linens, uniforms, special equipment rental, and any other needs.
- Forecast food and any special beverage needs; place orders.
- If alcohol is to be served, check on the local ordinances regarding age of the servers, licensing, and insurance requirements.
- Train employees, as needed, to carry out setup and service expectations.

These steps need to be taken in some form for all catering, even if it is just delivering coffee to a meeting.

> **Putting It Into Practice**
>
> 2. You have a new baker who is receiving many compliments. You decide to develop a brand for your bakery products that represent the home-made and healthy characteristics of her products. How would you market these products?

Supervising Cash Activities and Reports

The operation needs to have specific operating procedures for the cash register or POS (point of sale system). At the beginning of the work shift, the cashier should count the cash bank assigned to the register and verify the cash amount. During all cash counting operations, two people should be present: a cashier and a supervisor or Certified Dietary Manager. These two verify each other's work.

At the end of the shift, the cashier should complete applicable cashier records. A cashier and supervisor or manager count the cash, record the sum, and sign or initial the cash record. During the cafeteria operation, there may be times when the cashier must void a transaction or make other corrections. A manager or supervisor should authorize this. Standard operating procedures should be developed for handling issues such as these.

While cash-handling procedures vary by operation, some basic procedures generally apply:

- Keep the cash drawer closed when not in use.
- Give each new cashier his or her own bank (the base amount of change in the "till" used to open the cash register).
  - > The size of the bank should reflect the level of business that typically goes through the register during the cashier's shift.
  - > Cashiers should count and sign the cashier's log for receipt of the bank at the beginning of their shift.
- At the end of a shift, check out the cashier:
  - > Count the cash in the drawer.
  - > Set aside the defined bank amount.
    - The bank is the bank – do not short it to make the deposit whole.
    - The cashier should NOT know what the cash register records as the correct amount for the deposit.
  - > All remaining cash is the deposit.
  - > Document the checkout for cash, credit cards and department charges.
  - > Both the supervisor and cashier sign the cashier's log at the end of the shift. (See the *Supplemental Textbook Materials—Foodservice* for a sample cashier's log.)
- If credit cards or debits cards are accepted, ensure that the policies regarding data security are in place.
- Reconcile the cash deposits, credit card receipts and department charges to the cash register Z reading.
  - > Record any amount over or under on the cashier's log.
- Have policies and procedures in place for addressing discrepancies between cash in the drawer and actual sales
  - > Address the steps if the amount is significant.
  - > Address the steps if the cashier consistently makes errors in cash handling.
- Train each cashier on use of the system, and keep a reference or manual available.
- In a POS system, be sure that register buttons that are keyed to specific items match the menu, and that cashiers know on which key to enter each item.
- Be sure that pricing is up-to-date in the system.

Putting It Into Practice

3. The cash drawer has been short $5.00 the past three days. What steps would you take to address this?

Monthly Operating Statement and Variance Report

Overview and Objectives

Achieving department goals while staying within budget depends on setting realistic goals and understanding how funds are allocated. It also requires the flexibility to make adjustments in operations in response to changing budget performance. The department manager has the ongoing responsibility to review cost-saving principles, recommend efficient purchasing practices and analyze program changes based on actual cost versus budget. After completing this chapter, you should be able to:

✓ Review actual costs with budget estimate to identify problem areas

✓ Analyze the factors impacting financial performance

✓ Develop a variance report addressing actual costs versus budget

Financial Tools

Throughout the Business Operations unit, we have discussed how to prepare purchasing specifications, manage revenue generating services, and monitor the cost of food and labor. The information presented earlier in the textbook identified the financial control process by setting standards and measuring performance. Now it is time to complete the cycle by comparing performance with standards and taking corrective action. Let's examine some of the financial reporting tools available. See Figure 26.1 for an overview of common financial documents.

Figure 26.1 Comparisons of Financial Documents

BUDGET	BALANCE SHEET	OPERATING STATEMENT
A financial planning document that predicts where you want to be in the next year.	A snapshot showing assets, liabilities, and net assets on a given day in time—usually the last day of the financial period.	Shows your department's monthly financial performance compared to what was budgeted.

Balance Sheet

The balance sheet for a not-for-profit organization is a statement of the facility's assets, liabilities, and net assets (what is left after all bills are paid). A balance sheet showing for-profit financial activities would include investor or stockholder information. This financial statement presents a snapshot in time (on the day it was generated, usually the last day of the accounting period). Different facilities have different account periods; the most common are monthly, quarterly, semi-annually, and annually.

Operating Statement

Once a budget has been approved, tracking performance becomes a monthly activity. Use the budget as a tool to manage revenues and expenses in the department.

A number of reports help keep the pulse on finances. Where these reports come from varies by facility. The most common model uses a centralized accounting system, which is almost always managed on a computer. In a centralized process, the accounting functions are handled by one finance department office for the entire organization. What this means for a dining services department is that:

- Payroll, invoices for food, services, repairs, capital, and other items are paid by Accounting and tracked in specified department budget categories on a master ledger.

- As the payroll is processed each pay period, paycheck totals for the dining services department are entered into department budget categories for labor expenses. (Some employee benefits may also be entered in the department budget, or they may be handled through a separate budget for human resources. This varies by organization.)

- Any cash operations, such as dining rooms, cafeterias, Meals On Wheels®, day care meals, guest trays or vending, should deposit cash in the cashiers/accounting office. Accounting personnel transfer the deposit to a bank account, and credit the funds to a revenue category in the dining services department budget.

An advantage of this model is that financial managers responsible for the entire facility can keep track of the bottom line.

In this common model, the accounting office typically runs an operating statement for each department or cost center. Often, this is done shortly after the end of each month. So, on January 5, the department manager may receive an **operating statement** that is current through December. The operating statement is a report that shows financial performance (revenues and expenses), as compared with the budget. This statement may also be called a budget report, monthly responsibility statement, profit & loss statement.

From one facility to the next, specific formats for financial reports vary. The statement, or report, typically shows figures for a given period of time, along with a report for year to date. (Year-to-date means a cumulative total of revenues and expenses in each budget category for the portion of the fiscal year that has been completed so far.) Let's consider what this report may look like. Figure 26.2 provides an example.

In this example, several labels appear at the tops of columns. Here is a closer look at what they are and what they mean.

Figure 26.2 Sample Operating Statement (Monthly Budget Report)

RUN DATE: 04 I 02 I 17
RUN TIME: 12:59 PM
Dept Code:51 0

510 Food Operations

A MEDICAL CENTER
OPERATING STATEMENT
ACTUAL TO BUDGET COMPARISON
PERIOD ENDING:MARCH 31,2017

Data for the Month				Year to Date			
ACTUAL	BUDGET	VAR	DESCRIPTION	YTD ACTUAL	YTD BUDGET	VAR	BUDGET REMAINING
37	-	37	OUTPATIENT	150	-	150	-
37	-	37	TOTAL PATIENT REVENUE	150	-	150	-
31,407	31,962	(555)	CAFETERIA REVENUE	103,644	102,129	1,515	381,455
31,444	31,962	(518)	TOTAL OPERATING REVENUE	103,793	102,129	1,664	381,455
			OPERATING EXPENSE				
39,800	37,119	(2,681)	SALARIES	127,359	126,425	(935)	551,711
325	-	(325)	STAFF SERVICES	974	-	(974)	-
8,756	8,166	(590)	EMPLOYEE BENEFITS	28,019	27,266	(753)	121,376
48,881	45,285	3,596	LABOR	156,353	153,691	2,662	673,088
15,190	6,806	8,384	SUPPLIES-MEAT, FISH, POULTRY	47,091	20,750	26,341	74,700
15,394	25,091	(9,697)	SUPPLIES-OTHER FOOD	63,657	74,700	(11,043)	371,840
2,335	2,774	(439)	SUPPLIES-SUPPLEMENTS	7,471	7,968	(497)	33,200
(4,499)	(4,339)	(159)	SUPPLIES-FOOD TRANSFERS	(14,396)	(12,948)	(1,448)	(51,460)
(37)	35	(72)	SUPPLIES-OTHER MEDICAL	(117)	100	(217)	534
437	348	89	SUPPLIES-CLEANING PRODUCTS	1,398	1,029	368	3,637
363	429	(65)	SUPPLIES-MINOR NON-MEDICAL EQ	1,017	1,245	(228)	6,737
83	131	(48)	SUPPLIES-OFFICE & ADMIN	283	398	(116)	1,853
1,358	1,371	(13)	SUPPLIES-OTHER NON-MEDICAL	3,396	4,150	(754)	21,719
1,358	1,371	(13)	SUPPLIES-UNIFORMS	232	83	149	396
30,864	32,717	(1,853)	**SUPPLIES**	110,539	97,571	12,968	463,618
3,497	2,771	726	PURCHASED SERVICES	9,636	7,968	1,668	33,062
266	317	(51)	REPAIRS & MAINTENANCE	851	955	(104)	3,864
26	124	(97)	OTHER	87	365	(278)	1,479
1,379	1,831	(452)	DEPRECIATION/AMORTIZATION	4,412	4,980	(568)	22,581
18	17	1	RENTAL/LEASE	47	47	(1)	208
84,931	83,062	1,868	TOTAL OPERATING EXPENSE	281,923	265,577	16,347	1,164,837
(53,487)	**(51,100)**	**(2,387)**	**NET REVENUE OVER EXPENSES**	**(178,130)**	**(163,448)**	**(14,682)**	**(783,382)**
			STATISTICS				
2,517	2,807	290	TOTAL HOURS	7,298	8,128	(830)	33,003
2,061	2,188	(127)	PATIENT DAYS	6,596	6,784	(188)	25,783
8,621	9,257	(636)	MEALS	26,431	26,956	(525)	109,196

Data for the Month

This often has a title of current period and usually occupies the three columns on the left side of the table. This section totals expenses and revenues for the time period that was just completed, such as the month that just ended. On this sample report, the current period is identified in the report header as PERIOD ENDING MARCH 31, 2017. Under the current period heading are three columns: ACTUAL, BUDGET, and VAR for Variance.

- **Actual**: Identifies what revenues were actually received in each of these budget categories, and what expenses were actually paid out during the current period of March.

  Note: the term Actual is a little misleading as it refers to the amount Accounts Payable paid out during the month which does not exactly match the amount spent. Consider that the invoices for the 30th of the month are usually paid in the next month. Some finance departments estimate (accrue) the amount carried over from month to month.

- **Budget**: Shows what the monthly budget was for these accounting sub- categories for the reporting period. This budget was established in advance for this fiscal year. In this example, a one-month budget for any category is the annual budget divided by 12, in other settings the budget number may be based on the number of days in the month (Total divided by 365 days in the year times 31 days in the month of March).

- **Variance**: Shows how the actual figures compare with the budget as planned. A variance of zero means that the budget is precisely on target; there is no variance. For example, in the Revenue section for the current period in Figure 26.2, the total revenue is under budget by $518. This shows that the department received $518 less in revenue than anticipated for the month. Parentheses ( ) are used to show places where the actual values represent an operating loss for this budget category. Where was the revenue under budget? The detail shows that the cafeteria revenue was under performing for the month.

- Now, look at the Expenses section. Notice that the wages paid to employees during March exceeded the budget. Thus, the report shows a variance of $3,596.

- In the section related to Supplies, some sub-accounts are under budget and some are over budget. Overall, the cost of Supplies was under budget by ($1,853).

- Finally, looking at NET REVENUE OVER EXPENSES shows that the bottom line totals for the month were over budget by $2,387. Between less than budgeted revenue and higher than planned labor costs, the savings in supplies was not able to make up for the losses.

Year to Date

In the right-hand section of this report, we see a major heading called year to date. Beyond March, this section of the report is identifying how the revenue and expense categories of the budget total from the beginning of the fiscal year until now. It is showing cumulative figures. Under the year to date heading are three more columns, ACTUAL, BUDGET, and VAR. These are identical with the three labels explained above, except that they cover a different time period, giving a cumulative report on financial performance for the year to date. Many organizations also include a column for BUDGET REMAINING that helps the department manager know how much money is planned for the remaining months.

The example in Figure 26.2 shows that so far, the revenue has been $103,793, and this is $1,664 more than expected in the budget planning. This report also shows that even though the operation was over budget for expenses for March, in the cumulative year to date, the operation is over budget for expenses by an even larger amount: $14,682. In

Putting It Into Practice

1. How would you explain the difference between a budget and an operating statement? Which one would you use if you were told to reduce your labor costs?

reality, the $2,387 is below the average of the first two months of the year and demonstrates that efforts on the part of the manager are bringing costs into better budget compliance.

Net Revenue Over Expense

The bottom line at the end of the report, shows how revenues and expenses balance out. For example, the month shows a net loss of $2,387. With continued effort and financial control, the manager may be able to be at or below budget by the end of the fiscal year.

Statistics

Many facilities include a section at the end of the report that reflects the statistics that are tracked for the department. These statistics may also be referred to as Units of Measure (UOM) and are used as an indicator of the level of activity and productivity of the department.

Preparing and Using an Operating Systems Statement

Responsibility statements (monthly financial report, or operating statement, or profit & loss) are prepared by the finance department. As noted above, typically the supplies cost figures reflect the amount paid during the month by Accounts Payable and may not be consistent with what was purchased during that month. Bill payments are often 15-45 days out from the time the product is delivered and invoiced.

The Variance Report

The third column of data on most monthly operating reports is the VARIANCE. Simply stated, the Variance is the difference between Actual Expenses/Revenues and the Budget. If you have to write a monthly variance report, then this is the column of data that is of concern. This is where over or under is identified for the month or year to date.

The Finance Department may provide a guideline of what areas need to be addressed. Often, they are not concerned that small amounts over or under be explained, so they may specify that items with a variance more than $500 or 5% need to be explained. If you are tracking the numbers every month in a spend-down system or by steno pad (see Chapter 24) then you will know when you are over budget, and why, before the finance department sends out the monthly operating report.

The variance report is the opportunity to educate the senior leadership team on what the drivers are for the dining services department. They usually remember that December's food expense is going up with special meals and catering. But how many remember that May is Mother's Day and Hospital Week and Nurses Day and a legal holiday? How many understand that poultry is the number one group of products in healthcare and the 10% increase in chicken prices just destroyed the food budget, or that the freeze in California is related to the quality of salads in the dining room?

The variance report is also something to share with department staff. By including staff in the financial information, they become invested in the corrective actions that need to be taken and share the positive impacts of changes made.

How to write a variance report? Often, the finance department has a defined form they want all managers to submit. If a form is not available, consider designing one a that works as a running log that serves as a reference during the next budgeting cycle. Here are some basic steps:

Review

First, review the performance in each category and keep notes.

- Is it over or under budget? Do you know why (like the changing price of chicken)?
- Was there a new service started during the month?
- Was a unit closed for renovation?
- Was there a major holiday with increased catering?
- Was there a large dishware delivery during the month?

Compare

- Has the performance improved since the prior month or over the course of the last six months?
- Do the numbers match the expectations?
- Is the variance related to seasonal fluctuations?
- Or, are the numbers a surprise?

Ask Why

- Is there a clear reason for the variance?
- Do you know what is driving the costs?
- Sometimes unexpected jumps in business, such as increased catering or snack shop sales, can also generate increased expenses (to purchase more food and pay for more employee hours in order to honor increased service demands). This is not a bad thing. It can be a sign of business growth.
- The important figure to monitor in this situation is the net gain or loss.

Recommend Cost Saving Practices

- Is labor expense too high?
- Are overtime hours excessive?
    - > Look carefully at the schedules and find a way to cut back.
- Is the cafeteria showing a drop in revenue?
    - > Check the sales records, identify specific items on the menu for change.
    - > Update the menu mix, pricing, or other areas.

If you are over budget for expenses—or under budget for revenues—this can contribute to a cash flow issue for the facility. Either of these situations is potentially troublesome and represents an opportunity to analyze and change as quickly as possible. The primary responsibility in managing a budget is to help meet the financial objectives of the facility and maintain financial viability.

Putting It Into Practice

2. Your department operating statement shows the actual food costs are higher than what was budgeted. What steps would you take to address this variance?

Food Cost Report

Another report of value is a food cost report. Keep in mind that food costs represent a large portion of the budget. If a single distributor is the primary source of food and supply purchases, work with them to obtain a monthly Descending Dollar Report. When a computer order/entry system is available, this report may be accessible by the manager through the same software used for purchasing.

The descending dollar report lists all items purchased within the specified period of time in order of how much money was spent on each product. Review and verify the figures, compare them with expectations, and ask questions about significant trends. Comparing month to month can identify a sudden shift in pricing. Maybe a particular item is no longer covered by the purchasing agreement and the price per case jumped $3.89.

If the report is in a spreadsheet format (like Excel), the information can be sorted to look at the expenditures for meat, or dairy or frozen. The answers to the questions are not in these reports but they can expose pricing or cost changes that prompt the manager to dig deeper.

Review of the items should show a consistent pattern month to month and the absence of products the manager has decided to take off the menu. If ready-to-serve barbecue ribs are on the menu only one time but the cost is always in the top 25 of items purchased, maybe it is the price or maybe it is an easy theft item. It may be time for a menu change. Alternately, a foodservice menu computer system can provide cost control reports relative to the menu as planned.

Cost-Saving Purchasing Practices

In addition to reviewing food cost reports, the manager should be staying current with market trends. If there has been a freeze in Florida and orange juice is a daily menu item, review the product specifications to ensure that Florida is not specified as the only source for orange juice. Often, the vendors provide Weekly Product Updates that cover produce, fresh meats, seafood and the status of staples such as the upcoming peach pack for the next year. There are websites that can track market trends such as http://www.foodservice.com/marketprices. Figure 26.3 shows a sample of the information available from this website. When food costs are increasing, start monitoring the market trends for the most expensive items such as meat and produce, work with the vendors, and adjust the menu, the purchases and the individual products to get the best prices.

Figure 26.3 Weekly Produce Market Report

The weekly *Produce Market Report* is an online document providing information on all segments of food. The example below shows a list of produce. The report starts with a commentary, such as the paragraph below, followed by a substantial listing of foods, source of the food, how it is packed and the cost.

"Bell Peppers (Western): Sources from Baja California are very light and upcoming transitions in California aren't expected for another month, pressing markets higher as extreme demand exceeds supplies. From all indications, supplies will continue very short until the late summer/ fall crops start in southern California...."

FOOD	SOURCE	HOW PACKED		COST
Broccoli	California	Bunches 14s	Cartons	$19.50
Carrots	California	Medium-Large	Sacks 10-5 lb. bags	$22.00
Celery, Organic	California	30s	Cartons	$45.00
Kale Greens	California	24s	Cartons Bunches	$15.50
Onions—Dry, Yellow	Colorado	Medium-Large	50 lb. Sack	$15.00
Peppers—Bell Type, Green	North Carolina	Large	1/9 Bushel Cartons	$17.00

Source: www.foodservice.com/marketprices/ August, 29, 2015

Sales Report

Another report that can be extremely useful to a Certified Dietary Manager is a sales report for cash operations such as a cafeteria, a restaurant, a C-store (convenience store), or others. A sales report provides a pulse on daily revenues. In addition, it can provide a basis for comparison of food sold with food prepared.

A common way to receive a sales report is through the reporting feature of a point of sale (POS) system. This is a computer-based cash register system. It records transactions and maintains very detailed records of sales. Information may be reported by location, date, meal period, menu item, and much more. Most POS systems provide a broad range of reporting options. It is worthwhile to become familiar with the POS system in the facility, examine options, and specify the reports needed for review.

The Certified Dietary Manager has an important role in the control of sales generated from cash operations. For effective control, the manager needs to know what the amount of sales should be and needs to know what sales actually were. Any discrepancies need to be investigated and corrective action promptly taken..

Let's take a look at each of these control points.

1. **Know what the amount of sales should be**: In a cafeteria or dining room situation, there can be errors in portioning, errors in ringing up food, and other situations that lead to poor control. Regardless of whether mistakes are intentional or accidental, the impact on the dining services operation will be the same: sales revenues that should be collected will not be collected. To control cash in a dining services operation, a Certified Dietary Manager has to examine some basic information, and reconcile accordingly. Using a food usage record, as shown in Figure 26.4, is one way to do this.

Figure 26.4 Food Usage Record—Cafeteria

Date: _____ Serving Period: _____

Item	Quantity Issued				Amount Left	Total Used	Sales Income Per Pan	Total Income
	#1	#2	#3	Total				
Mashed Potatoes	.50 pan	.50 pan	.50 pan	1.50 pan	.25 pan	1.25 pan	$18.00	$22.50

Projected Income: _____ Actual Income: _____

This form provides a control mechanism because it shows what food has been issued to the serving area, what is left over, and what has actually been used. In this example, mashed potatoes is a menu item featured on the cafeteria line. As the line opened, one half-pan of potatoes was issued to the line. During the meal period, two additional half pans were sent to the line. A total of three half pans were issued. At the end of the meal period, only half of the half-pan remained. Therefore, two and a half of the half-pans have been used.

If each pan contained 30 servings, then the total number of servings that should have been sold is:

- 2.5 pans x 30 servings per pan = 75 servings

If each serving should have sold for $0.60, then total revenue that should have been collected for mashed potatoes is:

- 75 servings x $0.60 per serving = $45.00

So now, both an item count and a dollar figure have been calculated for the amount of mashed potatoes sent to the cafeteria for service.

2. **Know what actual sales were**: At the end of the serving period, the POS report lists what the real item count and dollar figures were for mashed potatoes for the same time period.

3. Compare expected with actual: For example:

Sales for Mashed Potatoes	Projected	Actual
# of Servings	75	68
Total Revenue @ $0.60	$45.00	$40.80
To Calculate the Over or Short of Actual Sales:		
Percentage $45.00 - $40.80 = $4.42 divided by $45.00 = 0.98 or 10%		

There is a 10% discrepancy. What might cause this?

- Perhaps the cook did not produce or obtain the intended yield from a recipe, and/or did not properly fill the pans before service.
- Perhaps the servers over-portioned the potatoes, giving a little too much to each person.
- Perhaps several servings were dropped and discarded.
- Perhaps, at checkout, a cashier neglected to notice potatoes on several plates and did not ring them up.

These are just a few examples of how discrepancies can occur in sales. To manage costs in the operation, investigate causes of discrepancies such as these and implement finer controls. To exert the greatest impact, focus on menu items with the highest costs, prices, and volume.

Realistically, these figures will not be perfect matches all the time. However, a Certified Dietary Manager needs to manage the service by:

- Establishing a standard for the variance that will be permitted (e.g., 2-3%)
- Making the routine comparisons.
- Investigating discrepancies.
- Making corrections as warranted.

Census Variations

Monitoring the census or client count is part of the key to sound financial management. Many of the operating costs are based on projected census or client figures. Revenues are often tied to the expected activity represented by census counts. As the census or client count changes, adjust the expenditures accordingly in order to keep the budget on track.

Consider this example:

- You work in a facility where the census may vary and has dropped from 200 to 160 (that is a 20% drop).
- The budget for both food and labor is based on a census of 200.
- Understand that with a lower census, the facility will be experiencing a decrease in revenues, because it will receive less reimbursement for services.
- Because the census dropped, so did the traffic in the cafeteria, therefore, cash revenues have decreased as well.
- To maintain a balanced bottom line, the cost factors related to food and labor need to be adjusted downward, either through budget control, cuts in services or system reductions, such as lay-offs.

In many dining services arenas, reimbursement is limited and even unpredictable. Expenses are managed with tight control. It is not uncommon for a facility that depends upon a census to experience budget cuts, even during a fiscal year whose budget has already been approved. For example, there may a push to reduced labor by eliminating overtime, leaving an open position unfilled, or cutting back hours for employees. A reduction-in-force (RIF) may be the final step.

A Certified Dietary Manager can keep control of the budget, and support the facility's financial goals at the same time, by working proactively to respond to changes in census. Figure 26.5 outlines a process for doing this.

Figure 26.5 Proactive Labor Adjustment

STEP	PROCEDURE	EXAMPLE
1	Determine the usual number of labor hours required in one work day. This is a total of all hours worked by all employees in one day.	You operate with 50 hours.
2	Determine your usual census.	Your census is 200.
3	Calculate a ratio of daily labor hours to census.	Your ratio is: 50 ÷ 200 = 0.25
4	Monitor census. When it changes significantly, determine an adjusted number of labor hours that will keep the ratio stable.	Your census has dropped to 150. To maintain a ratio of 0.25, multiply your new census by the ratio you established in Step 3: 0.25 x 150 = 37.5 hours.
5	Adjust labor	Now, adjust your daily schedules to use about 37.5 hours of labor per day, instead of your usual 50.

Putting It Into Practice

3. Your census has dropped significantly over the past month increasing the labor costs. The administrator has just informed each department that they have to cut one FTE. What steps would you take?

According to Kathleen Deckard, a Certified Dietary Manager, who has consulted across the U.S., this approach can prevent a situation where you are asked to eliminate positions.

Deckard also offers the following tips:

- Spread out the adjustments whenever possible, so that each employee works a little less. For example, let a breakfast cook leave early.

- Do not send night shift employees home early. Instead, bring them in a little later than usual.

- Take advantage of shift overlaps, when morning employees are near the end of their work days, and evening employees are just starting.

- Look for small parts of jobs that an employee can pick up, such as labeling nourishments.

- Explain to employees what you are doing and why. Ask for help. Let the staff be part of the solutions.

- Post a copy of the census and the calculations where employees can see them; let employees monitor figures as well.

Aside from labor, realize that with census changes, adjust the food production quantities. In particular, if census declines, scale the production forecast downwards to avoid food waste.

Cost Containment Techniques

The above approach is a very proactive method for controlling operational costs. In addition, a number of specific cost containment techniques can help to minimize costs. Here are some examples that were discussed earlier in greater detail within their respective chapters:

Menu

- Adjust menus seasonally to take advantage of food prices that fluctuate by time of year. For example, strawberries may be inexpensive in June, but very expensive in February.

- Cost each menu. Know the specifics and the averages.

- If serving multiple diets, consolidate menu offerings when appropriate to reduce the number of different items for production. Be careful of using one-pot recipe cooking as it becomes so restrictive, it compromises taste and quality for the liberal diets.

- Examine ways to consolidate items produced at any one meal for multiple service areas. For example, consider whether a soup produced for the dining room meal service may also be used for client service or a catered event at the same time.

- Perform a cost comparison of condiments that arrive pre-packaged in individual service units with condiments that are pre-portioned by employees. Also consider the portion size of each condiment that is pre-packaged in individual service units.

- Carefully evaluate make-versus-buy decisions, and determine the cost effectiveness of using convenience foods.

Labor

- Match scheduled labor to staffing needs.

- Design daily assignment tasks to maximize workflow and reduce back-tracking.

- Evaluate the labor cost of scratch made menu items to convenience product items.

- Flex the daily staffing level to reflect the census or client count.

Putting It Into Practice

4. How would you minimize costs if you are noticing an increase in food waste?

Food Purchasing

- Access a Group Purchasing Organization or obtain and use competitive bids for products.
- Examine opportunities for product rebates; track and obtain rebates.
- Ask a Registered Dietitian to help evaluate the use of nutritional supplements and tube feeding products. Determine whether supplementation is provided in the most cost effective manner.
- Research grade and quality for products carefully. Avoid specifying premium quality when it is not necessary for a particular recipe.

Receiving and Storage

- Verify that receiving procedures are being enforced so that deliveries match purchase orders.
- Check invoices to be sure they are correct.
- Monitor use of FIFO inventory rotation.
- Establish procedures for identifying inventory shrinkage.
- Practice security measures to protect inventory from theft.
- Ensure that perishable foods are put away quickly.
- Monitor storage conditions, such as temperature, to maximize product shelf life.
- Monitor food that is wasted due to spoilage, and intervene to prevent waste.
- Evaluate purchasing schedules for perishable foods such as fresh fruit. If needed, adjust the schedule or the quantities purchased.
- Evaluate the purchase unit of any product not fully used before part of it spoils.

Food Production and Service

- Cost each recipe.
- Take the time to calculate the labor element for each recipe to obtain a more refined analysis of cost.
- Monitor compliance with portion control guidelines:
- Examine ingredients in recipes. Ask whether a similar ingredient could also work. Compare costs. (Example: Which is less expensive for the recipe: ketchup or tomato paste?)
- Forecast production quantities:
  - > Monitor leftovers and make adjustments.
  - > Use leftovers for other points of service when possible to avoid food waste.
- Scale standardized recipes to required needs on an ongoing basis.
- Monitor compliance with standardized recipes.
- Analyze time-intensive tasks in production and seek alternative methodologies.
- Evaluate the value and options for providing move self-service items to reduce labor requirements.
- Examine service and delivery systems for efficiency and streamline, if possible.
- Analyze ordering processes or individual menu systems for efficiency and streamline, if possible.

Non-Food Supplies

- Check to be sure all chemical products are being used in proper amounts and concentrations.
- Investigate use of alternative products; compare costs per usage unit.
- Cost the use of disposable products against the cost of reusable products.
- Ensure that disposable containers are not oversized for their intended uses.
- Check storage and display of disposable products.
- Train staff about when to use (or not use) disposable products.
- Examine dispensers for paper goods to make sure they easily distribute a single-use item without waste.

Using these cost containment techniques, a Certified Dietary Manager can positively contribute to the financial success of the facility.

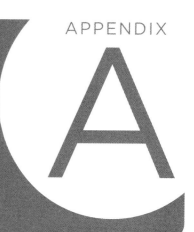
Chapter References and Resources

CHAPTER 1

Aladdin Temp-Rite®	aladdintemprite.com
Carter Hoffmann®	carter-hoffmann.com
The Joint Commission (TJC)	jointcommission.org
World Health Organization (WHO)	who.int
Centers for Medicare & Medicaid Services (CMS)	cms.gov
Culture Change in Dining and Regulatory Compliance	Handy, Linda, *Dietary Manager Magazine*, June, 2010, pgs. 14-19
Schoeneman, Karen. *The Pioneer Network Culture Change*, project of alternative words for bibs, elderly	pioneernetwork.net/culturechange/language

CHAPTER 2

Dietary Guidelines for Americans 2015	health.gov/dietaryguidelines/2015/default.asp
MyPlate	choosemyplate.gov
USDA DRI (Daily Reference Intakes)	fnic.nal.usda.gov
Recommended Dietary Allowances (RDAs)	fnic.nal.usda.gov/dietary-guidance/dietary-reference-intakes
U.S. Department of Agriculture (USDA)	cnpp.usda.gov/sites/default/files/nutrition_insights_uploads/Insight32.pdf usda.gov/factbook/chapter2.pdf
Nutrition Standards School Meals	fnsusda/gov/school-meals/nutrition-standards-school-meals
Food for Fifty	Molt, Mary, Pearson Education, Inc.
Centers for Medicare & Medicaid Services (CMS)	cms.gov
Ohio Codes	codes.ohio.gov/oac/3701-17-60

CHAPTER 3

Alaska Seafood Marketing Institute	alaskaseafood.org
The Foodservice Tune Up	Toczek, Wayne & Bauman, Tim

Continued...

CHAPTER 3 (continued)

Food Values of Portions Commonly Used Portions	Bowes and Church
USDA National Nutrient Database	nal.usda.gov/fnic/pubs/foodcomp.pdf
NutritionistPro®	
Nutri-Base®	
TheFood Processor®	
Food for Fifty	Molt, Mary, Pearson Education, Inc.
Academy of Nutrition and Dietetics	eatright.org
USDA *Standard Portion Sizes*	cnpp.usda.gov/sites/default/files/nutrition_insights_uploads/Insight22.pdf
Food Resources For Consumers	www.fda.gov/Food/ResourcesForYou/Consumers/ucm079311.htm
FDA	FDA.gov
WebMD	www.WebMD.com
Food Allergy	Foodallergy.org
A Brief History of Health Care Quality Assessment	http://www.ncbi.nlm.nih.gov/pmc/articles/PMC1022402/pdf/westjmed00067-0065.pdf

CHAPTER 4

American Egg Board	aeb.org/food-manufacturers/eggs-product-overview/functional-properties
Goat World	goatworld.com/articles/goatmanagement.shtml
I Love Cheese	ilovecheese.com/cheeses.asp?Search=A-C
Food for Fifty	Molt, Mary, Pearson Education, Inc.
Team Nutrition	teamnutrition.usda.gov/HealthierUS/wholegrainresource.pdf
National Association of Meat Purveyors (NAMP) *Meat Buyer's Guide*	namp.com/namp/default.asp
FDA Food Code	fda.gov
F&N Training Paks® 1998	The Grossbauer Group
Nutrition411.com *Leftover Food Usage Policy*	nutrition411.com/content/left-over-usage
The Diamond Approach to Quality Improvement in Food Service	Eck Mills, Linda S., *Dietary Manager,* May 2010, pg 25-27
Service Disney Style	Disney Institute, disneyinstitute.com

CHAPTER 5

Nutrition411.com *Performance Improvement Worksheet*	nutrition411.com/content/performance-improvement-worksheet
Becky Dorner	beckydorner.com
FDA Food Code	fda.gov

CHAPTER 5 (continued)

Commercial Building Energy Cost Per Square Foot & Restaurant Energy Use	sustainablefoodservice.com/cat/energy-efficiency.htm
Energy Saving Tips	Fisher-Nickel, Inc., fishnick.com/saveenergy/energytips/

CHAPTER 6

Nutrition411.com *Enteral Feeding Formulary*	nutrition411.com/content/enteral-feeding-formulary
Centers for Medicare & Medicaid Services (CMS) *F-tags*	cms.gov/Regulations-and-Guidance/Regulations-and-Guidance.html
Nutrition411.com *Between Meal Feedings*	nutrition411.com/content/between-meal-feedings-snacks
Ohio Codes	codes.ohio.gov/oac/3701-17-60

CHAPTER 7

Hospital Consumer Assessment of Health-care Providers and Systems Survey (HCAHPS)	cms.gov/Regulations-and-Guidance/Regulations-and-Guidance.html
Sample Customer Survey Tool	Press Ganey, pressganey.com/ourSolutions/patient-voice/census-based-surveying.aspx

CHAPTER 8

Centers for Medicare & Medicaid Services (CMS) Hospital	
Consumer Assessment of Healthcare Providers and Systems Survey (HCAHPS)	cms.gov/Medicare/Quality-Initiatives-Patient-Assessment-Instruments/HospitalQualityInits/HospitalHCAHPS.html
The Institute for Healthcare Improvement *Plan, Do, Check, Study Tool*	ihi.org
Food for Fifty	Molt, Mary, Pearson Education, Inc.
FDA Food Code	fda.gov
The Joint Commission (TJC)	jointcommission.org
Centers for Medicare & Medicaid Services (CMS)	cms.gov

CHAPTER 10

U.S. Equal Employment Opportunity Commission (EEOC) Oversight and Coordination Policies	eeoc.gov
State of Michigan, Michigan Department of Civil Rights, Lansing, Mic. Pre-Employment Inquiry Guide	
U.S. Equal Employment Opportunity Commission (EEOC) Uniform Guidelines on Employee Selection Procedures	uniformguidelines.com
	ncbi.nlm.nih.gov/pmc/articles/PMC1022402/pdf/westjmed00067-0065.pdf

CHAPTER 11

F&N Training Paks© 1998	The Grossbauer Group
Health Insurance Portability and Accountability Act (HIPAA) *HIPAA Inservice Training*	dk Foodservice Solutions, LLC, dkfsolutions.net
FDA Food Code	fda.gov
	blink.ucsd.edu/safety/resources/training/food.html
	krex.k-state.edu/dspace/bitstream/2097/806/1/RobertsFPTApr2008.pdf

CHAPTER 12

Fair Labors Standards Act, Controlling Overtime	dol.gov/whd/flsa/

CHAPTER 13

USDA Standard Operating Procedures	sop.nfsmi.org/sop_list.php
Social Media Policy and Procedure	itbusinessedge.com/cm/docs/DOC-2014
Social Media Policy and Procedure	danielhoang.com/2009/02/21/social-media-policies-and-procedures/
Alcohol and the Workplace	pubs.niaaa.nih.gov/publications/aa44.htm
Alcohol and the Workplace	pubs.niaaa.nih.gov/publications/economic-2000/index.htm
25 Ways to Reward Employees	hrworld.com/features/25-employee-rewards/
Nutrition411.com *Performance Improvement Plan*	nutrition411.com/content/performance-evaluation-tips
Turnover Rate	compensationforce.com/
ANFP *Pride in Foodservice Week*	anfponline.org/
Nutrition411.com *Job Satisfaction Survey*	nutrition411.com/content/job-satisfaction-survey-employees

CHAPTER 14

S.M.A.R.T. Goals and Objectives	smart-goals-guide.com/smart-goal.html
Maslow's Hierarchy of Needs	1954, Maslow
A 1954 Motivation and Personality New You	Maslow, NY Harper, pg. 91
	smartcommunities.ncat.org/buildings/gbprinc.shtml
KPI Key Performance Indicators	en.wikipedia.org/wiki/Performance_indicator
	unc.edu/world/Action%20Plan%20Booklet.pdf
	hrworld.com/features/25-employee-rewards
	pubs.niaaa.nih.gov/publications/aa44.htm
	niaaa.nih.gov/publications/economic-2000/index.htm
	humanresources.about.com/od/meetingmanagement/a/meetings_work_3.htm

CHAPTER 15

	humanresources.about.com/od/meetingmanagement/a/meetings_work_3.htm
Association of Nutrition Foodservice Professionals (ANFP) *Standards of Practice*	anfponline.org/news-resources/standards-of-practice
Association of Nutrition Foodservice Professionals (ANFP) *Code of Ethics*	anfponline.org/docs/default-source/legacy-docs/docs/codeethics.pdf
The Academy of Nutrition and Dietetics (Academy) *Code of Ethics*	eatrightpro.org/resources/career/code-of-ethics
Five Star Teamwork—How to Achieve Success Together	Ventura, Steve and Templin, Michelle

CHAPTER 16

	workplace-communication.com/four-types-communication.html
Change Management	en.wikipedia.org/wiki/Change_management

CHAPTER 17

FDA Food Code	fda.gov
U.S. Equal Employment Opportunity Commission (EEOC)	eeoc.gov
American with Disabilities Act *Rights of Employees*	ada.gov
Foodservice Employee Safety Rules	Leon County School
OSHA Occupational Safety & Health Administration	osha.gov
	osha.gov/SLTC/etools/hospital/dietary/dietary.html
	blink.ucsd.edu/safety/resources/training/food.html
	roughnotes.com/rnmagazine/2006/october06/10p026.htm
OSHA Safety Data Sheets	osha.gov/Publications/OSHA3514.html
OSHA Ergonomic Hazards and Solutions	osha.gov/SLTC/etools/hospital/dietary/dietary.html
Ergonomically Sound Techniques	The Grossbauer Group
	blink.ucsd.edu/safety/occupational/ergonomics/awareness.html
U.S. Department of Labor *Strains and Sprains*	osha.gov/SLTC/youth/restaurant/strains_foodprep.html

CHAPTER 18

U.S. Department of Agriculture (USDA) *Grading Standards*	ams.usda.gov/grades-standards
U.S. Department of Agriculture (USDA) *Inspection Standards*	fsis.usda.gov/wps/portal/fsis/topics/food-safety-education/get-an-swers/food-safety-fact-sheets/production-and-inspection
Group Purchasing Organizations (GPOs)	en.wikipedia.org/wiki/Group_purchasing_organization
	clemson.edu/fyd/food_safety.htm
	ehs.ucsd.edu/ergo/mcergo/backinj.pdf

CHAPTER 19

U.S. Food and Drug Administration (FDA)	foodsafety.gov/news/fsma.html
Centers for Disease Control and Prevention *Food Safety*	cdc.gov/foodsafety/
FDA Food Code	fda.gov
Hazard Analysis Critical Control Point (HACCP)	fda.gov/Food/GuidanceRegulation/HACCP/

CHAPTER 20

FDA Food Code	fda.gov
National Sanitation Foundation (NSF) International Mark of Approval	nsf.org
Underwriters Laboratories (UL) *Electrical Safety Standards*	ul.com
OSHA *Occupational Hazard Communication Standard*	osha.gov
OSHA *Safety Data Sheets*	osha.gov/Publications/OSHA3514.html
Blink	blink.ucsd.edu/safety/occupational/ergonomics/awareness.html

CHAPTER 21

U.S. Department of Labor Collective Bargaining	dol.gov/dol/topic/labor-relations/collbargaining.htm

CHAPTER 22

Return on Investment	en.wikipedia.org/wiki/Return_on_investment
Cost Benefit Analysis	https://en.wikipedia.org/wiki/Cost%E2%80%93benefit_analysis

CHAPTER 23

Foodservice Technology Center (FSTC) *Energy Wise Foodservice Equipment Rebates*	fishnick.com/saveenergy/rebates/
Foodservice Technology Center (FSTC) *Life-Cycle & Energy Cost Calculators*	fishnick.com/saveenergy/tools/calculators/
Consortium for Energy Efficiency (CSS)	http://www.cee1.org/
U.S. Green Building Council *Leadership in Energy and Environmental Design* (LEED)	
Janitorial Storage, Restrooms, Lounge Areas, Space Allocation	Knight, John B., Purdue University
University of Mississippi *Guidelines for Equipment to Healthy Meals*	National Food Service Management Institute
Smart Communities Network *Creating Energy Smart Communities*	smartcommunities.ncat.org/buildings/gbprinc.shtml
Sustainable Foodservice *Efficient Commercial Kitchen Equipment*	sustainablefoodservice.com/cat/equipment.htm

CHAPTER 24

USDA *Commercial Item Descriptions*	ams.usda.gov
Food for Fifty	Molt, Mary, Pearson Education, Inc.
Group Purchasing Organizations (GPOs)	en.wikipedia.org/wiki/Group_purchasing_organization
Anti-Kickback Safe Harbors	oig.hhs.gov/compliance/safe-harbor-regulations/index.asp
Environmentally Preferable Purchasing (EPP) *Green Cafeterias*	epa.gov/epp/pubs/case/cafeteria.htm

CHAPTER 25

Theme Day or Party Ideas	stylecaster.com/101-theme-party-ideas
Catering Menus	dk Foodservice Solutions, LLC
Meridian Public Schools Food Service Sample School Foodservice Catering Form	images.pcmac.org/Uploads/MeridianPS/MeridianPS/Departments/PagesLevel1/Documents/Special.Function.Req.Form%201.pdf
USDA *Healthier School Day Tips*	fns.usda.gov/healthierschoolday/tools-schools

CHAPTER 26

Monthly Budget Report	dk Foodservice Solutions, LLC
Marketprices	foodservice.com/marketprices

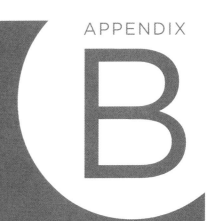
Commonly Referenced Food Temperatures

Activity	Temperature
Cooking	
Beef or Pork Roasts	145°F (4 minutes)
Beef Steak	145°F (surface temperature on top and bottom)*
Poultry, Game, Stuffed Foods	165°F (15 seconds)
Chopped or Ground Meat	155°F (15 seconds)
Fish and Seafood	145°F (15 seconds)
Eggs, Cooked to Hold	155°F (15 seconds)
Eggs, Single serving, Cooked to Order	145°F (15 seconds)
Fruits and Vegetables	135°F
Food in Microwave	165°F (2 minutes standing time after cooking)
Reheating Food	165°F (Within two hours)
Washing	
Handwashing, Water Temperature	100°F
Dishwashing, Manual—Wash Water	110°F - 120°F
Dishwashing, Mechanical—Wash Water	
• Stationary Rack, single temperature	165°F
• Stationary Rack, dual temperature	150°F
• Single Tank, conveyor, dual temperature	160°F
• Multi-tank, conveyor, multi-temperature	150°F
Sanitizing	
With Hot Water	171°F (a minimum of 30 seconds)
Chemical Sanitizer, Water Temperature	
• Iodine	70° - 120°F
• Chlorine	75°F - 100°F
• Quats	75°F minimum
Dishwashing, Mechanical	
• Stationary Rack, single temperature	165°F
• Stationary Rack, dual temperature	180°F
• Single Tank, conveyor, dual temperature	180°F
• Multi-tank, conveyor, multi-temperature	180°F

* Not recommended for highly susceptible populations. Needs to be at minimum of 150°F

Continued...

Activity	Temperature
Holding	
Hot Holding	Above 135°F (Check local regulatory authority if different requirements and follow the most stringent.)
Cold Holding	Below 41°F
Cooling	
PHF/TCS Cooling from Hot	135°F to 70°F within two hours, then 70°F to 41°F in four hours or less, for a total of no more than six hours.
PHF/TCS Cooling from Room Temperature	70°F to 41°F in 4 hours
Thawing	
Under Refrigeration	41°F or below
Under Running Water	70°F or below
Receiving	
PHF/TCS (Refrigerated)	41°F or below
PHF/TCS (Frozen)	0°F or below
Ice Cream	6°F - 10°F
Storage	
Dry Storage	50°F - 70°F
Refrigerated	41°F or below
Deep Chill	26°F - 32°F
Frozen	0° or below
Utensil Storage Between Uses	135°F water
Hazard Zone	**41°F - 135°F**

Reviewed and updated 8-2015

Management Math and Formulas

by Susan Davis Allen, MS, RD, CHE

Management Math	Formula	Example
Edible Yield Factor Used to calculate edible yield from produce or meat	Edible portion (EP) ÷ As purchased (AP)	16 lbs. of broccoli (AP) After cleaning yields 13 lbs.: 13 ÷ 16 = 81% yield
FTE Full Time Equivalent	One person @ 8 hrs./day x 5 days/wk x 52 wks/yr. = 2080 hrs	If you have six employees who work full-time, you have 6 FTEs; if you have 10 employees, two work full-time, two work 3/4 time; and six work 1/2 time, how many FTEs and hours are there? 2 x 1 FTE = 2 x 2,080 = 4,160 hours 2 x .75 FTE = 1.5 x 2,080 = 3,120 hours 6 x .5 FTE = 3 x 2,080 = 6,240 hours Total FTEs = 6.5 x 2,080 = 13,520 hours
Inventory Valuation The value of all of your inventory	Number of purchase units on hand x product price, then added together	In a cooler: 1 bag lettuce x $8/bag = $ 8.00 10 lbs. carrots x .39/lb. = 3.90 25# onions x .25/lb. = 6.25 Inventory Valuation = $ 18.15
Productivity Rate Used to measure the productivity of foodservice employees	A measure of work such as trays assembled ÷ measure of time	14 trays assembled in seven minutes 14 ÷ 7 = 2 minutes/tray
Recipe Cost Used to determine the cost of a standardized recipe	List of ingredients with price per amount of ingredient, added together ÷ by the recipe yield = price per portion	Recipe: Scrambled Eggs for 12 clients: 18 eggs @ $1.50/doz. ($1.50 ÷ 12 = $.125/egg); 18 x .125 = **$2.25 for 18 eggs** 1/4 cup milk @ $4.00/gal (16 cups/gal and four 1/4 cups/cup) $4.00 ÷ 16 = $.25/cup ÷ 4 = **$.0625 for 1/4 cup milk** **Total cost/client = $2.25 + .0625 = $2.31 ÷ 12 = .19/ client**
Scaling a Recipe Used when increasing or decreasing the amount a recipe serves	Divide the New yield by the Original yield. Remember it by the fact that N comes before O in the alphabet so the formula is always N/O to get the conversion factor. Then multiply the ingredients in the recipe by the conversion factor.	Let's use the Scrambled Eggs above. You want to increase this recipe to serve 50 people. 1. Determine the conversion factor: 50 ÷ 12 = **4.167** 2. Multiply that by each ingredient: 18 eggs x 4.167 = **75 eggs** .25 cup milk x 4.167 = **1 cup milk** *Continued...*

Management Math	Formula	Example
Tray Accuracy Used to determine the number of errors in assembling trays	1. Count the total numbers of items on the menu ticket 2. Count the number of errors you discover on one tray 3. Divide the number of errors by the total number of items	For today's noon meal, there are seven items including drink and condiments. You discover two errors. $2 \div 7 = .29 \times 100 = 29\%$
Monthly Food Cost Used to determine food cost for the month	1. Record beginning inventory valuation 2. Add total purchases for the month 3. Subtract ending inventory valuation	For the month of June: 1. Inventory valuation as of June 1: $7,456 2. Purchases for the month of June: + 10,914 3. Subtract ending inventory on the 30th - 9,002 Monthly Food Cost: $9,368
Monthly Food Cost Percent A percentage used to track food costs and may be used to determine meal prices	1. Record the monthly food cost 2. Divide by the sales for the month (or the raw food cost PPD x number of clients)	June monthly food cost $9,368 Sales for the month: 27,398 Food cost % for June: $\$9,368 \div \$27,398 = .342 \times 100$ or 34.2%
Turnover Rate Used as a measure of stability in the foodservice department	1. List the number of employees who have left over a defined period of time 2. Divide this by the total number of positions you have	Turnover rate for 2017: 1. 12 employees have left the department in 2017 2. The total number of positions is 99 3. $12 \div 99 = .12 \times 100 = 12\%$
Raw Food Cost (PPD) Per Patient Day Used as a financial measurement for tracking and benchmarking	[(Monthly Food Cost from above ÷ total days in the month ÷ total) clients]	June monthly food cost $[(\$9,368 \div 30 \text{ days}) \div 74 \text{ clients}] = \$4.16/\text{day}$
Raw Food Cost per Meal The cost of the raw ingredients to produce a meal	[(Monthly Food Cost from above ÷ ((the number of meals served in the month, for example: the client count x 3 meals a day x (30 days))]	June monthly food cost: $[\$9,368 \div ((74 \text{ clients} \times 3 \text{ meals}) \times 30 \text{ days})] =$ Cost per Meal $[\$9,368 \div ((222 \text{ meals}) \times 30 \text{ days})] =$ Cost per Meal $(\$9,368 \div 6,660 \text{ meals}) = \$1.40$ per Meal
Meals per Labor Hour Used as a measure of productivity and for tracking and benchmarking	Total meals served ÷ total hours worked (Note total meals served includes regular meals plus any catering)	June meals: 1. Regular meals: 30 days x 3 x 74 clients = 2,220 meals 2. Catering meals: (total food cost ÷ average meal cost) = $648 ÷ $4.16 = 156 additional meals 3. Total meals: 2,220 + 156 = 2,376 meals ÷ 485 hours = 14 meals per labor hour

Management Math	Formula	Example
COLA Adjustment Calculating budget increase for COLA (cost of living adjustment)	1. Current budget x proposed cost of living adjustment percentage. 2. Current budget + figures from #1 above = proposed budget increase	Proposed COLA is 3.4%. Current labor budget is $78,650 per month. $78,650 x .034 = $2,674 $78,650 + $2,674 = $81,234 for next month that includes adjustment for COLA
Labor Cost per Meal Served Used as a financial measurement for tracking and benchmarking	Total labor costs ÷ total meals served	Using the example from above for total meals: 2,376 Total labor costs for June: $6,305 6,305 ÷ 2,376 = $2.65/meal

Frequently Used Conversions

How to Calculate Percentages	Cross multiply and divide June monthly food cost $9,368 Sales for the month: $27,398	Food cost % for June: $\frac{\$9,368}{?}$ $\frac{\$27,398}{100}$ = [(9,368 x 100) ÷ 27,398] = 34.2%
Liter → Ounces Conversions	Quick conversions to keep in mind	1 liter = 100 cc's = 1000 ml's 30 ml = 1 oz. 240 ml = 8 oz. = 1 cup
How Many Ounces IN:	Quick conversions to keep in mind	1 gallon = 128 oz. 1 gallon = 4 quarts = 16 cups 1 quart = 4 cups = 32 oz. 1 cup = 8 oz.
How Many Meat Portions in a Pound	Quick conversions to keep in mind	1 lb. of raw meat = 16 oz. A standard protein portion is 4 oz. raw or 3 oz. cooked 1 lb. of meat = four portions
How Many Portions in a #10 Can	Quick conversions to keep in mind	A #10 can = 12 - 13 cups of product A typical serving is 1/2 cup A #10 can = approximately 25 - 1/2 cup servings
Calculate the Scoop Size	Quick conversions to keep in mind	The scoop size is equal to the number of scoops in a quart (32 oz.) There are eight half-cups in a quart (#8 scoop) There are 12 one-third cups in a quart (#12 scoop)

Index

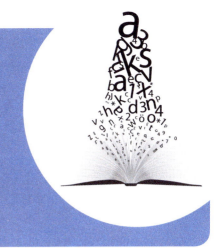

V

W

Y